Quality and Safety in Women's Health

Quality and Safety in Women's Health

Edited by

Thomas Ivester MD MPH
Professor, Division of Maternal—Fetal Medicine, Department of Obstetrics and Gynecology, University of North Carolina School of Medicine &
Chief Medical Officer / Vice President for Medical Affairs, University of North Carolina Hospitals, Chapel Hill, NC, USA

Patrice M. Weiss MD FACOG
Chair, Department of Obstetrics and Gynecology, Virginia Tech University Carilion Clinic, Roanoke, VA, USA

Paul A. Gluck MD
Associate Clinical Professor, Department of Obstetrics and Gynecology, University of Miami Miller School of Medicine, Miami, FL, USA

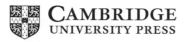

CAMBRIDGE
UNIVERSITY PRESS

University Printing House, Cambridge CB2 8BS, United Kingdom

One Liberty Plaza, 20th Floor, New York, NY 10006, USA

477 Williamstown Road, Port Melbourne, VIC 3207, Australia

314–321, 3rd Floor, Plot 3, Splendor Forum, Jasola District Centre, New Delhi – 110025, India

79 Anson Road, #06-04/06, Singapore 079906

Cambridge University Press is part of the University of Cambridge.

It furthers the University's mission by disseminating knowledge in the pursuit of
education, learning and research at the highest international levels of excellence.

www.cambridge.org
Information on this title: www.cambridge.org/9781107686304
DOI: 10.1017/9781139505826

First published 2018

Printed in the United Kingdom by TJ International Ltd. Padstow Cornwall

A catalogue record for this publication is available from the British Library

Library of Congress Cataloging-in-Publication Data
Names: Ivester, Thomas, editor. | Weiss, Patrice M., editor. | Gluck, Paul A., editor.
Title: Quality and safety in women's health / edited by Thomas Ivester, Patrice M. Weiss, Paul A. Gluck.
Description: Cambridge, United Kingdom ; New York : Cambridge University Press, 2018. |
Includes bibliographical references and index.
Identifiers: LCCN 2017049396 | ISBN 9781107686304 (paperback)
Subjects: | MESH: Women's Health Services | Patient Safety |
Maternal Health Services | Quality of Health Care
Classification: LCC RA564.85 | NLM WA 309.1 | DDC 613/.0424–dc23
LC record available at https://lccn.loc.gov/2017049396

ISBN 978-1-107-68630-4 Paperback

Contents

Notes on Figures and Tables

The Publishers would like to thank the following for permission to reproduce copyright material.

Table 2.2, p. 9 Macones GA, Hankins GD, Spong CY, Hauth J, Moore T. The 2008 National Institute of Child Health and Human Development workshop report on electronic fetal monitoring: update on definitions, interpretations, and research guidelines. © 2008 by The American College of Obstetricians and Gynecologists, Wolters Kluwer Health Inc.

Figure 3.3, p. 31 Elliott M, Yisi Lui. 'The nine rights of medication administration'. Reproduced by permission © 27 March 2013 by British Journal of Nursing, www.magonlinelibrary.com/doi/10.12968/bjon.2010.19.5.47064

Figure 3.4, p. 32 Hickner JM, et al. 'Issues and Initiatives in the Testing Process in Primary Care Physician Offices'. Journal on Quality and Patient Safety © Feb 2005 Elsevier.

Figure 13.1, p. 118 Koh HK, Berwick DM, Clancy CM, et al., New federal policy initiatives to boost health literacy can help the nation move beyond the cycle of costly "crisis care." ' Health Affairs 1 February 2012 © Project Hope.

Table 13.1, p. 121 The Universal Patient Compact™ Principles for Partnership © 2011, National Patient Safety Foundation. Reprinted with permission. All rights reserved.

Figure 20.1, p. 180 Grobman WA1, Hornbogen A, Burke C, Costello R. 'Development and implementation of a team-centered shoulder dystocia protocol.'

© 2010 Society for Simulation in Healthcare, Wolters Kluwer Health Inc.

Figure 21.1, p. 188 Institute for Healthcare Improvement. © 'Cause and Effect Diagram.' www.ihi.org/resources/Pages/Tools/CauseandEffectDiagram.aspx

Figure 23.2, p. 206 Philip Aspden, Janet M. Corrigan, Julie Wolcott, Shari M. Erickson, Editors, Committee on Data Standards for Patient Safety. 'Patient Safety: Achieving a new standard for care.' National Academies Press, © 2004, The National Academies Press.

Table 24.1, pp. 213–214 Brian M Wong, Wendy Levinson, Kaveh G Shojania. 'Quality improvement in medical education: current state and future directions' Medical Education, 13 Dec 2011 © John Wiley and Sons.

Table 24.2, pp. 215–216 Sachdeva AK, Philibert I, Leach DC, Blair PG, Stewart LK, Rubinfeld IS, Britt LD. 'Patient safety curriculum for surgical residency programs: results of a national consensus conference.' Surgery. © 2007 Elsevier.

Table 24.3, p. 217 Brian M Wong, Wendy Levinson, Kaveh G Shojania. 'Quality improvement in medical education: current state and future directions' Medical Education, 13 Dec 2011 © John Wiley and Sons.

Every effort has been made to trace all copyright holders, but if any have been inadvertently overlooked, the Publishers will be pleased to make the necessary arrangements at the first opportunity.

Contributors

Michael E. Barfield
General Surgery Residency Training Program, Department of Surgery, Duke University Medical Center, Durham, NC, USA

Diana Behling
OB Right Program Manager, Sentara Healthcare, Norfolk, VA, USA

Angela Brenner
Pharmacy Clinical Lead – Women and Children, Ministry-St Joseph's Hospital, Marshfield, WI, USA

Hans P. Cassagnol
Vice President of Quality, Chief Quality Officer, Assistant Dean of Quality, Associate Clinical Professor of Obstetrics & Gynecology, Associate Clinical Professor of Public Health & Preventive Medicine, SUNY Upstate Medical University Health System, Syracuse, NY, USA

Nancy Chescheir
Professor of Maternal Fetal Medicine, Department of Obstetrics and Gynecology, University of North Carolina School of Medicine, Chapel Hill, NC, USA

Bonnie Dattel
Associate Director, Maternal Fetal Medicine, and Medical Director, Labor and Delivery, Eastern Virginia Medical School, Norfolk, VA, USA

Shad Deering
Professor and Chair, Department of Obstetrics and Gynecology, Uniformed Services University of the Health Sciences, Bethesda, MD, USA

Mark S. DeFrancesco
Assistant Clinical Professor, Department of Obstetrics and Gynecology, University of Connecticut, Farmington, CT, USA and Treasurer/Board Member, Accreditation Association of Hospitals and Health Systems (AAHHS), Chicago, IL, USA

Alan M. Dulit
Vice-President of Medical Affairs, OB Hospitalists Group, Inc., Mauldin, SC, USA

Allison R. Durica
Division of Maternal Fetal Medicine, Carilion Clinic Department of Obstetrics and Gynecology, and Assistant Professor, Virginia Tech Carilion School of Medicine, Roanoke, VA, USA

Ty B. Erickson
Rosemark, Idaho Falls, ID, USA

Bruce B. Ettinger
Consulting for Regulatory and Accreditation Compliance in Health Services, Santa Monica, CA, USA

Maggie M. Finkelstein
Stevens & Lee, Philadelphia, PA, USA

Karen Frush
Professor of Pediatrics, Duke University School of Medicine, and Chief Patient Safety Officer, Duke University Health System, Durham, NC, USA

Edmund F. Funai
Associate Dean of Administration, Ohio State University College of Medicine, and Chief Operating Officer, Ohio State University Health System, Columbus, OH, USA

Joseph C. Gambone
Clinical Professor of Obstetrics and Gynecology, Western University of Health Sciences, Pomona, CA, USA

William A. Grobman
Professor of Obstetrics and Gynecology, Department of Obstetrics and Gynecology and Center for Healthcare Studies, Feinberg School of Medicine, Northwestern University, Chicago, IL, USA

John P. Keats
Assistant Clinical Professor of Obstetrics and Gynecology, David Geffen School of Medicine at UCLA, Los Angeles, CA, USA

Sandra Koch
Carson Medical Group, Carson City, NV, USA

Abraham Lichtmacher
Chief of Women's Services, Lovelace Health System, Albuquerque, NM, USA

Amber D. Masse
Nurse Practitioner, Idaho Falls, ID, USA

Harry Mateer
Director of Obstetrics and Gynecology, Geisinger Health System, Danville, PA, USA

Elizabeth S. McCuin
Section Chief, OB/GYN Generalist Division, Carilion Clinic Department of Obstetrics and Gynecology, and Assistant Professor, Virginia Tech Carilion School of Medicine, Roanoke, VA, USA

David Miller
University of Southern California Keck School of Medicine, Los Angeles, CA, USA

Dotun Ogunyemi
Clinical Services Professor, David Geffen School of Medicine at UCLA, Los Angeles, CA, USA

Mark D. Pearlman
Associate Chief of Clinical Affairs and Professor, Department of Obstetrics and Gynecology, University of Michigan Hospital and Health Systems, Ann Arbor, MI, USA

Christian M. Pettker
Assistant Professor, Department of Obstetrics, Gynecology, and Reproductive Sciences, Yale University School of Medicine, and Medical Director, Labor and Birth Unit, Yale-New Haven Hospital, New Haven, CT, USA

Holly S. Puritz
Private Practice, Norfolk, VA, USA

Steve Rad
Maternal Fetal Medicine Fellow, Cedars Sinai Medical Center, Los Angeles, CA, USA

Roseann Richards
Pharmacy Clinical Specialist – Women and Children, WakeMed Health and Hospitals, Raleigh, NC, USA

James W. Saxton
Stevens & Lee, Philadelphia, PA, USA

Pamela K. Scarrow
American College of Obstetrics and Gynecology, Washington, DC, USA

Peter A. Schwartz
Department of Obstetrics and Gynecology, Reading Hospital, Reading, PA, USA

Roger Smith
Director of Quality Improvement and Assistant Professor, Department of Obstetrics and Gynecology, University of Michigan Hospital and Health Systems, Ann Arbor, MI, USA

Margaret Sturdivant
Administrative Director, Duke University Health System Patient Safety Office, Durham, NC, USA

Christopher C. Swain
Founder and President, OB Hospitalists Group, Inc., Mauldin, SC, USA

Fidel A. Valea
Department of Obstetrics and Gynecology, Duke University Medical School, Raleigh, NC, USA

John S. Wachtel
Clinical Professor, Stanford University Medical School, Stanford, CA, USA

Preface

In healthcare today, "variation," "standardization," "quality improvement," and "patient safety" have become buzzwords. The past several years have seen tremendous growth in interest and activity around quality improvement and patient safety. Staff positions and new titles dedicated to patient safety and quality improvement have been created in countless organizations. Committees and councils have been formed, and numerous initiatives have been undertaken. We have entered an era where transparency of performance data and comparison with peers is becoming commonplace, and our competitiveness and financial stability depend upon our responses. Furthermore, the welfare of our patients requires nothing less.

The reality is that "standardization," "quality improvement," and "patient safety" are not just buzzwords. Nor are they necessarily goals to be achieved or short-term initiatives to be undertaken. They are not effective as tactical responses to a focused area of poor performance. Instead, they represent a powerful set of tools and strategies that underlie a culture of quality and safety that we all must embrace. It is not the job of a subcommittee, or of one or a few designated persons. It is not a checklist, or a protocol, or a drill, or a guideline. Instead, it is a deeply embedded culture – the way of doing things every day. It is the job of *everyone* in the organization. It isn't always easy – but it is necessary and most often rewarding.

In this book, we present a highly practical guide for introducing a culture of quality and safety through case presentations of everyday situations that we each face as providers of women's health care, and include in-depth discussion of underlying factors in underperformance and methods for improving them. Though many topics focus on a specific clinical area, the principles are universal and can be applied across many settings. As such, these practices should not be applied in isolation. In doing so, the likelihood for short-term implementation and long-term sustainability is nil. Rather, they should be undertaken as a component of a more comprehensive approach to improving quality and safety, and engaging stakeholders at all levels. Applied in this context, they will serve as important building blocks for the foundation of a culture of quality.

There are a number of methods available for adoption as part of a strategy to improve quality and safety. Among the more prominent quality improvement (QI) methods are Six Sigma, Lean, Kaizen, and the Model for Improvement. For patient safety, common strategies from the Agency for Healthcare Research and Quality (AHRQ) include Team Strategies to Enhance Performance and Patient Safety (Team STEPPS) and Comprehensive Unit-based Safety Program (CUSP). Other promising initiatives include the Partnership for Maternal Safety and the Safety Program in Perinatal Care, a Team STEPPS based program sponsored by AHRQ. No single methodology has proven itself superior to others. They are perhaps best used in combination, while being adapted to local contexts.

For those looking to build a culture of quality and safety, this book alone will not get you there, but it can serve as a valuable tool with immediate relevance to many clinical and operational challenges we face, and as a building block in the march to build that quality culture.

Several important elements are critical to the success and sustainability of a quality and safety program. Some or all of these may be present at your institution, but many will lack at least some of these. Early efforts must emphasize certain foundational elements, which we will outline below. Certainly, having embedded clinicians and staff formally trained in CQI and safety methods is important, but key aspects of the culture are deeper and more extensive. Ultimately, the formula for quality is simple: *Structure + Process = Outcomes.*

Implementation and sustainability of patient safety initiatives is often difficult and requires a receptive organizational culture. Leadership, measurement, and engagement are necessary components of this culture.

Leadership that is engaged, present, and involved is perhaps the single most important factor in the successful deployment of any QI or safety program, and in building the culture. Failed efforts to establish QI in any setting can, in the majority of cases, be traced directly to this aspect of culture. Yet it remains overlooked or underemphasized all too commonly. Instead, QI efforts are often relegated to isolated subcommittees or individuals, who often suffer from limited influence and even further limited resources. Leadership at all levels simply must be meaningfully engaged in these endeavors. They cannot be merely complicit.

Measurement is similarly given short shrift in many programs. This may be due to budgetary constraints, limited personnel, or information technology resources. In some cases, it is simply not seen as necessary or important. However, we would very strongly argue that measurement and evaluation are absolutely necessary to the success of any quality program. In the absence of effective measurement, how will teams and stakeholders truly know if they are making a difference, if the investment is worthwhile, or even where, what, and how to improve? Without evidence of impact or cost-effectiveness, efforts and investment will wane, and an opportunity to develop a culture may be lost. Finally, measurement can be a very powerful motivator for staff and teams engaged in QI and safety efforts.

Nearly equally important as the "whys" to collect data is the "what." Data collection can suffer in either direction – collecting too little or incorrect data, or collecting too much data and thus creating clutter, confusion, and consuming unnecessary resources. Measurement should be carefully considered, and should extend beyond those measures required for report to outside agencies. Data collection and analysis should serve the specific and overall goals of your quality program, the pillars of which comprise structural elements, clinical and operational processes, immediate outcomes, and ultimately impact. Use of some simple tools, such as logic models, driver diagrams, or process maps can help with planning measurement and evaluation.

Engagement and empowerment of all staff and relevant stakeholders is critical. The multitude of processes that impact patient safety, clinical excellence, and the patient experience do not take place in a boardroom or administrative office, nor do most of them occur in silos. Rather, they are the culmination of the coordinated efforts of many individuals who comprise a healthcare team. These are happening at the point of care as well as countless interrelated processes taking place behind the scenes.

We hope that you will embrace this book as a valuable set of tools in guiding and developing local efforts in quality and safety, or boosting and tailoring those already functioning. It is targeted to anyone involved in delivering healthcare to women, including leaders, clinicians, and staff in community hospitals, private practices, health departments, and tertiary and academic medical centers. Within the text, you will find many examples of cases representative of our daily practices and challenges. Most chapters have been organized as a relevant case presentation, followed by an in-depth exploration of key factors and suggested responses. Though some may prefer to read the text in its entirety, it is organized in a way that readers may also go directly to a section or even a chapter of specific relevance, and gain the specific perspective of an expert fellow clinician as well as a review of pertinent evidence or experience.

Clinical and system level patient safety topics include obstetrics, gynecology, health policy, office practice, labor and delivery, regulatory issues, quality improvement, and medical education. Within, you will find guidance on surgical safety, obstetrical emergencies, and use of health information technology. There is also a comprehensive chapter on fetal monitoring, given its prominent role in patient safety, and two chapters addressing the incorporation of quality and safety into medical education programs.

Office Safety

Ty B. Erickson and Amber D. Masse

The clinician's office has continued to evolve in scope and complexity – both increase the risk of failed systems and reduced patient safety. The growth in office-based invasive procedures has resulted from a number of variables including technology innovation, economic and time pressures, and patient convenience. However, clinicians need not fail to provide a safe environment. Consider the following scenario.

> *After a careful history, physical and imaging workup for a patient with menometrorrhagia you elect, with the patient's consent, to proceed with an endometrial ablative technique. You discuss the options of an in-office versus hospital setting and the patient elects for the office procedure. The following week she arrives at the office and your staff prepares her and the procedure room for the ablation. You have administered an oral anxiolytic, NSAID, and an intramuscular injection of a narcotic. This "cocktail" template was provided by the representative from the equipment manufacturer for your procedure; you were told that the template is being used by many offices. You administer a paracervical block while waiting for the equipment to be prepared. Shortly thereafter the patient has a seizure, respiratory arrest, and codes. Mayhem erupts and people scramble to find the crash cart. Someone yells to call 911. You are in the middle of the procedure and are asking a medical assistant to find the oxygen tank for the patient, while you try to remove the equipment and move the patient from the lithotomy position to supine. No one is managing the airway.*

This scenario identifies core concerns in the following areas relating to in-office procedures: economic incentives, leadership, competency and assessment, anesthesia safety, and teamwork. A scenario such as this introduces the opportunity to emphasize practical corrective measures in advance, such as checklists, timeouts, and mock drills.

Why did you decide to perform the ablation in the office? Common responses could include patient familiarity, cost savings for the patient and her insurance company, or time savings in avoiding the hassles of checking into the hospital with its attendant inefficiencies. However, the most likely but often less-discussed reason for providing more in-office procedures is the financial incentive to you and your practice; the fee is not distributed to the hospital. This financial incentive for in-office procedures should be disclosed to the patient, and ethically your practice should not drive procedures to your office merely for economic gain.

Carefully select the right setting for the patient, taking into consideration risk elements such as health history, BMI, airway management risk, pain tolerance, etc. What governance do you have in your practice to determine the protocols and procedures you plan to incorporate in your office? Have you considered formal certification such as the American College of Obstetricians and Gynecologists Safety Certification in Outpatient Practice Excellence (SCOPE) program? This voluntary certification process, which can be reviewed at www.scopeforwomenshealth.org, has a robust pre- and post-evaluation of your office systems to assure improved safety with opportunities to have outside independent review. Another excellent opportunity to increase patient safety during in-office procedures is available at www.aaahc.org/en/accreditation. The Accreditation Association for Ambulatory Health Care has published a tool kit available for purchase titled "Accreditation Guidebook for Office-Based Surgery." As the leader in your practice, you should recommend accreditation from an outside body. Visit with your insurance carrier, as they may provide financial support with premium discounts to offset the cost. Also consider reinvesting some of the additional profit from performing the procedure in the office to accreditation, staff training, upgrading safety equipment (e.g., monitoring capabilities), updating your crash cart, and other safety initiatives.

The scenario above also demonstrates concerns regarding the competency of you and your staff. As you integrate more invasive procedures into the office setting, safety initiatives must include the promotion of training and teamwork. Before bringing new technology into your office, verify individual competency by performing enough of the cases in the hospital environment under more careful supervision. A weekend course is simply not sufficient for your own credentialing. State regulatory agencies will continue to encroach on your office domain as more complications surface in the mass introduction of more and more invasive procedures. Create a core team of staff who understand the procedure you plan to perform. Even though they are not the actual clinician performing the procedure, they will be of greater value as a team if they have been instructed in the pathophysiology of the disease process, the actual equipment being utilized, and most importantly the risks of complications and how to mobilize as a team to manage such complications. Enlist assistance from the scheduling team to assure that all patients are advised of an absolute need for a driver with any procedure requiring sedation. By the same token, engage the manufacturer's representative to provide ongoing in-service on the equipment, maintenance, sterilization techniques, troubleshooting unusual case reports, etc. The company generally receives revenue from the disposables and they should be expected to become more engaged with your office training as part of their relationship with you. Leadership also includes the facilitation of an internal credentialing process for clinicians in your office with the same rigor a hospital medical staff would require.

Anesthesia risks are critical in the office environment. Oral administration of agents can create the same levels of patient anesthesia as parenteral usage. It is unethical to try and circumvent conscious sedation policies with an attempt at an oral cocktail. A decision tree allows you essentially two options. Door number one: choose to become fully competent in administration of anesthetics to your patients through training including comprehensive airway management, advanced cardiovascular life support (ACLS), and other specific pathways. Examine the elements that anesthesia personnel use in their profession including monitoring equipment, emergency medications, and ongoing training, and verify that you can provide comparable care. Door number two: create a collaborative relationship with an anesthesia group with experience in the office setting. These individuals often will bring all the equipment to your office and

provide a full service program. This allows you as the surgeon to perform your procedure knowing a second individual is managing the airway, pain control, and providing a second eyes and ears to your team, helping to avoid any catastrophes. They can often bill the insurance company separately while still keeping rates below hospital costs.

Finally, how do you avoid the tension, yelling, and disorder when an emergency arises? Two extremely important tools are available – checklists and mock drills. The lead author of this article has extensive experience with checklists as a general aviation pilot. Prior to every flight a checklist must be followed to evaluate all the elements for a safe flight. This checklist is followed every time, and every element of the list must be checked off prior to flight. There are checklists for routine flight and in-flight emergencies and even the airplane has its own annual checklist for the mechanic. These checklists reduce the risk of a disaster in the air. Comparatively, clinicians will stave off numerous disasters and near-misses with the utilization of checklists for seemingly routine processes in the office. A critical component of the checklist is a timeout; pause and review identification of the correct patient with the correct procedure. Review consents, pertinent labs and diagnostics to assure safety and accuracy before beginning the procedure. For a complete source of checklist components, go to ACOG.org and review, under the heading Task Force and Work Group Reports, 2010 Report of the Presidential Task force on Patient Safety in the Office Setting. Mock drills are discussed later in the chapter.

Consider the following scenario.

A 25-year-old female presents for her routine OB appointment. While speaking to billing personnel, she develops chest pain and shortness of breath. She states she is just having an anxiety attack. The patient returns to the waiting room. Minutes later, the receptionist hears a call for help from another patron. The staff walks to the waiting room and finds the pregnant patient lying on the floor in respiratory arrest. After a rocky hospital course she finally recovers. Your malpractice company completes a risk-assessment profile of your office and identifies you need to establish an emergency response protocol. In particular, the protocol needs to guide staff on how to proceed in a medical emergency and specifically on the use of a crash cart and automated external defibrillator (AED). It is also recommended that periodic emergency drills be conducted and documented.

Emergency response protocols in the office setting are imperative to patient safety. Patients perceive the office setting to be a safe environment where all personnel, both clinical and non-clinical, will have knowledge of how to handle any medical situation. Any delays in emergency treatment may be perceived as negligence. When performing in-hospital surgical procedures, clinicians are much more prepared to handle emergencies with clinical personnel at the bedside to respond. In contrast, an office emergency could be witnessed by any employee, including the receptionist or billing staff.

The roles and expectations of members in the response team are important. Empower staff to identify signs of impending emergency. Post signs at the check-in area for staff to identify common emergency symptoms including chest pain, shortness of breath or changes in breathing, pale skin, sweating, or profuse bleeding.

An overhead intercom system may be utilized to announce the location of the emergency. The clinic may want to apply a unique phrase to an emergency to reduce distress and flow amongst the other patrons in the clinic. Utilization of an emergency button, a simple doorbell installed at the receptionist's desk, may also aid in the early recognition of an emergency.

Basic CPR is a simple tool you can provide to your staff that provides extraordinary rewards. Not only will your staff be more empowered on how to respond to an emergency in the office, they can utilize those tools on a personal level when responding to emergencies in their homes and community settings. Other more advanced practitioners including physicians should be current in ACLS.

Keep a 911 card present at each work station or post information on the back of the employee badge. This emergency information should have the address and phone number of your clinic and the number of the nearest Emergency Department (ED). When calling 911, it is important to identify local landmarks by your location. For instance, "Our address is 101 Lincoln Ave; we are the first turn after the bridge on the right side of the road. We will meet you at the back of the building." When activating 911, the operator asks a list of standard questions which may include the name and age of the patient, the problem, and any current set of vital signs. Make your office staff aware of those questions and how to answer them accurately and quickly.

Develop a more integrative relationship with acute care facilities including the Emergency Department as a safety net for emergencies. Authorize the phone scheduler to routinely educate patients: "If your symptoms worsen or change prior to your appointment, please do not hesitate to go to the Emergency Department." Encourage your patients to be proactive in an emergency situation. For instance, when we review the acronym ACHES (abdominal pain, chest pain, headache, eye changes, shortness of breath) after starting women on oral contraceptives, for any positive response we advise the patient to go to the ED or contact EMS immediately rather than have them wait two days until an appointment is available. New federal meaningful-use standards encourage patients to receive a care summary. Encourage patients to carry portions of their healthcare record to improve safety particularly regarding medication concerns. A portable healthcare record or "passport" (even a simple note card) may be provided with update capabilities for an ongoing list of medical problems, medications, allergies, etc.

The goal of the written Emergency Response Protocol must describe the expected roles of each of the team members. Ideally, these expectations would be utilized and reviewed during a regular mock drill. Mock drills in the hospital setting have helped improve the handling of emergencies. Integrating such drills in the office is a natural extension of this tool. Develop an in-office protocol and conduct mock drills so the staff has clear expectations of their role during an emergency. Utilize the guidelines from www.justculture.org, which promote a workforce culture with a safe atmosphere [1]. Practice simulations will enhance team confidence and improve performance during office emergencies.

Practical suggestions on development of drills include focusing on a single issue such as respiratory arrest. Multiple system failures will be identified. Conduct drills in a limited time (e.g., 10–30 minutes). Have outside members of the staff, not included in the drill, take notes for debriefing and consider multimedia devices to record the event for playback. Emphasize learning and process analysis rather than criticizing team members. Allow time for feedback and discussion by all participants. The protocol will also vary depending on the amount of support staff available. Finally, the protocol will depend on environmental factors such as locale of the office to the ED. Many offices become complacent about their emergency response plan because of their close proximity to the ED or rapid EMS response times. The assignment of roles during an emergency will aid in the execution of an organized emergency response team.

Therefore, the following roles are suggested.

- **Reporter**: The person who initially identifies the emergency and verifies 911 has been called either directly or through the designated personnel.
- **Leader**: Designated clinical team member (usually a clinician). Each clinician within the practice must respond to the emergency. One will be designated as the leader. Each provider may be able to provide additional assistance including patient history and advanced skill sets including ACLS.
- **Nursing staff**: Obtains emergency kit, supplemental oxygen supply, AED, assists with CPR, acquires vital signs, prepares drugs for administration and completes Emergency Occurrence Report.
- **Recorder**: Keeps chronological log of events.
- **Runner**: Traffic control of other patients and responders within the clinic. Meets EMS and escorts them to patient.

Clear communication amongst the team members is crucial for success and cannot be understated. Guidelines from ACOG's Report of the Presidential Task Force on Patient Safety in the Office Setting outline each member's duty to call out their assumed roles and responsibilities [2]. After the emergency is recognized, call for help, and notify the front desk about the incident. Identify who will call 911, and who will meet EMS at the door. Often times, the person who has identified the emergency has the most information about the patient (reporter); however, they are usually the best suited to be at the site of the emergency. Have that person specifically give report to the runner to notify EMS personnel of the situation.

One of the authors of this article worked at a hospital with the addition of a new Emergency Department and Intensive Care Unit. The remodel also included a medical office building (MOB). Physicians were incentivized to move their practices. One day, a code blue was called on the overhead system in the MOB. There was no emergency response protocol established so EMS was activated and hospital staff attempted to respond to the emergency. Many problems ensued during the course of this incident. The hospital staff was not familiar with the layout and did not know where to go. EMS arrived and attempted to take the elevator. However, the gurney would only fit if the head of the bed was elevated, but the patient was not stable enough to elevate the head of the bed.

A mock drill done prior to the incident would have easily identified these problems.

Review the Emergency Occurrence Form at the end of the drill. Components of the Emergency Occurrence Form include review of roles assigned to each of the members who respond to the emergency and assessment of clear communication amongst them. Was there any confusion or panic over roles and responsibilities assigned? Was equipment available to handle the emergency? Are there any modifications to the plan that would have assisted in the emergency?

Create a specific Emergency Response Kit. Simply having the medications and supplies available is not sufficient. The inherent increase in situational anxiety when an emergency occurs can contribute to disorganization. A regular review of the contents and use of mock drills is imperative. A checklist format including contents and expiration dates will make staff more familiar with the kit and will ease use during an emergency. The checklist should also include reporting on the functionality of equipment. When considering the contents of the kit, never include instruments or medications that the provider is not comfortable using. By the same token, never include medications within the kit for which you cannot monitor or manage the potential side effects. Store supplies in a central location. Depending on the size of the clinic, a single room may be designated for procedures. Ideally, however, the emergency kit must be as mobile as the emergency itself, as they may occur at various locations within the office.

Consider the following scenario.

A patient presents to the office with suboptimal rise of HCG levels from 5700 mIU/ml to 5800 mIU/ml over a 48-hour time interval. A transvaginal ultrasound is negative for an intrauterine pregnancy. You elect to use an injection of methotrexate. The patient signs a consent form and the nurse injects the dose. Fourteen days later the patient arrives in the ER in hypovolemic shock with a ruptured ectopic pregnancy. A root-cause analysis is performed at your office and you detect that an adequate medical history was not taken. You also identify that your new nurse had misread the label on the methotrexate bottle and had administered an excessive dose of methotrexate. You promptly fire the nurse and remind the remaining staff that such gross negligence will not be tolerated.

A key safety discussion from this scenario centers on the process of patient tracking and follow-up. The use of methotrexate is off-label but appropriate for ectopic pregnancy. Patient follow-up is a subset of the more global discussion regarding tickler files and data tracking. A robust tickler file system must be in place to track data and patient appointment follow-up including referrals to specialists. This process may be either physical or a computer system; the filing system must manage all paper or electronic inputs from internal and outside sources. If an "in basket" is utilized, time should be allocated for placement into the chart or scanned electronically. Reminder systems for appointments or follow-up test results should have elements such as pop-up windows or built in alarms. They may also include auto-generated email or text capability. If such automatic reminders are not available, then an external calendar and time clock reminder system should be established. The office should task a specific individual to monitor the tracking system. There should also be a back-up individual when someone is on vacation or leave. The delay of a week or even a long weekend may result in patient harm if someone is not clearly assigned to review the tickler files in the absence of the primary responsible party. This core concept holds particular validity with providers. Notification of a partner concerning a patient being treated for an ectopic and as in this case with levels that would suggest a higher than average failure rate is important to prevent the patient from hitting the ER with a ruptured ectopic. The responsibility of scheduling a follow-up visit rested not solely with the nurse but also with the clinician and checkout team, who should routinely verify if a follow-up visit is indicated. Additional elements of the data-tracking system should include:

- Sign-offs: All results including consults should be reviewed, initialed, and dated by the designated provider. Electronic medical records have capabilities to auto-perform this function; however, there is a risk of an electronic signature being completed without a follow-up assignment for an abnormal result.
- Verification of file management: Office managers should monitor the process and timely execution of the tickler system. You cannot simply assume once a process is memorialized that it will flow according to design. The oversight personnel should frequently review the tickler file and assign staff to verify timely and accurate handling of the data.
- Documentation evidence of patient contact: Always remember the end of the chain

is the patient. Not only should they be contacted, but clear evidence of their understanding of the action plan and a method to verify compliance until resolution of all elements of the tracked data.

During your root-cause analysis you review the consent form that your staff had the patient sign. You observe it was hand-written on a generic form but did not include elements specific to the risk of off-label use of methotrexate. The consent process (we use the word *process* not *form*) is an important educational tool for your patients. This process helps define specifically the purpose of proposed intervention in your patient's life and well-being. Invasive procedures are planned, and a thorough review of all the pertinent elements in an understandable format will help the patient not only give consent but also become a part of the procedure including the recovery; for example, have the patient circle a mole on their body that they want you to remove. Review the purpose of the in-office sterilization or ablative procedure you propose with a robust dialogue of permanency. The educational steps you utilize (e.g., handouts, drawings, video or internet media) all contribute to the consent process. Memorializing this in written form protects you against future liability risks, but the process is more important than the form. It is imperative that you, the provider, engage in this process. Some elements can be delegated to staff, but the core discussion must come from the provider who will perform the invasive procedure or authorize the methotrexate injection as in this case.

It was noble that you used a root-cause analysis to evaluate where the system failed. A root-cause analysis includes the following elements:

- Intensely analyze the error
- Redesign system
- Test new design
- Educate staff on changes
- Follow-up on the new design
- Monitor over time as the staff and processes change in the office

Most errors in patient safety can be identified through effective examination such as a root-cause analysis. The primary purpose centers on identification of process or systems-level error and using the team approach to identify and implement changes going forward. This will provide a more permanent behavior change and will lead to improved safety practices

[3]. However, you failed to establish a just culture for your office. Unfortunately, we live in a society where people look to blame others for failures. The media screams "who is to blame?" Our world is filled with short sound bites; we live in a quick-paced environment wherein people want the blame to happen immediately – even before a thorough analysis of the problems emerges. You must restrain this temptation in your office. Teams will get nowhere with this culture of blame. A careful and thorough analysis with all members of the team will lead to a correct understanding of the process failure. Each office personnel should feel safe to honestly express their thoughts and concerns against a backdrop of protection for expression.

Beginning in 1976, as a result of a fatal accident in Washington, DC, the United States via the Aviation Safe Reporting System (ASRS) has been collecting confidential voluntary reports of near-misses from pilots, flight attendants, and air traffic controllers. The reports are provided to NASA, which acts as a neutral body with no enforcement power. An important cornerstone of this safety reporting system is the immunity and confidentiality provided to the person generating a report. This allows the aviation industry to review safety trends and create better systems for the aviation community. The Association of Perioperative Registered Nurses has implemented a similar concept called Safety Net covering near-miss reporting of medication, wrong site, communication, technology and consent issues. The Patient Safety Reporting System (PSRS) developed by the Department of Veterans Affairs encourages patient safety through voluntary confidential reports to NASA similar to the aviation industry.

In your office you need to create such a just culture of safety where your staff can report near-misses in a confidential protected environment [1]. As you collect near-miss data you will observe trends of risk and adapt processes to change the methods that will improve the safe transit of a patient through your office. We encourage you and your team to review the power of a just culture. ACOG's December 2009 *Committee Opinion 447* [4] discusses the importance of a just culture where mistakes may be admitted and corrected with an emphasis on non-punitive action. There will be the rare exception where an office employee harms a patient with disregard or has multiple near-misses that may require termination inasmuch as there is zero tolerance for reckless actions. Yet the primary emphasis centers on systems-thinking rather than attempting to assign individual blame.

Patient safety in the office or any setting requires the full cooperation of the entire team, but ultimately, you the reader of this book must light the torch and lead the way through the dark abyss ahead.

References

1 Marx D. *Patient Safety and the "Just Culture": A Primer for Health Care Executives*. New York, NY: Trustees of Columbia University in the City of New York. 2001. Retrieved from www.mers-tm.org/support/Marx_Primer.pdf

2 The American Congress of Obstetricians and Gynecologists. (2010). *Report of the Presidential Task Force on Patient Safety in the Office Setting*. Retrieved from www.acog.org/Resources_And_Publications/Task_Force_and_Work_Group_Reports

3 Erickson, T.B. (2012). Office procedures: Practical and safety considerations. *Clinical Obstetrics and Gynecology*, 55(3), 620–634.

4 Patient Safety in Obstetrics and Gynecology. (2009). ACOG Committee Opinion No. 447. The American Congress of Obstetrics and Gynecologists. Retrieved from www.acog.org/Resources_And_Publications/Committee_Opinions/Committee_on_Patient_Safety_and_Quality_Improvement/Patient_Safety_in_Obstetrics_and_Gynecology

Electronic Fetal Monitoring and Patient Safety

David Miller

Introduction

Electronic fetal heart rate monitoring (EFM) was introduced into clinical practice during an era in which intrapartum fetal hypoxia was thought to be the primary cause of cerebral palsy (CP). Based on this assumption, EFM offered the hope of detecting intrapartum fetal oxygen deprivation so that early intervention could prevent CP [1]. When EFM replaced the traditional practice of intermittent auscultation in the 1970s, a series of non-randomized studies reported significantly lower perinatal mortality rates in electronically monitored patients [2–12]. However, subsequent randomized trials failed to demonstrate consistent improvements in either perinatal morbidity or mortality when the new technology was compared to intermittent auscultation summarized in Table 2.1 [13–24].

Randomized Trials of EFM versus Intermittent Auscultation

In 2006, a Cochrane review of these studies concluded that EFM was associated with an increased rate of cesarean delivery compared with intermittent fetal heart rate (FHR) auscultation during labor [25]. In the 1970s, four randomized trials compared EFM to intermittent auscultation during labor [13–16]. Together, these four trials included 2,027 patients, and each of the four trials demonstrated a significantly higher rate of cesarean birth in the electronically monitored groups. Subsequently, seven randomized trials were published on the same topic, six of which included data regarding overall cesarean rates [17–19,21–23]. These six trials included a total of 20,640 patients. None of the trials published after 1980 demonstrated a higher rate of cesarean delivery in women managed with EFM compared with those managed with intermittent auscultation.

To date, no randomized controlled trial has confirmed the original assumption that EFM can prevent CP. Retrospective studies have demonstrated that more than 90% of CP cases may have no identifiable link to intrapartum hypoxia. Such cases cannot reasonably be expected to be detectable or preventable by refinements in the management of labor, including interpretation and management of intrapartum EFM [26,27]. The false-positive rate of EFM for predicting CP has been reported to exceed 99%, yielding a positive predictive value of less than 1% [28,29]. Potential explanations for this imprecision include the relative rarity of intrapartum hypoxic neurologic injury, the mitigating interventions that frequently are triggered by FHR "abnormalities," the amount of time that separates EFM from the later diagnosis of CP, and finally, EFM is a screening test rather than a diagnostic test. Despite these limitations, some form of intrapartum fetal monitoring is necessary, even in low-risk pregnancies. The only form of intrapartum fetal monitoring that has been demonstrated in randomized trials to be equivalent to EFM in safety and efficacy is intermittent auscultation conducted under research protocols employing one-on-one nursing care. No study has demonstrated that such an approach is as cost-effective as EFM, much less more cost-effective. Therefore, principles of patient safety dictate that future efforts should focus on standardization and simplification of EFM as it is used in contemporary clinical practice. These efforts should include promulgation of standardized definitions, simplification of interpretation and development of practical, evidence-based approaches to management.

The Evolution of Standardized FHR Definitions

Electronic FHR monitoring was introduced into clinical practice before consensus was achieved regarding standardized definitions of FHR patterns. This resulted in wide variations in the description and interpretation of common FHR observations. In 1995

Table 2.1 Randomized trials of EFM versus intermittent auscultation.

Author [Reference] Year of publication	Number of patients	EFM impact on:					
		Cesarean rate	Perinatal mortality	Apgar scores	Umbilical cord blood pH	NICU admissions	Neonatal neurologic abnormalities
Haverkamp et al. [13] 1976	483	Increase	No difference	No difference	No difference	No difference	No difference
Renou et al. [14] 1976	350	Increase	No difference	No difference	Higher cord pH in EFM group	Fewer NICU admissions in EFM group	Fewer neonatal neurologic abnormalities in EFM group
Kelso et al. [15] 1978	504	Increase	No difference	No difference	No difference	No difference	No difference
Haverkamp et al. [16] 1979	690	Increase	No difference	No difference	No difference	No difference	No difference
Wood et al. [17] 1981	989	No difference	No difference	No difference	No difference	No difference	No difference
MacDonald et al. [18] 1985	12,964	No difference	No difference	No difference	No difference	No difference	Fewer neonatal seizures in EFM group
Neldam et al. [19] 1986	969	No difference	No difference	No difference	No difference	No difference	No difference
Luthy et al. [21] 1987	246	No difference	No difference	No difference	No difference	No difference	No difference
Vintzileos et al. [22] 1993	1,428	No difference	No difference	No difference	No difference	No difference	No difference
Herbst & Ingemarrson [23] 1994	4,044	No difference	No difference	No difference	No difference	No difference	No difference

and 1996, the National Institute of Child Health and Human Development (NICHD) convened a workshop to develop "standardized and unambiguous definitions for fetal heart rate tracings" [30]. In 2005 and 2006, the NICHD definitions were endorsed by the American College of Obstetricians and Gynecologists (ACOG), The Association of Women's Health, Obstetric and Neonatal Nurses (AWHONN), and the American College of Nurse Midwives (ACNM) [31–33]. In 2008, a second NICHD consensus panel was convened to review and update the standardized definitions published in 1997 and to reach consensus regarding basic principles of FHR interpretation [34]. The standardized NICHD FHR definitions published in 2008 are summarized in Table 2.2.

The 2008 NICHD Consensus Report

In addition to clarifying and reaffirming the standardized FHR definitions proposed in the 1997 NICHD consensus report, the 2008 report recommended a simplified system for classifying FHR tracings using baseline rate, variability and decelerations to group FHR tracings into three categories as summarized in Table 2.3.

The proposed FHR categories represent a shorthand method of defining FHR tracings. Category II, in particular, includes a very wide range of FHR tracings with variable clinical significance. Consequently, categories alone do not provide sufficient information for accurate communication of FHR patterns. Categories specifically do not replace a full description of baseline rate, variability, accelerations, decelerations, and changes or trends over time. The 2008 NICHD consensus report also made recommendations regarding uterine activity. Normal uterine contraction frequency was defined as five or fewer contractions in a 10-minute window averaged over 30 minutes. Contraction frequency of more than five in 10 minutes averaged over 30 minutes was defined as tachysystole.

Table 2.2 Standard fetal heart rate definitions.

Pattern	Definition
Baseline	The mean FHR rounded to increments of 5 beats/min during a 10-min segment, excluding accelerations, decelerations, and periods of marked FHR variability The baseline must be for a minimum of 2 min (not necessarily contiguous) in any 10-min segment, or the baseline for that segment is defined as "indeterminate"
Tachycardia	Baseline FHR greater than 160 beats per min
Bradycardia	Baseline FHR less than 110 beats per min
Baseline variability	Fluctuations in the FHR baseline that are irregular in amplitude and frequency. Variability is measured from the peak to the trough of the FHR fluctuations and is quantified in beats/min. Variability is classified as follows. Absent – amplitude range undetectable Minimal – amplitude range detectable but ≤ 5 beats/min Moderate – amplitude range 6–25 beats/min Marked – amplitude range > 25 beats per min No distinction is made between short-term variability (or beat-to-beat variability or R-R wave period differences in the electrocardiogram) and long-term variability because in actual practice they are visually determined as a unit
Acceleration	A visually apparent abrupt increase (onset to peak < 30 sec) in the FHR from the baseline At 32 weeks of gestation and beyond, an acceleration has a peak at least 15 beats/min above baseline and duration of at least 15 sec but less than 2 min Before 32 weeks of gestation, an acceleration has peak at least 10 beats/min above baseline and a duration of at least 10 sec but less than 2 min Prolonged acceleration lasts ≥ 2 min but < 10 min If an acceleration lasts ≥ 10 min, it is a baseline change
Early deceleration	In association with uterine contraction, a visually apparent, gradual (onset to nadir ≥ 30 sec) decrease in FHR with return to baseline. In general, the nadir of the deceleration occurs at the same time as the peak of the contraction
Late deceleration	In association with a uterine contraction, a visually apparent, gradual (onset to nadir ≥ 30 sec) decrease in FHR with return to baseline. In general, the onset, nadir, and recovery of the deceleration occur after the beginning, peak, and end of the contraction, respectively
Variable deceleration	An abrupt (onset to nadir < 30 sec) visually apparent decrease in the FHR below the baseline The decrease in FHR is at least 15 beats/min and lasts at least 15 sec but less then 2 min
Prolonged deceleration	Visually apparent decrease in the FHR at least 15 beats/min below the baseline lasting at least 2 min but less than 10 min from onset to return to baseline
Periodic deceleration	Accompanies a uterine contraction
Episodic deceleration	Does not accompany a uterine contraction
Sinusoidal pattern	Visually apparent, smooth, sine wave-like undulating pattern in FHR baseline with a cycle frequency of 3–5 per minute which persists for ≥ 20 min

Adapted from: Macones GA, Hankins GD, Spong CY, Hauth J, Moore T. The 2008 National Institute of Child Health and Human Development workshop report on electronic fetal monitoring: update on definitions, interpretations, and research guidelines. Obstet Gynecol. 2008 Sep,112(3):661–666 [34].

The terms hyperstimulation and hypercontractility have been defined inconsistently in the literature; therefore, the consensus report recommended that they be abandoned [34]. Contraction frequency alone is a partial assessment of uterine activity. Other factors such as duration, intensity, and relaxation time between contractions are equally important in clinical practice. Finally, the 2008 NICHD report introduced for the first time in consensus form two key statements that form the basis for standardized EFM interpretation: (1) moderate variability reliably predicts the absence of metabolic acidemia at the time it is observed, and (2) accelerations reliably predict the absence of metabolic acidemia at the time they are observed. These recommendations are summarized in ACOG Practice Bulletins 106 and 116 [29,35].

Table 2.3 Fetal heart rate categories.

Category I requires all of the following:
Baseline rate: 110–160 bpm
Variability: Moderate
Accelerations: Present or absent
Decelerations: No late, variable, or prolonged decelerations
Category II
Any FHR tracing that does not meet criteria for classification in Category I or Category III
Category III requires at least one of the following:
Absent variability with recurrent late decelerations
Absent vaiability with recurrent variable decelerations
Absent variability with bradycardia for at least 10 minutes
Sinusoidal pattern for at least 20 minutes

NICHD Definitions – General Considerations

The standardized definitions proposed by the NICHD in 1997 and reaffirmed in 2008 apply to the interpretation of FHR patterns produced by a direct fetal electrode detecting the fetal electrocardiogram (ECG), or by an external Doppler device detecting fetal cardiac motion using the autocorrelation technique. Autocorrelation, used in modern FHR monitors, is a computerized method of minimizing the artifact associated with Doppler ultrasound calculation of the FHR. Patterns are categorized as baseline, periodic, or episodic.

- Baseline patterns include baseline rate and variability.
- Periodic and episodic patterns include FHR accelerations and decelerations.
- Periodic patterns are those associated with uterine contractions.
- Episodic patterns are those not associated with uterine contractions.
- A number of FHR characteristics are dependent upon gestational age, so gestational age must be considered in the full evaluation of the pattern.
- In addition, the FHR tracing should be evaluated in the context of maternal medical condition, prior results of fetal assessment, medications, and other factors.
- FHR patterns do not occur alone and generally evolve over time.
- A full description of an FHR tracing requires assessment of uterine activity as well as a

qualitative and quantitative description of all components, including baseline rate, variability, accelerations, decelerations, and changes or trends over time.

Baseline

Baseline FHR is defined as the approximate mean FHR rounded to increments of 5 bpm during a 10-minute segment, excluding accelerations, decelerations, and periods of marked variability. Baseline rate is defined as a single number (for example, 145 bpm), not as a range (for example "140–150 bpm" or "140s"). In any 10-minute window the minimum baseline duration must be at least 2 minutes (not necessarily contiguous) or the baseline for that period is deemed indeterminate. If the baseline during any 10-minute segment is deemed indeterminate, it may be necessary to refer to previous 10-minute segment(s) for determination of the baseline.

Fetal Heart Rate Variability

Variability is defined as fluctuations in the baseline FHR that are irregular in amplitude and frequency. Variability is quantitated in beats per minute and is measured from the peak to the trough in beats per minute. No distinction is made between "short-term" ("beat-to-beat") variability and "long-term" variability because in actual practice they are visually determined as a unit. Standardized NICHD nomenclature classifies variability as absent, minimal, moderate, or marked. Variability is defined as absent when the amplitude range of the FHR fluctuations is undetectable to the unaided eye. Variability is defined as minimal when the amplitude range is detectable but less than or equal to 5 beats per minute. When the amplitude range of the fluctuations is 6–25 beats per minute, variability is defined as moderate (Figure 2.1). Finally, variability is defined as marked when the amplitude range is greater than 25 beats per minute.

Acceleration

Acceleration is defined as an abrupt (onset to peak < 30 sec) increase in FHR above the baseline. The peak is at least 15 bpm above the baseline and the acceleration lasts at least 15 sec from the onset to return to baseline. Before 32 weeks of gestation, an acceleration is defined as having a peak at least 10 bpm above the baseline and a duration of at least 10 sec. An acceleration lasting at least 2 min but less than 10 min is

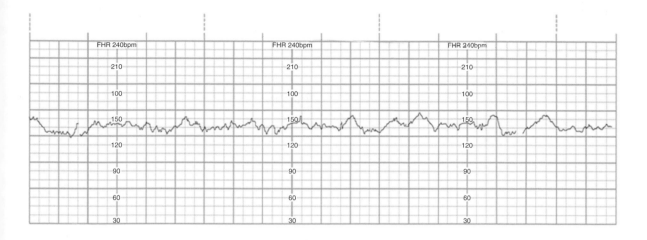

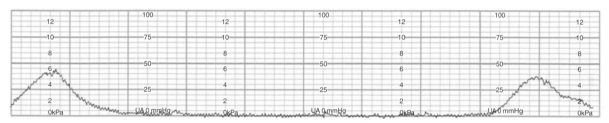

Figure 2.1 Moderate fetal heart rate variability.

defined as a prolonged acceleration. An acceleration lasting 10 min or longer is defined as a baseline change. Accelerations that are provoked by fetal stimulation have the same clinical significance as spontaneous accelerations [34].

Decelerations

Decelerations in the FHR are categorized as early, late, variable, or prolonged and are quantitated by depth in bpm below the baseline and duration in minutes and seconds. An abrupt deceleration reaches its nadir in less than 30 sec. A gradual deceleration reaches its nadir in ≥ 30 sec. Decelerations that occur with at least 50% of uterine contractions in a 20-min period are defined as recurrent. Decelerations occurring with fewer than 50% of contractions in a 20-min period are defined as intermittent. Decelerations may be accompanied by other characteristics such as slow return of the FHR after the end of the contraction, biphasic decelerations, tachycardia following variable deceleration(s), accelerations preceding and/or following decelerations (sometimes called shoulders or overshoots), and fluctuations in the FHR in the trough of the deceleration. The clinical

significance of these characteristics requires further research investigation; therefore, they are not included in standard NICHD terminology. Classification of decelerations as "mild," "moderate," or "severe" has not been shown to correlate with metabolic acidemia or newborn outcome independent of known confounding factors such as baseline rate, moderate variability, accelerations, and frequency of decelerations. Therefore, such classification is not included in standardized NICHD terminology [34].

Early Deceleration

Early deceleration is defined as a gradual (onset to nadir < 30 sec) decrease in FHR from the baseline and subsequent return to baseline associated with a uterine contraction (Figure 2.2). The onset, nadir, and recovery of the deceleration occur at the same time as the beginning, peak, and end of the contraction, respectively.

Late Deceleration

Late deceleration of the FHR is defined as a gradual (onset to nadir ≥ 30 sec) decrease of the FHR from the

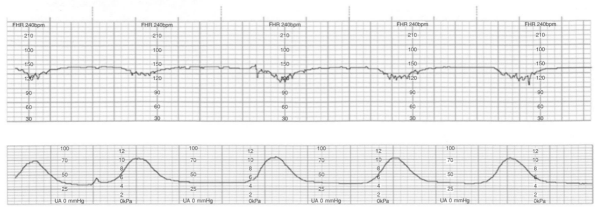

Figure 2.2 Fetal heart rate trace showing early deceleration.

baseline and subsequent return to the baseline associated with a uterine contraction (Figure 2.3). In most cases the onset, nadir, and recovery of the deceleration occur after the beginning, peak, and ending of the contraction, respectively.

Variable Deceleration

Variable deceleration of the FHR is defined as an abrupt (onset to nadir < 30 sec) decrease in FHR below the baseline (Figure 2.4). The decrease is at least 15 bpm below the baseline and the deceleration lasts at least 15 sec and < 2 min from onset to return to baseline. Variable decelerations can occur with or without uterine contractions.

Prolonged Deceleration

Prolonged deceleration of the FHR is defined as a decrease (either gradual or abrupt) in FHR at least 15 bpm below the baseline lasting at least 2 min from onset to return to baseline. According to NICHD terminology, a prolonged deceleration lasting 10 min or longer is defined as a baseline change.

Sinusoidal Pattern

The sinusoidal pattern is a smooth, sine wave-like undulating pattern in FHR baseline with a cycle frequency of 3–5/min that persists for at least 20 min (Figure 2.5). It is specifically excluded from the definition of variability. The sinusoidal pattern can be distinguished from variability because it is characterized by fluctuations in the baseline that are regular in amplitude in frequency.

Physiology of Fetal Heart Rate Patterns

Many factors interact to regulate the FHR, including cardiac pacemakers, the cardiac conduction system, autonomic innervation (sympathetic, parasympathetic), humoral factors (catecholamines), extrinsic factors (medications), and local factors (calcium, potassium). Fluctuations in PO_2, PCO_2, and blood pressure are detected by chemoreceptors and baroreceptors located in the aortic arch and carotid arteries. Signals from these receptors are processed in the medullary vasomotor center, possibly with regulatory input from higher centers in the hypothalamus and cerebral cortex. Sympathetic and parasympathetic signals from the medullary vasomotor center modulate the FHR in response to moment-to-moment changes in fetal PO_2, PCO_2, and blood pressure.

Baseline Fetal Heart Rate

Fetal bradycardia may be seen in association with maternal beta-blocker therapy, hypothermia, hypoglycemia, hypothyroidism, fetal heart block, or interruption of fetal oxygenation. Fetal tachycardia may be associated with fever, infection, medications, maternal hyperthyroidism, fetal anemia, arrhythmia, or interruption of fetal oxygenation.

Variability

With every heartbeat, slight corrections in the heart rate help to optimize fetal cardiac output and maximize the distribution of oxygenated blood to the fetal tissues resulting in observed FHR variability. The 2008

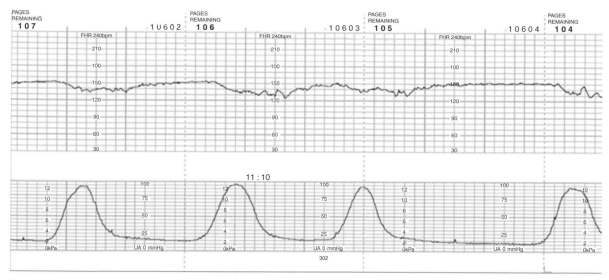

Figure 2.3 Fetal heart rate trace showing late deceleration.

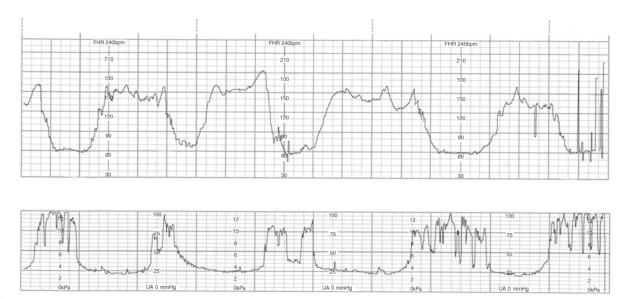

Figure 2.4 Fetal heart rate trace showing variable deceleration.

NICHD consensus report stated that moderate variability reliably predicts the absence of fetal metabolic acidemia at the time it is observed [34]. However, the converse is not true. Minimal or absent variability alone do not confirm the presence of fetal metabolic academia [34]. Other conditions potentially associated with minimal or absent variability include fetal sleep cycle, arrhythmia, medications, extreme prematurity, congenital anomalies, or pre-existing neurologic injury. It is important to note that most of the literature regarding "decreased" variability does not differentiate between absent variability (amplitude range undetectable) and minimal variability (amplitude range detectable but ≤ 5 bpm). Therefore, it is not possible to draw valid conclusions regarding the relative clinical significance of these two categories. The significance of marked variability is not known. Possible explanations include a normal variant or an exaggerated autonomic response to transient interruption of fetal oxygenation.

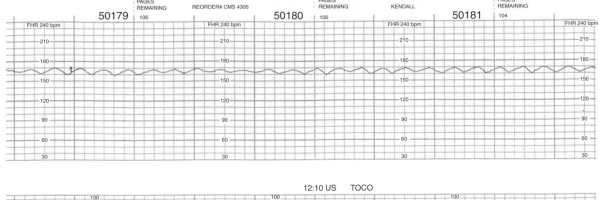

Figure 2.5 Fetal heart rate trace showing sinusoidal pattern.

Accelerations

Accelerations in FHR frequently occur in association with fetal movement, possibly as a result of stimulation of peripheral proprioceptors, increased catecholamine release, and autonomic stimulation of the heart. Another suspected mechanism of FHR acceleration is transient compression of the umbilical vein, resulting in decreased fetal venous return and a reflex rise in heart rate. The 2008 NICHD consensus report stated that FHR accelerations variability reliably predict the absence of fetal metabolic acidemia at the time they are observed [34]. However, the converse is not true. The absence of accelerations does not confirm the presence of fetal metabolic acidemia [34]. Other conditions potentially associated with the absence of accelerations include fetal sleep cycle, arrhythmia, medications, extreme prematurity, congenital anomalies, fetal anemia, and pre-existing neurologic injury.

Early Deceleration

Although the precise physiologic mechanism is not known, early decelerations are considered to represent a fetal autonomic response to changes in intracranial pressure and/or cerebral blood flow caused by intrapartum compression of the fetal head during uterine contractions. Early decelerations are not correlated with adverse outcome and are considered clinically benign. Appropriately designed case-control studies have failed to identify any measure of uterine activity as an independent risk factor for cerebral palsy [26,36–41]. The notion that fetal brain injury can be caused by mechanical forces of labor is further challenged by level II evidence from a large cohort study comparing neonatal outcomes of more than 380,000 spontaneous vaginal deliveries to those of more than 33,000 cesarean deliveries without labor [42]. Neonates who were exposed to uterine contractions of sufficient frequency and intensity to result in vaginal delivery had no higher rates of mechanical brain injury, in the form of intracranial hemorrhage, than those exposed to no contractions at all.

Late Deceleration

A late deceleration is a reflex fetal response to transient hypoxemia during a uterine contraction [43]. Myometrial contractions can compress maternal blood vessels traversing the uterine wall and reduce maternal perfusion of the intervillous space of the placenta. Reduced delivery of oxygenated blood to the intervillous space can reduce the diffusion of oxygen into the fetal capillary blood in the chorionic villi, leading to a decline in fetal PO_2. If the fetal PO_2 falls below the normal range (approximately 15–25 mmHg in the umbilical artery), chemoreceptors detect the change and signal the medullary vasomotor center in the brainstem to initiate a protective autonomic reflex response. Initially, sympathetic outflow causes peripheral vasoconstriction, shunting oxygenated blood flow away from non-vital vascular beds and toward vital organs such as the brain, heart, and adrenal glands. The resulting increase in fetal blood pressure is detected by baroreceptors, which trigger a parasympathetic reflex slowing of the heart rate to reduce cardiac output and return the blood pressure to normal. After the contraction, fetal oxygenation is restored, autonomic reflexes subside, and the FHR gradually returns to baseline. This combined sympathetic–parasympathetic reflex response to transient interruption of fetal oxygenation, summarized in Figure 2.6, has been confirmed in animal studies [43–52].

Occasionally, fetal oxygenation can be interrupted sufficiently to cause metabolic acidemia. In that event, a late deceleration may result from direct

Uterine contraction impedes maternal perfusion
of the placental intervillous space

⇩

Transient fetal hypoxemia

⇩

Chemoreceptor stimulation

⇩

Reflex sympathetic outflow

⇩

Peripheral vasoconstriction, preferentially shunting
oxygenated blood away from peripheral
tissues and toward central vital organs
(brain, heart, adrenal glands, placenta)

⇩

Increase in fetal peripheral
resistance and blood pressure

⇩

Baroreceptor stimulation

⇩

Reflex parasympathetic outflow

⇩

Gradual slowing of the FHR

⇩

Late deceleration

⇩

After the contraction, these reflexes subside
and the FHR gradually returns to baseline

Figure 2.6 The combined sympathetic–parasympathetic reflex response to transient interruption of fetal oxygenation.

hypoxic myocardial depression [43]. Since this mechanism requires metabolic acidemia, it can be excluded by the observation of moderate variability or accelerations [34].

Variable Deceleration

A variable deceleration represents a fetal autonomic reflex response to transient mechanical compression of the umbilical cord [53–62]. Initially, compression of the umbilical cord occludes the thin-walled, compliant umbilical vein, decreasing fetal venous return and triggering a baroreceptor-mediated reflex rise in FHR (previously described as a "shoulder"). Further compression occludes the umbilical arteries, causing an abrupt increase in fetal peripheral resistance and blood pressure. Baroreceptors detect the abrupt rise in blood pressure and signal the medullary vasomotor center in the brainstem which, in turn, triggers an increase in parasympathetic outflow and an abrupt decrease in heart rate. As the cord is decompressed, this sequence of events occurs in reverse.

Prolonged Deceleration

If the physiologic mechanisms responsible for late or variable decelerations persist, a deceleration can last 2 min or longer. A deceleration lasting 2 min but less than 10 min is defined as a prolonged deceleration. A deceleration lasting 10 min or longer is defined as a baseline change.

Sinusoidal Pattern

Although the pathophysiologic mechanism is not known, this pattern classically is associated with severe fetal anemia. Variations of the pattern have also been described in association with administration of narcotic analgesics and chorioamnionitis.

Interpretation

Intrapartum FHR monitoring is intended to assess the adequacy of fetal oxygenation during labor. Fetal oxygenation involves the transfer of oxygen from the environment to the fetus along a pathway that includes the maternal lungs, heart, vasculature, uterus, placenta, and umbilical cord. Fetal oxygenation also involves the fetal physiologic response to interruption of the oxygen pathway, including the sequential progression from fetal hypoxemia, to fetal hypoxia, metabolic acidosis and finally, metabolic acidemia.

Interruption of Oxygen Transfer from the Environment to the Fetus

Oxygen is carried from the environment to the fetus by maternal and fetal blood along a pathway that includes the maternal lungs, heart, vasculature, uterus, placenta and umbilical cord (Figure 2.7).

Interruption of the oxygen pathway at one or more points can result in a FHR deceleration. For example, interruption of the oxygen pathway by compression of the umbilical cord can result in a variable deceleration [29,53]. A late deceleration can result from reduced placental perfusion during a uterine contraction [43]. Interruption at any point along the pathway can result in a prolonged deceleration. Examples at each point are illustrated in Table 2.4.

Variable, late, and prolonged decelerations all share a common initiating event: interruption of the oxygen pathway at one or more points. *The first principle of standardized intrapartum FHR interpretation is that all FHR decelerations that have potential clinical significance (variable, late, or prolonged) reflect interruption of the pathway of oxygen transfer from the environment to the fetus at one or more points.*

Interruption of fetal oxygenation has the potential to result in hypoxic neurologic injury. The pathway from normal fetal oxygenation to potential hypoxic injury includes a series of sequential physiologic steps. The first step, hypoxemia, is defined as decreased oxygen content in the blood. Hypoxemia can lead to reduced oxygen content in the tissues, termed hypoxia. Tissue hypoxia can trigger anaerobic metabolism, lactic acid production, and metabolic acidosis

Table 2.4 Examples of potential causes of prolonged deceleration.

Oxygen pathway	Potential cause
Maternal lungs	Maternal apnea during a convulsion
Heart	Acute reduction in cardiac output due to arrhythmia
Vasculature	Accute hypotension due to regional anesthesia
Uterus	Uterine rupture or excessive uterine activity
Placenta	Placental abruption
Cord	Umbilical cord compression or prolapse

in the tissues. Eventually, the blood pH can fall, causing metabolic acidemia. The 2008 NICHD Research Planning Workshop identified two FHR characteristics that reliably predict the absence of fetal metabolic acidemia [34]. *The second principle of intrapartum FHR interpretation is that moderate variability or accelerations reliably predict the absence of fetal metabolic acidemia at the time they are observed.*

Criteria for Hypoxic Neurologic Injury

In 1999 and 2003, the International Cerebral Palsy Task Force, ACOG, and the American Academy of Pediatrics (AAP) published consensus statements that significant fetal metabolic acidemia (umbilical artery pH < 7.0 and base deficit ≥ 12 mmol/l) is an essential precondition to acute intrapartum hypoxic neurologic injury in the form of cerebral palsy. Other criteria are summarized in Tables 2.5 and 2.6.

The third principle of intrapartum FHR interpretation is: acute intrapartum interruption of fetal oxygenation does not result in neurologic injury (cerebral palsy) in the absence of significant fetal metabolic acidemia. Intrapartum FHR monitoring interpretation can be summarized in three central principles that are illustrated in Figure 2.8.

A Simplified, Standardized Approach to Management

The ability to distill intrapartum FHR monitoring into three evidence-based principles of interpretation permits the development of a simplified, standardized approach to management [63]. The management

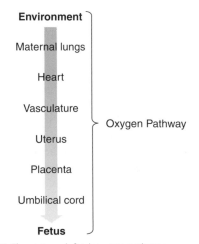

Figure 2.7 The maternal–fetal oxygen pathway.

Table 2.5 Essential criteria that define an acute intrapartum event sufficient to cause cerebral palsy (must meet all four).

1. Umbilical cord arterial blood pH < 7 and base deficit ≥ 12 mmol/l
2. Early onset of severe or moderate neonatal encephalopathy in infants born at 34 or more weeks of gestation
3. Cerebral palsy of the spastic quadriplegic or dyskinetic type
4. Exclusion of other identifiable etiologies such as trauma, coagulation disorders, infectious conditions, or genetic disorders

Table 2.6 Criteria that collectively suggest the event occurred within 48 hours of birth.

1. A sentinel hypoxic event immediately before or during labor
2. A sudden and sustained fetal bradycardia or the absence of FHR variability in the presence of persistent late or variable decelerations, usually after a hypoxic sentinel event when the pattern was previously normal
3. Apgar scores of 0–3 beyond 5 minutes
4. Onset of multisystem involvement within 72 hours of birth
5. Early imaging study showing evidence of acute non-focal cerebral abnormality

algorithm described below incorporates standard FHR definitions and simplified principles of interpretation. It does not include adjunctive tests of fetal status, which are not commonly used in the United States, such as fetal scalp blood sampling, fetal pulse oximetry, or fetal ST-segment analysis. The management recommendations are consistent with those proposed by ACOG in November, 2010 [35].

Confirm Fetal Heart Rate and Uterine Activity

The objective of standardized EFM management is to identify and minimize potential sources of preventable error. The first step is to confirm that the monitor is recording the FHR and uterine activity adequately to permit informed management decisions (Figure 2.9). If external monitoring does not provide adequate information, placement of a fetal scalp electrode and/or intrauterine pressure catheter should be considered.

Evaluate Five FHR Components

Thorough evaluation of a fetal monitor tracing includes assessment of uterine contractions along with five FHR components: baseline rate, variability, accelerations, decelerations, and changes or trends

over time. If a tracing meets criteria for inclusion in Category I, it is considered normal. In low-risk patients, the FHR tracing should be reviewed at least every 30 minutes during the active phase of the first stage of labor and at least every 15 minutes during the second stage [29,64,65]. In high-risk patients, the corresponding frequency of review is at least every 15 minutes during the active phase of the first stage and at least every 5 minutes during the second stage. As recommended by ACOG and the AWHONN, documentation should be performed periodically [29,65,66]. The content and frequency of documentation should be determined by the clinical scenario and applicable institutional policies.

If an FHR tracing does not meet criteria for classification in Category I, a systematic "ABCD" approach can help ensure that important considerations are not overlooked and that decisions are made in a timely fashion (Table 2.7).

A: Assess the Oxygen Pathway and Consider Other Causes of FHR Changes

Intrapartum FHR monitoring is used to assess the adequacy of fetal oxygenation during labor. A Category I FHR tracing indicates normal fetal oxygenation. A tracing that moves beyond Category I raises the possibility of interruption of fetal oxygenation at one or more points along the oxygen pathway. Therefore, when a tracing moves beyond Category I, the oxygen pathway should be assessed systematically (Table 2.7). In addition, several factors can affect the FHR tracing by mechanisms other than interruption of oxygenation. The factors summarized in Table 2.8 should be identified and addressed as clinically indicated.

B: Begin Corrective Measures as Indicated

Interruption of the oxygen pathway should be addressed with appropriate conservative corrective measures [35,63–66]. Table 2.7 summarizes common measures to consider at each level.

Re-evaluate the FHR tracing

After beginning conservative corrective measures, the FHR tracing should be re-evaluated within a reasonable time frame. If the tracing returns to Category I, surveillance can be resumed. If the tracing progresses to Category III despite corrective measures, expedited delivery should be considered. Tracings that remain in Category II require additional evaluation. If there is moderate variability and/or accelerations without

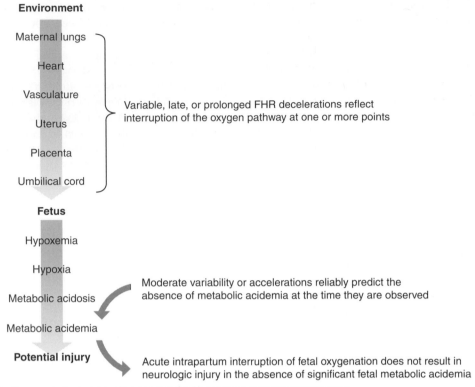

Figure 2.8 The three central principles of intrapartum fetal heart rate monitoring interpretation.

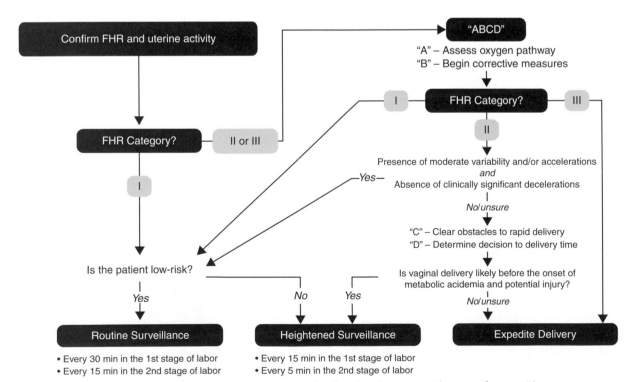

Figure 2.9 Scheme illustrating standardized EFM management to identify and minimize potential sources of preventable error.

significant decelerations, continued surveillance is appropriate (Figure 2.9). However, some Category II tracings are more difficult to interpret, and the clinical team might not always agree on the level of risk. One example is a Category II tracing with a normal baseline rate, minimal variability, no accelerations but no decelerations. Some clinicians might be concerned by the lack of moderate variability or accelerations, while others might be comforted by the absence of decelerations. A standardized approach to management can minimize the controversy generated by confusing Category II tracings. If any member of the healthcare team has any question about the presence of moderate variability, the presence of accelerations or the significance of any observed decelerations, the safest and easiest approach is to proceed to the next step.

C: Clear Obstacles to Rapid Delivery

If conservative measures do not correct the FHR tracing to the satisfaction of the clinicians involved, it is prudent to plan ahead for the possible rapid delivery. This does not constitute a commitment to a particular time or method of delivery. It simply serves as a reminder of common sources of unnecessary delay so that they can be addressed in a timely manner. Because many of the considerations summarized in Table 2.7 are viewed by clinicians as "common

Table 2.7 A standardized "ABCD" approach to intrapartum EFM management.

	"A" Assess oxygen pathway	"B" Begin corrective measures *if indicated*		"C" Clear obstacles to rapid delivery	"D" Determine decision to delivery time
Lungs	Airway and breathing	Supplemental oxygen	Facility	OR availability Equipment	Facility response time
Heart	Heart rate and rhythm	Position change Fluid bolus Correct hypotension	Staff	Consider notifying: Obstetrician Surgical assistant Anesthesiologist Neonatologist Pediatrician Nursing staff	Consider staff: Availability Training Experience
Vasculature	Blood pressure Volume status		Mother	Consider: Informed consent Anesthesia options Laboratory tests Blood products Intravenous access Urinary cathether Abdominal prep Transfer to OR	Surgical considerations (prior abdominal or uterine surgery) Medical considerations (obesity, hypertension, diabetes, SLE) Obstetric considerations (parity, pelvimetry, placental location)
Uterus	Contraction strength Contraction frequency Baseline uterine tone Exclude uterine rupture	Stop or reduce stimulant Consider uterine relaxant	Fetus	Consider: Fetal number Estimated fetal weight Gestational age Presentation Position	Consider factors such as: Estimated fetal weight Gestational age Presentation Position
Placenta	Placental separation				
Cord	Vaginal exam Exclude cord prolapse	Consider amnioinfusion	Labor	Consider IUPC	Consider factors such as: Arrest disorder Protracted labor Poor expulsive efforts

Table 2.8 Several maternal and fetal factors can influence the appearance of the FHR tracing but are not specifically related to fetal oxygenation.

Factor	Reported FHR associations
Fever/infection	Increased baseline rate, decreased variability
Medications	Effects depend upon specific medication and may include changes in baseline rate, frequency and amplitude of accelerations, variability and sinusoidal pattern
Hyperthyroidism	Tachycardia, decreased variability
Prematurity	Increased baseline rate, decreased varibaility, reduced frequency and amplitude of accelerations
Fetal anemia	Sinusoidal pattern, tachycardia
Fetal heart block	Bradycardia, decreased variability
Fetal tachyarrhythmia	Variable degrees of tachycardia, decreased variability
Congenital anomaly	Decreased variability, decelerations
Pre-existing neurologic abnormality	Decreased variability, absent accelerations
Sleep cycle	Decreased variability, reduced frequency and amplitude of accelerations

sense," they may be overlooked, potentially jeopardizing patient safety and inviting criticism. One way to address this problem is to use a simple checklist that organizes potential sources of unnecessary delay into major categories and arranges them in non-random order (see Table 2.7).

D: Decision-to-delivery Time

After appropriate conservative measures have been implemented, it is sensible to take a moment to estimate the time needed to accomplish delivery in the event of a sudden emergency. This step should be addressed by the clinician ultimately responsible for performing operative delivery should it become necessary. The time between decision and delivery can be estimated systematically by considering individual characteristics of the facility, staff, mother, fetus, and labor (Table 2.7).

Delivery

Management steps A, B, C, and D are relatively uncontroversial, readily amenable to standardization, and represent the majority of decisions that must be made during labor. These steps do not replace clinical judgment. On the contrary, they encourage the systematic, timely application of clinical judgment.

Once steps A, B, C, and D are completed, the clinician must decide whether to await spontaneous vaginal delivery or to expedite delivery by other means. This decision balances the estimated time until vaginal delivery against the estimated time until the onset of metabolic acidemia and potential injury. The former estimate is guided by usual obstetric considerations, including power, passenger, and passage. The latter is guided by limited data suggesting that with normal antecedent FHR, metabolic acidemia usually does not appear suddenly, but can evolve gradually over a period of approximately 60 minutes [67]. The inherent imprecision of these estimates can make the decision difficult. Despite the difficulty, a decision must be made using the best-available information. If a decision is made to expedite delivery, the rationale should be documented and the plan implemented. If a decision is made to wait, the rationale and plan should be documented and the decision should be revisited after a reasonable period of time. One of the most common preventable errors at this point is to postpone a clinically necessary but difficult decision in the hope of spontaneous resolution. It is important to recognize that "deciding to wait" is distinctly different from "waiting to decide." The former reflects clinical judgment, while the latter suggests procrastination.

Adjunct Methods of Intrapartum Fetal Monitoring

Fetal Pulse Oxymetry

Intrapartum reflectance fetal pulse oxymetry is a modification of transmission pulse oxymetry that indirectly measures the oxygen saturation of hemoglobin in fetal blood [68]. An intrauterine sensor placed in contact with fetal skin uses the differential absorbtion of red and infrared light by oxygenated and deoxygenated fetal hemoglobin to provide continuous estimation of fetal oxygen saturation. Sensors have been reported to obtain reliable signals 45–60% of the time [69]. In fetal sheep, normal aerobic metabolism is maintained at oxygen saturations above 30% [70,71]. Below that level, metabolic acidosis, and eventually metabolic acidemia, may develop.

The inconclusive and inconsistent results of a number of randomized trials (references from above) led the manufacturer of the fetal pulse oxymeter to announce that it would no longer distribute the sensors needed for the monitors, effectively withdrawing it from the market.

S-T Segment Analysis

Study of the fetal electrocardiogram (ECG) has produced some promising results. The S-T segment of the fetal ECG represents myocardial repolarization. Myocardial hypoxia can lead to elevation of the S-T segment and T wave secondary to catecholamine release, β-adrenoceptor activation, glycogenolysis, and tissue metabolic acidosis [72–74]. These observations led to the development of technology to analyze the fetal ECG plus the S-T waveform (STAN) [75,76].

A recent meta-analysis of four studies, including 9,829 women, concluded that adjunctive S-T segment analysis was associated with significantly fewer cases of severe metabolic acidemia at birth, fewer cases of neonatal encephalopathy, and fewer operative vaginal deliveries [77]. However, there were no significant differences in cesarean delivery rates, low 5-minute Apgar scores, or NICU admissions. This meta-analysis suggests that S-T segment analysis might prove to be a useful adjunct to standard EFM, but it needs further study before it can be recommended for widespread use. However, a very recent multi-center randomized trial in the USA (published as an abstract as of this writing), including over 11,000 women, showed no significant differences in perinatal outcomes or operative delivery rates [78].

Summary

The greatest strength of intrapartum EFM is its ability to predict the absence of metabolic acidemia and hypoxic neurologic injury with an extremely high degree of reliability. Its greatest weakness is its inability to predict the presence of these conditions with any clinically relevant accuracy. The false-positive rate of EFM for predicting CP has been reported to exceed 99%, yielding a positive predictive value of less than 1% [28,29]. Reasonable management decisions cannot be based on the results of a test that it is virtually always wrong. On the other hand, the negative predictive value of EFM is near 100%. A test that is virtually always right is the ideal foundation for rational decision-making. The interpretation and management method described in this chapter uses the exceptional negative predictive value of EFM to formulate a structured, systematic, nonrandom approach to intrapartum care. Standardization of FHR definitions and simplification of interpretation and management promote safety by reducing unnecessary complexity and minimizing reliance on random recall, consistent with basic principles of patient safety. Standardization and checklists can improve outcomes and reduce liability by providing a framework for clinicians of all educational backgrounds to apply and articulate a plan of management that is evidence-based, factually accurate, and reasonable [79,80].

References

1 Quilligan EJ, Paul RH. Fetal monitoring: is it worth it? *Obstet Gynecol.* 1975;45(1):96–100.

2 Chan WH, Paul RH, Toews J. Intrapartum fetal monitoring: maternal and fetal morbidity and perinatal mortality. *Obstet Gynecol.* 1973;41(1):7–13.

3 Kelly VC, Kulkarni D. Experiences with fetal monitoring in a community hospital. *Obstet Gynecol.* 1973;41(6):818–824.

4 Tutera G, Newman RL. Fetal monitoring: its effect on the perinatal mortality and caesarean section rates and its complications. *Am J Obstet Gynecol.* 1975;122(6):750–754.

5 Sibanda J, Beard RW. Influence on clinical practice of routine intra-partum fetal monitoring. *Br Med J.* 1975;3(5979):341–343.

6 Shenker L, Post RC, Seiler JS. Routine electronic monitoring of fetal heart rate and uterine activity during labor. *Obstet Gynecol.* 1975;46(2):185–189.

7 Koh KS, Greves D, Yung S, Peddle LJ. Experience with fetal monitoring in a university teaching hospital. *Can Med Assoc J.* 1975;112(4):455–456, 459–460.

8 Lee WK, Baggish MS. The effect of unselected intrapartum fetal monitoring. *Obstet Gynecol.* 1976;47(5):516–520.

9 Paul RH, Huey JR Jr, Yaeger CF. Clinical fetal monitoring: its effect on cesarean section rate and perinatal mortality: five-year trends. *Postgrad Med.* 1977;61(4):160–166.

10 Amato JC. Fetal monitoring in a community hospital. A statistical analysis. *Obstet Gynecol.* 1977;50(3):269–274.

11 Johnstone FD, Campbell DM, Hughes GJ. Has continuous intrapartum monitoring made any impact on fetal outcome? *Lancet.* 1978;1(8077):1298–1300.

12 Hamilton LA Jr, Gottschalk W, Vidyasagar D, Horn C, Wynn RM. Effects of monitoring high-risk pregnancies

and intrapartum FHR monitoring on perinates. *Int J Gynaecol Obstet*. 1978;15(6):483–490.

13 Haverkamp AD, Thompson HE, McFee JG, Cetrullo C. The evaluation of continuous fetal heart rate monitoring in high-risk pregnancy. *Am J Obstet Gynecol*. 1976;125(3):310–320.

14 Renou P, Chang A, Anderson I, Wood C. Controlled trial of fetal intensive care. *Am J Obstet Gynecol*. 1976;126(4):470–476.

15 Kelso IM, Parsons RJ, Lawrence GF, Arora SS, Edmonds DK, Cooke ID. An assessment of continuous fetal heart rate monitoring in labor. A randomized trial. *Am J Obstet Gynecol*. 1978;131(5):526–532.

16 Haverkamp AD, Orleans M, Langendoerfer S, McFee J, Murphy J, Thompson HE. A controlled trial of the differential effects of intrapartum fetal monitoring. *Am J Obstet Gynecol*. 1979;134(4):399–412.

17 Wood C, Renou P, Oats J, Farrell E, Bleischer N, Anderson I. A controlled trial of fetal heart rate monitoring in a low-risk obstetric population. *Am J Obstet Gynecol*. 1981;141(5):527–534.

18 MacDonald D, Grant A, Sheridan-Pereira M, Boylan P, Chalmers I. The Dublin randomized controlled trial of intrapartum fetal heart rate monitoring. *Am J Obstet Gynecol*. 1985;152(5):524–539.

19 Neldam S, Osler M, Hansen PK, Nim J, Smith SF, Hertel J. Intrapartum fetal heart rate monitoring in a combined low- and high-risk population: a controlled clinical trial. *Eur J Obstet Gynecol Reprod Biol*. 1986;23(1–2):1–11.

20 Leveno KJ, Cunningham FG, Nelson S, et al. A prospective comparison of selective and universal electronic fetal monitoring in 34,995 pregnancies. *N Engl J Med*. 1986;315(10):615–619.

21 Luthy DA, Shy KK, van Belle G, et al. A randomized trial of electronic fetal monitoring in preterm labor. *Obstet Gynecol*. 1987;69(5):687–695.

22 Vintzileos AM, Antsaklis A, Varvarigos I, Papas C, Sofatzis I, Montgomery JT. A randomized trial of intrapartum electronic fetal heart rate monitoring versus intermittent auscultation. *Obstet Gynecol*. 1993;81(6):899–907.

23 Herbst A, Ingemarsson I. Intermittent versus continuous electronic fetal monitoring in labour: a randomised study. *Br J Obstet Gynaecol*. 1994;101(8):663–668.

24 Grant A, O'Brien N, Joy MY, Hennessy E, MacDonald D. Cerebral palsy among children born during the Dublin randomized trial of intrapartum monitoring. *Lancet*. 1989;2(8674):1233–1236.

25 Alfirevic Z, Devane D, Gyte GM. Continuous cardiotocography (CTG) as a form of electronic fetal monitoring (EFM) for fetal assessment during labour. *Cochrane Database Syst Rev*. 2006;(3):CD006066.

26 Nelson KB, Ellenberg JH. Antecedents of cerebral palsy: multivariate analysis of risk. *N Engl J Med*. 1986;315:81–86.

27 Blair E, Stanley FJ. Intrapartum asphyxia: a rare cause of cerebral palsy. *J Pediatr*. 1988;112:515–519.

28 Nelson KB, Dambrosia JM, Ting TY, Grether JK. Uncertain value of electronic fetal monitoring in predicting cerebral palsy. *N Engl J Med*. 1996;334(10):613–618.

29 American College of Obstetricians and Gynecologists. ACOG Practice Bulletin number 106: intrapartum fetal heart rate monitoring: nomenclature, interpretation, and general management principles. *Obstet Gynecol*. 2009;114:192–202.

30 Electronic fetal heart rate monitoring: research guidelines for interpretation. National Institute of Child Health and Human Development Research Planning Workshop. *Am J Obstet Gynecol*. 1997;177(6):1385–1390.

31 American College of Obstetricians and Gynecologists. ACOG practice bulletin. Clinical management guidelines for obstetricians-gynecologists, number 70, December 2005 (replaces practice bulletin number 62, May 2005). Intrapartum fetal heart rate monitoring. *Obstet Gynecol*. 2005;106:1453–1461.

32 Association of Women's Health, Obstetric and Neonatal Nurses. *Fetal Heart Monitoring: Principles and Practices*. 3rd ed. Washington, DC: Association of Women's Health, Obstetric and Neonatal Nurses; 2005.

33 American College of Nurse-Midwives. *Position Statement: Standardized Nomenclature for Electronic Fetal Monitoring*. Silver Spring, MD: American College of Nurse-Midwives; 2006.

34 Macones GA, Hankins GD, Spong CY, Hauth J, Moore T. The 2008 National Institute of Child Health and Human Development workshop report on electronic fetal monitoring: update on definitions, interpretation, and research guidelines. *Obstet Gynecol*. 2008;112(3):661–666.

35 Management of intrapartum fetal heart rate tracings. Practice Bulletin No. 116. American College of Obstetricians and Gynecologists. *Obstet Gynecol*. 2010;116:1232–1240.

36 US Preventive Services Task Force Procedure Manual. AHRQ Publication No. 08-05118-EF, July 2008.

37 Kułak W, Okurowska-Zawada B, Sienkiewicz D, Paszko-Patej G, Krajewska-Kułak E. Risk factors for cerebral palsy in term birth infants. *Adv Med Sci*. 2010;55(2):216–221.

38   Walstab J, Bell R, Reddihough D, et al. Antenatal and intrapartum antecedents of cerebral palsy: a case-control study. *Aust N Z J Obstet Gynaecol*. 2002;42(2):138–146.

39   Nelson KB, Ellenberg JH. Antecedents of cerebral palsy. Univariate analysis of risks. *Am J Dis Child*. 1985;139(10):1031–1038.

40   Badawi N, Kurinczuk JJ, Keogh JM, et al. Intrapartum risk factors for newborn encephalopathy: the Western Australian case-control study. *Br Med J*. 1998;317:1554–1558.

41   Suvanand S, Kapoor SK, Reddaiah VP, Singh U, Sundaram KR. Risk factors for cerebral palsy. *Indian J Pediatr*. 1997;64:677.

42   Towner D, Castro MA, Eby-Wilkens E, Gilbert WM. Effect of mode of delivery in nulliparous women on neonatal intracranial injury. *N Engl J Med*. 1999;341(23):1709–1714.

43   Martin CB Jr, de Haan J, van der Wildt B, Jongsma HW, Dieleman A, Arts TH. Mechanisms of late decelerations in the fetal heart rate. A study with autonomic blocking agents in fetal lambs. *Eur J Obstet Gynecol Reprod Biol*. 1979;9(6):361–373.

44   Ball RH, Espinoza MI, Parer JT. Regional blood flow in asphyxiated fetuses with seizures. *Am J Obstet Gynecol* 1994;170:156–161.

45   Ball RH, Parer JT, Caldwell LE, Johnson J. Regional blood flow and metabolism ovine fetuses during severe cord occlusion. *Am J Obstet Gynecol*. 1994;171:1549–1555.

46   Cohn HE, Sacks EJ, Heymann MA, Rudolph AM. Cardiovascular response to hypoxemia and acidemia in fetal lambs. *Am J Obstet Gynecol*. 1974;120:817–824.

47   Field DR, Parer JT, Auslander RA, Cheek DB, Baker W, Johnson J. Cerebral oxygen consumption during asphyxia in fetal sheep. *J Dev Physiol*. 1990;14:131–137.

48   Itskovitz J, LaGamma EF, Rudolph AM. The effect of reducing umbilical blood flow on fetal oxygenation. *Am J Obstet Gynecol*. 1983;145:813–818.

49   Jensen A, Roman C, Rudolph AM. Effects of reducing uterine blood flow on fetal blood flow distribution and oxygen delivery. *J Dev Physiol*. 1991;15:309–323.

50   Peeters LL, Sheldon RD, Jones MD, Makowski EL, Meschia G. Blood flow to fetal organs as a function of arterial oxygen content. *Am J Obstet Gynecol*. 1979;135:637–646.

51   Reid DL, Parer JT, Williams K, Darr D, Phermaton TM, Rankin JHH. Effects of severe reduction in maternal placental blood flow on blood flow distribution in the sheep fetus. *J Dev Physiol*. 1991;15:183–188.

52   Richardson BS, Rurak D, Patrick JE, Homan J, Carmichael L. Cerebral oxidative metabolism during prolonged hypoxemia. *J Dev Physiol*. 1989;11:37–43.

53   Itskovitz J, LaGamma EF, Rudolph AM. Heart rate and blood pressure responses to umbilical cord compression in fetal lambs with special reference to the mechanism of variable deceleration. *Am J Obstet Gynecol*. 1983;147:451–457.

54   Itskovitz J, LaGamma EF, Rudolph AM. The effect of reducing umbilical blood flow on fetal oxygenation. *Am J Obstet Gynecol*. 1983;145:813–818.

55   Itskovitz J, LaGamma EF, Rudolph AM. Effect of cord compression on fetal blood flow distribution and O_2 delivery. *Am J Physiol*. 1987;252:H100–H109.

56   James LS, Yeh MN, Morishima HO, et al. Umbilical vein occlusion and transient acceleration of the fetal heart rate. Experimental observations in subhuman primates. *Am J Obstet Gynecol*. 1976;126:276–283.

57   Lee CY, Di Loreto PC, O'Lane JM. A study of fetal heart rate acceleration patterns. *Obstet Gynecol*. 1975;45:142–146.

58   Lee ST, Hon EH. Fetal hemodynamic response to umbilical cord compression. *Obstet Gynecol*. 1963;22:553–562.

59   Mueller-Heubach E, Battelli AF. Variable heart rate decelerations and transcutaneous PO_2 during umbilical cord occlusion in fetal monkeys. *Am J Obstet Gynecol*. 1982;144:796–802.

60   Siassi B, Wu, PY, Blanco C, Martin CB. Baroreceptor and chemorecephtor responses to umbilical cord occlusion in fetal lambs. *Biol Neonate*. 1979;35:66–73.

61   Towell MD, Salvador HS. Compressionof the umbilical cord. In: Crasignoni P, Pardi G, eds. *An Experimental Model in the Fetal Goat, Fetal Evaluation During Pregnancy and Labor*. New York, NY: Academia Press; 1971: 143–156.

62   Yeh MN, Morishima HO, Niemann WE, James LS. Myocardial conduction defects in association with compression of the umbilical cord. Experimental observations on fetal baboons. *Am J Obstet Gynecol*. 1975;121:951–957.

63   Miller DA, Miller LA. Electronic fetal heart rate monitoring: applying principles of patient safety. *Am J Obstet Gynecol*. 2012;206(4):278–283.

64   American Academy of Pediatrics, *American College of Obstetricians and Gynecologists: Guidelines for Perinatal Care*. 6th ed. Washington, DC: American Academy of Pediatrics; 2007.

65   ACOG and Association of Women's Health, Obstetric and Neonatal Nurses. *Fetal heart monitoring (Position Statement)*. Washington, DC: Author; 2008.

66 Simpson KR, James DC. Efficacy of intrauterine resuscitation techniques in improving fetal oxygen status during labor. *Obstet Gynecol.* 2005;105:1362–1368.

67 Parer JT, King T, Flanders S, Fox M, Kilpatrick SJ. Fetal acidemia and electronic fetal heart rate patterns. Is there evidence of an association? *J Matern Fetal Neonatal Med.* 2006;19(5):289–294.

68 Dildy GA, Clark SL, Loucks CA. Intrapartum fetal pulse oximetry: past, present, and future *Am J Obstet Gynecol.* 1996;175(1):1–9.

69 Dildy GA, Clark SL, Loucks CA. Preliminary experience with intrapartum fetal pulse oximetry in humans. *Obstet Gynecol.* 1993:81:630–635.

70 Oeseburg B, Ringnalda BEM, Crevels J, et al. Fetal oxygenation in chronic maternal hypoxia: what's critical? *Adv Exp Med Biol.* 1992:317:499–502.

71 Nijland R, Jongsma HW, Nijhuis JG, et al. Arterial oxygen saturation in relation to metabolic acidosis in fetal lambs. *Am J Obstet Gynecol.* 1995:172:810–819.

72 Widmark C, Jansson T, Lindecrantz K, Rosén KG. ECG waveform, short term heart rate variability and plasma catecholamine concentrations in response to hypoxia in intrauterine growth retarded guinea pig fetuses. *Dev Physiol.* 1991;15:161–168.

73 Rosén KG, Dagbjartsson A, Henriksson BA, Lagercrantz H, Kjellmer I. The relationship between circulating catecholamine and ST waveform in the fetal lamb electrocardiogram during hypoxia. *Am J Obstet Gynecol.* 1984;149:190–195.

74 Hökegård KH, Eriksson BO, Kjellemer I, Magno R, Rosén KG. Myocardial metabolism in relation to electrocardiographic changes and cardiac function during graded hypoxia in the fetal lamb. *Acta Physiol Scand.* 1981;113:1–7.

75 Lilja H, Karlsson K, Lindecrantz K, Rosén KG. Microprocessor based waveform analysis of the fetal electrocardiogram during labor. *Int J Gynecol Obstet.* 1989;30:109–116.

76 Arulkumaran S, Lilja H, Lindecrantz K, Ratnam SS, Thavarasah AS, Rosén KG. Fetal ECG waveform analysis should improve fetal surveillance in labour. *J Perinatal Med.* 1990;18:13–22.

77 Neilson JP. Fetal electrocardiogram (ECG) for fetal monitoring during labour. *Cochrane Database of Systematic Reviews.* 2006; 3. Art. No.: CD000116. DOI: 10.1002/14651858.CD000116.pub2.

78 Saade G. Fetal ECG analysis of the ST segment as an adjunct to intrapartum fetal heart rate monitoring: a randomized clinical trial. *Am J Obstet Gynecol.* 2015;212(1):S2.

79 Clark SL, Belfort MA, Byum SL, Meyers JA, Perlin JB. Improved outcomes, fewer cesarean deliveries, and reduced litigation: results of a new paradigm in patient safety. *Am J Obstet Gynecol.* 2008;199(2):105e1–7.

80 Pettker CM, Thung SF, Norwitz ER, et al. Impact of a comprehensive patient safety strategy on obstetric adverse events. *Am J Obstet Gynecol.* 2009;200(5):492. e1–e8.

Chapter 3

Patient Safety in the Outpatient Setting

Roger Smith and Mark D. Pearlman

Introduction

After the landmark 1999 publication of the Institute of Medicine's report, "To Err is Human: Building a Safer Health System," increased attention and resources were devoted to improve safety in hospitals [1]. More recently, the safety focus has broadened to include outpatient care as well [2]. The pace of research and of quality initiatives in the ambulatory setting has not kept up to that of the inpatient environment [3]. The type of errors that harm inpatients and outpatients are mostly similar, but they have some unique aspects as well. Errors of diagnostic testing (test ordering, running the test, results follow up), errors in treatment (medication errors, surgical complications, misdiagnoses), errors in prevention (failure to prophylax, failure to follow up), communication failures; systems errors, and process failures are common to both the inpatient and outpatient areas. However, errors in the inpatient setting tend to be errors of commission, while those in the outpatient setting tend to be errors of omission [3]. Emerging standards have begun to guide practices and practitioners on areas of focus in the Ob/Gyn ambulatory setting [2].

There are many factors that influence both the nature of errors in the office, and the ability of the practitioner to mitigate them. The high volume of patients seen in the office is one important factor. The high patient volume consequently increases the number of medications prescribed and tests ordered which require follow-up. Resources available to outpatient practices to tackle error measurement and mitigation are beginning to emerge, and practices should assure that they pay attention to the increasing need to create systems of safety in the office.

There are accrediting agencies that provide ambulatory and outpatient practices self-assessment processes to assess practice structure and function. They can guide the development of tools to measure the quality of care being provided. The Accreditation Association for Ambulatory Health Care and the American Association for Accreditation of Ambulatory Surgery are two of many such accrediting bodies.

Because healthcare has moved toward the management of increasingly serious conditions in the office, surgical procedures that were once only performed in an inpatient hospital setting are now routinely performed in an ambulatory surgery setting, and increasingly in an office setting. Because oversight is often less robust in the ambulatory or office setting, careful attention to standard safety practices may not always occur. It is reasonable for patients to expect that such procedures should be as safe in the office setting as they were previously in the inpatient setting. If this cannot be assured, they should not be performed in the office.

Recognizing these trends, ACOG is attempting to address these important themes. Many of its efforts are cited in this chapter, including its "Report of the Presidential Task Force on Patient Safety in the Office Setting" [2]. In 2011, ACOG launched an initiative called Safety Certification for Outpatient Practice Excellence (SCOPE) [4]. This voluntary program intends to help individual practices to measure their quality and institute new processes to mitigate error and enhance safety.

This chapter will discuss strategies to reduce errors in three areas of particular concern in the office setting. Office procedures, the patient visit, and ordering and follow-up of diagnostic tests will be covered. Finally, the last section will offer a framework from which to build quality measurement and improvement initiatives.

Office Procedures

Case #1

A 32-year-old presents for office hysteroscopic sterilization. As a paracervical block with 1% lidocaine is being administered, she complains of a metallic taste in her mouth, ringing in her ears, and feeling dizzy. She develops a rapid respiratory rate, has seizure-like activity, followed by a loss of consciousness. Help is summoned. After some delay, the emergency kit is finally found but noted to have all expired medications.

Case #2

A 27-year-old undergoes LEEP in the office under local anesthetic. An unusual amount of bleeding occurs. Neither large cotton swabs nor gauze 4 × 4 sponges can clear the conization bed adequately to allow visualization of the source of bleeding. Cautery and Monsel's solution fail to slow the heavy bleeding. Suction is unavailable. The only suture available is 3-0 or 4-0 Monocryl. A needle driver cannot be found. Unable to control the bleeding, the vagina is packed and she is transported by ambulance to the hospital for management.

Case #3

A 37-year-old nulligravid woman has failed to get pregnant in two prior IVF cycles, and is undergoing her last attempt. Egg retrieval is scheduled for Saturday morning. At the time of her arrival, it is discovered that she had coffee and yogurt 2 hours prior. She pleads to avoid having her procedure canceled or postponed, and the team acquiesces. The retrieval is very painful to her, despite 3 mg of midazolam and IV fentanyl. She receives repeated doses of fentanyl, for a total of 200 μg. During recovery, her oxygen saturation falls, and she becomes unresponsive. She is given naloxone and requires brief bag-mask ventilation. Upon waking, she vomits. She remains awake and alert, but has increasing difficulty with shortness of breath and eventually is diagnosed with aspiration pneumonia.

Discussion

Increasing numbers of procedures are being performed in the office. A number of factors are driving this, including both patient and provider preference, and financial incentives. More complex procedures with increasing options for analgesia and sedation are being offered. The office realm, once a poorly monitored "wild west," is receiving more scrutiny and being required to sharpen its focus on patient safety (see Chapter 12 on regulatory and legal implications). The case scenarios illustrate that even minor procedures, which gynecologists may do frequently

and routinely, can result in complications and harm. Achieving the best outcomes requires competence, teamwork, effective communication, adherence to carefully defined standards and protocols, and emergency preparedness.

Case #1 describes a patient that displayed symptoms of lidocaine toxicity due to an inadvertent intravascular injection. Metallic taste sensations are not uncommon while administering paracervical blocks. Mild lightheadedness and "funny feelings" occur, and can be minimized by injecting slowly, drawing back on the syringe to avoid intravascular injection, and offering reassurance. However, these mild symptoms are similar to those that occur prior to vasovagal syncope and may also be early symptoms of anaphylaxis or systemic toxicity. Without directly injecting into a vascular channel, severe systemic toxicity is rare [5]. Allergies associated with local anesthetics are rarely due to the amide anesthetic, but rather to contained preservatives. Anaphylaxis is also rare [6]. Offices which perform simple procedures without sedating medications should have team members trained in BLS and should maintain an emergency kit that contains airway management equipment, oxygen, and non-expired medications to treat anaphylaxis. Communication plans with protocols for activating 911 services should be established. Personnel should be assigned to check expiration dates periodically, and replace expired medications.

Case #2 illustrates the importance of being prepared for unusual complications. Portable suction can be invaluable to help identify bleeding sources. Having the correct supplies and instruments to manage complications is a necessity, but even managing the common elements that go into carrying out a routine procedure can be challenging. Providers have different preferences, and personnel change. Just as it is done in the hospital, "pick lists" should be used to help gather supplies, and checklists should be used to aid in safely carrying out the procedure. Other practices can help reduce errors and improve efficiency such as a standardized system to pull supplies in to replace stock when they are used or expire. Organizing supplies and instruments decreases set-up time and speeds up supply procurement in emergencies. Running mock emergencies can help the team improve its performance.

Case #3 illustrates that as procedures become more complex, and anesthesia goes from light to moderate, training standards need to be more rigorous, and adherence to safety guidelines needs to be very strict. Providing sedation for office procedures carries significantly more risk. It is especially in this realm that office procedures must adopt a set of standards and protocols that is similar to those of the hospital [2]. ACOG's "Report of the Presidential Task Force on Patient Safety in the Office Setting" [2] is an excellent resource which discusses the elements of safe office surgery. This report serves as a guide for the high-level outline for safe office surgery presented here. The elements that offices should address while setting up their office surgical suite are briefly addressed.

Medical Director

Initial and ongoing coordination of all of the elements for the safe performance of office surgery should be overseen by a medical director. This person has to be familiar with all of the procedures that will be performed in that setting. The director's job includes: (1) verifying that all members of the surgery team are qualified; (2) planning and executing setting up the space; (3) managing the acquisition of equipment and supplies; and (4) performing ongoing appraisal of surgical activity and outcomes.

Credentialing, Training, and Privileging

Procedures that are performed in the ambulatory or office setting require a process to assure that providers have the background, training, and ongoing competency to perform those procedures. The medical director coordinates training of staff to help with procedures, and should verify their competency. It is natural that, once comfort is established with performing a procedure in the hospital or ambulatory surgical center, physicians migrate the venue of certain procedures to the office. It may be logical to tie privileging of office procedures to hospital privileges. ACOG's report offers sample office privileging forms [2].

Anesthesia

Performing increasingly complex office procedures may involve offering an increasing depth of anesthesia. The office unit must decide what level of anesthesia it wants to manage safely. Levels 1 or 2 are appropriate for the office. The levels are defined by the degree of sedation:

- **Level 1**: Minimal sedation. Local anesthesia and minimal oral anxiolysis.
- **Level 2**: Moderate sedation. Usually managed with IV narcotics and benzodiazepines.

The patient is sleepy and responds to verbal commands or light stimulation. Ventilatory, cardiovascular, and airway reflexes are intact, but may become compromised.

- **Level 3**: Deep sedation. Patient is sleeping and requires deep stimulus to arouse. Ventilatory and airway reflexes may be impaired.
- **Level 4**: Anesthesia.

At the authors' health system, gynecologists who administer moderate sedation must demonstrate competency and be privileged to do so. Moderate sedation privileges require maintaining BLS, ACLS, or ATLS certification, and completion of a moderate sedation course and test every two years. Delivery of moderate sedation requires both a physician or a physician designee (nurse practitioner or physician assistant) with moderate sedation privileges, and also a Sedation Analgesia Professional (typically a nurse). This staff delivers medications and monitors the patient before, during, and after the procedure – until discharge. For any office offering moderate sedation, ACOG recommends that at least one person with ACLS expertise is on site. In our health system, moderate sedation is administered in clinics with close proximity to an emergency department and/or code teams. Fader and Johnson offer a logical approach for deciding whether the office surgical teams need ACLS or BLS training (Figure 3.1) [7]. The approach is based on the finding that the highest rate of hospital discharge after cardiac arrest occurred when BLS started within 4 minutes of arrest, and ACLS with defibrillation occurred within 8 minutes [8]. So, offices doing surgery should gauge whether to train on-site personnel in ACLS or whether the Emergency Medical System can arrive within 8 minutes to help manage cardiac arrest.

Equipment

Offices performing procedures with Level 1 analgesia should have personnel trained in BLS present and equipment in a "Red Bag" to support BLS and treatment of anaphylaxis. This kit includes:

- Oxygen tank
- Airway supplies
- Automatic External Defibrillator
- IV supplies and solution
- First-aid supplies
- Stethoscope and sphygmomanometer
- Drugs: epinephrine, atropine, nitroglycerin, aspirin, glucagon

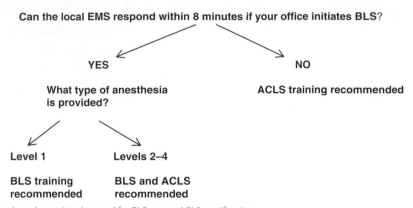

Figure 3.1 An approach to determine the need for BLS versus ACLS certification.
(Modified from: Fader DJ, Johnson TM. Medical issues and emergencies in the dermatology office. *J Am Acad Dermatol.* 1997; 36: 1–16.)

Sites that administer moderate sedation should have a crash cart (arrest cart). The contents of crash carts vary between hospitals and ambulatory surgery sites. The general contents include:

- Suction and suction supplies
- Defibrillator and its supplies
- Ambu bag, masks, oxygen
- Stethoscope, laryngoscope and blades, endotracheal tubes, airways
- Gloves, tape, tourniquet, syringes, needles
- I.V. fluid, tubing, catheters
- ACLS medications (atropine, adenosine, calcium, epinephrine, dexamethasone, digoxin, diltiazem, diphenhydramine, naloxone, glucagon, amiodarone, sodium bicarbonate, nitroglycerine, dopamine, furosemide, magnesium sulfate)

Transfer Guideline

Whatever the complexity of surgery performed – or depth of analgesia offered – the office needs to have a plan for efficient transport of a patient from the office to the hospital. This includes a communication plan of who will call for emergency help (e.g., front desk personnel) so that providers can stay with the patient. Clear instructions with repeat back should be part of the communication process (e.g., "I will call 911 and wait for them outside to direct them to the room").

Organization

Offices' supply areas need to be organized, with obvious visual cues to identify item location and depletion. The entire team should know where everything is, not just the staff members who do the stocking of supplies. Applying the "visual workplace" approach developed by Toyota has been successful in the health care setting [9,10]. The medical director should assure that a systematic approach to stocking allows rapid identification and retrieval of emergency supplies by any personnel who participate in these procedures.

Protocols

Protocols should be written for every procedure performed. These should be kept as the office's Policy and Procedure Manual and readily accessible. The roles of the team members should be specified. The steps of the procedure – from set-up to patient discharge – should be spelled out. Pick lists and checklists both improve efficiency and encourage a safer office environment for the patient. Application of the WHO Surgical Checklist improves patient outcomes [11]. Pick lists and procedure packs help make sure everything the surgeon needs is available.

- Pre-op checklists should include:
    - Patient identification and procedure verification
    - Patient education
    - Informed consent
    - Pre-procedure Time Out (following WHO's Surgical Safety Checklist) [12]
- For moderate sedation procedures, an anesthesia record should be kept during the procedure.
- Post-op checklists should include:
    - Recovery from anesthesia
    - Post-op instructions
    - Follow-up plan

- De-briefing
- Procedure note
- Record of complications

Mock Drills

The ACOG Report on Patient Safety in the Office Setting suggests several drills than an office may run to practice complication management [2]. It offers templates for running a drill and for assessing competence for seven complications: vasovagal episode, local anesthetic complication, cardiac event, allergic reaction, uterine hemorrhage, respiratory arrest, and excessive sedation. Figure 3.2 shows the mock drill for a vasovagal episode.

Quality Assessment and Quality Improvement

Complications should be reviewed and rates of complications should be tracked. These efforts can mirror the quality improvement efforts which hospitals have established.

Patient Visit

Case #4

A 37-year-old presents for follow-up two weeks after an emergency room visit, which concluded with suction curettage for an incomplete spontaneous abortion of a nine-week embryonic demise. The medical assistant in the office has never met her before. The patient is called back by her first name and prepared for a return prenatal visit. She is greeted enthusiastically with questions such as, "how are you feeling now?" and "are you feeling the baby move, yet?" The medical assistant has mistaken the patient for another with the same first name.

Case #5

During a typically busy day, the obstetrician tells her medical assistant, "Room 2 needs Rhogam before she leaves." Rhogam is brought into the room of a 55-year-old patient waiting for an influenza vaccination.

Case #6

A 27-year-old presents for a gynecologic health maintenance examination. She wants to resume prescription contraception. She is counseled and given a prescription for a combined oral contraceptive. The pharmacist calls later to tell the doctor about a potential drug interaction with the patient's carbamazepine.

Patient Identification Error

The high volume of patients in the office setting creates several problems. Among them are managing patient flow efficiently while maintaining contextual continuity. The office environment can be chaotic. Errors in identification and context are minimized, in part, by patients who are typically alert and oriented and able to effectively advocate for themselves. Simple routine practices by the healthcare team can further minimize mistakes in identification. The error in Case #4 is one of mistaken identity. Health systems have policies for rigorous patient verification prior to the performance of critical tasks. For instance, before medication administration, phlebotomy, or surgeries, multiple patient identifiers are checked. However, calling a patient back for an appointment is frequently treated with less attention to these critical details. Often, this is because patients and staff are familiar. However, the error of mistaken identity should be mitigated with standardization of the process of patient admission to the office visit. Such up-front verification does reduce errors that might be more critical, such as with medication administration. This is most successfully accomplished by applying a uniform verification procedure to every patient encounter. Two patient identifiers should be verified (e.g., name and date of birth) prior to an office visit, prior to medication administration, or prior to a procedure [13].

Electronic records, despite their benefits, introduce another opportunity for identification error. In some "paperless" offices, neither a chart nor any paperwork accompanies a patient during her visit. There might be multiple occasions for accessing the electronic care episode, by different team members logging in to the record. Consistent patient identification at each login can reduce errors.

Medication Safety

Adverse drug reactions make up the most frequently cited category of hospital medical errors [14]. Medication errors in the outpatient setting have been studied less, but certainly carry a huge burden of risk [15]. Case #5 illustrates several errors: in medication ordering; in communication; and in medication delivery.

Description: A vasovagal episode typically manifests itself with symptoms of dizziness and signs of hypotension. It may progress to syncope, which is usually transient.

Signs and Symptoms:

- Dizziness, light-headed feeling

- Loss of consciousness

- Nausea, emesis

- Weakness

- Cool, clammy, or pale skin

- Hypotension, bradycardia

Treatment:

- Place patient in supine position; elevate legs

- Maintain airway

- Evaluate and record pulse and blood pressure

- Fluid resuscitate

- Assess for allergic reactions to medications, treat by ACLS protocol as needed

- Assess level of consciousness, reassure patient

Disposition:

- When the patient can sit and then stand without adverse symptoms, discharge is appropriate. The appropriate triggers for seeking medical help should be specified.

- If cardiac or neurologic pathology is suspected, that evaluation should be initiated.

- If the patient displays swelling, loss of consciousness, or convulsions, then CPR should be administered and emergency response activated.

Approved by: _____ Date: _____

(From: Report of the Presidential Task Force on Patient Safety in the Office Setting. Washington DC. ACOG, 2010 P 11.)

Figure 3.2 Mock drill – vasovagal episode.

(From: Report of the Presidential Task Force on Patient Safety in the Office Setting. Washington, DC: ACOG, 2010, p. 11.)

Medication Administration

Reducing errors in mediation use in the office should start by emulating the process of ordering and administering medications established in the hospital setting. If verbal orders are to be practiced in the office, communication tools such as repeat-backs can reduce mistakes and should be routinely practiced. The system of ordering and delivering medication in the office should be standardized. The system should include physical documentation of the order and documentation of the drug administration. Nurses have used the "five rights" of medication administration to guide safe use. The five rights have been expanded to 7 and 9 rights [16] (Figure 3.3).

Number 7, "right action," refers to inviting staff to help verify that the medication makes sense for the patient's condition. Number 9 refers to monitoring the patient for the appropriate time to observe adverse reactions (e.g., monitoring after an HPV immunization is administered in the office).

Medication Reconciliation

Case #6 describes a failure to take an adequate medication history, and a failure to reconcile the patient's current medication regimen. Carbamazepine, a cytochrome P450 enzyme-inducing drug, may decrease the bioavailability of hormones in the oral contraceptive, and subsequently decrease the pill's efficacy. Reducing medication errors, and specifically improving the practice of medication reconciliation, is a focus of both AHRQ [17] and The Joint Commission (2018 Ambulatory Health Care National Patient Safety Goals) [18]. Medication reconciliation is a process that should be practiced at every patient encounter, both inpatient and outpatient. Specifically, the medication list should be updated whenever a patient experiences a change in healthcare venue, has a change in health status, is prescribed a new drug, or has a drug discontinued. AHRQ outlines the process:

- Obtaining, verifying, and documenting the patient's current prescriptions, including over-the-counter medications, herbs, and supplements.
- Considering the patient's regular medications when ordering new ones or instituting a new therapy or discontinuing therapy (i.e., drug–drug interaction, or loss of medication pregnancy protection while on a Category X drug).
- Verifying the patient's medication list and discussing and resolving unintended discrepancies. For example, a certain medication

1.	Right patient	6.	Right documentation
2.	Right drug	7.	Right action
3.	Right route	8.	Right form
4.	Right time	9.	Right reaction
5.	Right dose		

Figure 3.3 The nine rights of medication administration. (Reproduced by permission of British Journal of Nursing)

has been recommended to her, but the patient does not take it.
- Providing an updated mediation list at each encounter, or at least each time the list changes.

Electronic medical records and electronic prescribing can provide multiple tools to provide a source of truth for a patient's medication list, and to check for possible drug–drug interactions.

Follow-up of Patient Data and Tests

Case #7

A 52-year-old experiences postmenopausal spotting. Her endometrial echo is 8 mm, so an endometrial biopsy is performed. At her 3-month return visit, she reports experiencing monthly episodes of light spotting. There is no record of a biopsy having been performed. A biopsy is repeated and shows endometrial cancer.

Case #8

A 26-year-old presents to a routine prenatal care visit at 25 weeks' gestation with increased frequency of urination, and crampy pelvic pain. Her examination is normal. A urinalysis does not suggest cystitis, but a urine culture is sent. No treatment is initiated, pending the result of the culture. She presents a week later in labor, with pyelonephritis. The urine culture was positive for *Escherichia coli*, but it was not reviewed by the ordering doctor, who was out of town.

Case #9

A 28-year-old has a Pap test performed at her routine gynecologic health maintenance exam. She phones the office six weeks later to inquire about the result. The result is negative. However, she is concerned and disappointed that she had not received anything in the mail.

Discussion

Much focus has been placed on critical value reporting in the inpatient venue. Outside the hospital, lab results with values that would be considered "critical" occur less commonly. However, the factors that affect the testing process in the office setting can be more complex and difficult to manage. Some tests rely on patient compliance in order for them to be initiated. Some practices, due to various payer rules, send specimens to multiple different testing laboratories. The volume of radiology, pathology, and laboratory test results to review can be very high.

The scenarios illustrate that errors can result from failure of different components of the testing and follow-up process. Hickner et al. analyze errors in testing by dividing it into three phases. They are the preanalytic phase, the analytic phase, and the postanalytic phase [19]. An error-free testing process requires successful performance through each phase (Figure 3.4). The case scenarios illustrate failures in the preanalytic and postanalytic phases. Errors in the analytic phase – the actual running of the test – are uncommon [20]. Errors seem to occur more in the parts of the process under the practitioner's control. The preanalytic and postanalytic phases can be depicted graphically as in Figure 3.4.

Preanalytic Phase

This phase requires correct ordering and implementing of a test. The process of tracking the test also begins here. In Case #7, an error may have occurred among the many steps necessary to get the pathology specimen from the office to pathology. The specimen or the histological report may have been mishandled by pathology, but failure by the office to recognize the lost test missed the opportunity to correct the error.

Ordering and Implementing

Errors in ordering can occur because of poor communication with nurses and medical assistants. Employing "read-back" or "repeat-back" communication tools can reduce misunderstanding of verbal orders. Errors may also be reduced by using standard processes for requisition completion, specimen labeling, identifier verification, and specimen handling. Electronic medical records that embed the ordering process within the documentation of an encounter can reduce errors and subsequently serve in tracking results. Clinical decision support built into some electronic records can help avoid both the omission of tests, and may reduce over-testing. Standard order sets, or "smart sets," can prompt a provider to order or perform a test that is considered standard in a particular clinical scenario, or remind providers when a patient is due for screening tests. These order sets can tailor orders to particular problems, and avoid extra or unnecessary testing.

Tracking

ACOG endorses tracking systems to reduce the chance of missed diagnoses [21]. Office practices should establish simple, reliable, standardized, transparent processes which keep the care episode "open" or "incomplete" until the test is received and the patient is notified. Much of this work takes place in the postanalytic phase, but to be effective, tracking must begin with test ordering. The ACOG Committee Opinion *Tracking and Reminder Systems* [21] suggests that Ob/Gyn practices should track:

- Cervical cytology
- Mammography
- All laboratory and radiology studies
- Pathology
- Tests initiated outside of the office (e.g., while caring for patients on-call)

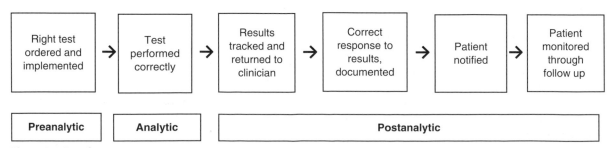

Figure 3.4 Error-free testing process.

(From: Hickner JM, et al. Issues and Initiatives in the Testing Process in Primary Care Physician Offices. *Journal on Quality and Patient Safety Feb* 2005; 31(2):81–89.)

Tracking systems may be manual or electronic. Electronic tracking of test results may offer improved outcomes [22]. A manual tracking system marks a testing episode "open" during the order and implementation of the test. Key information needs to be attached to the "open" order:

- Patient identifiers
- Date ordered
- Clear test description (or procedure, or consultation)

This process can be accomplished in many ways. Data can be entered onto a list or into a database. The requisitions used to order and accompany the test can be copied and filed. The "open" order can be subsequently "closed" by staff during the postanalytic phase of testing. To assure appropriate follow-up, the tracking system would not consider the test completed until the patient is notified of the result. The most robust process keeps the order "open" until the medical record reflects that appropriate follow-up has occurred. In Case #7, the ideal system would keep the patient's endometrial biopsy testing encounter "open" until the physician documented discussing the result with the patient and hysterectomy and staging for uterine cancer were completed. The notification and follow-up pieces of the process are discussed subsequently.

Postanalytic Phase

The postanalytic phase of testing involves receiving and responding to the result, notifying the patient and a plan, documenting this information in the medical record, and following up the subsequent treatment. Successful error reduction in this phase hinges on initiating tracking at the time of ordering the test.

Return and Response Errors

This category involves returning the result to the ordering practitioner or his designee, and responding to it. The response should be in a manner and timeframe appropriate to the result. It should also be appropriate to the nature of the test, and to the patient's expectations. Case #8 displays an inappropriate delay in treatment due to failure to respond quickly enough to the positive urine culture. The most successful tracking system will not only alert the provider to the failure to receive a test result that was ordered, it would also alert the provider to a missing result at the time the result was expected. Once a result becomes available, it must be triaged and assigned a priority for action.

The volume of test results that return to an Ob/Gyn practice, and the busy schedule of the typical physician, require systems to alert the provider to critical values. While the more routine and less-critical results can be managed when time allows, the most important results require attention even in the middle of a busy day. These are *critical* results.

Critical Values

A group of Massachusetts hospitals collaborated to develop a reliable and timely system for communicating critical results to ordering providers [23]. They developed a checklist for the development of a highly reliable reporting system, and they defined a "starter set" of critical test values which everyone could agree on. Although critical values requiring immediate attention to optimize patient outcome may be more prevalent in the hospital setting, they do occur in the ambulatory setting. For example, a sodium reading of 120 mEq/l or a potassium reading of 6.0 mEq/l require immediate alert and immediate attention. A lower extremity Doppler positive for thrombosis or an ultrasound suggestive of ectopic pregnancy require immediate notification. And although it seems true that few tests returning to the office will be "critical," a system of priority should be established to make sure the results are managed in the appropriate timeframe. There are results that should be managed on the same day, some that should be managed within a few days, and others that may appropriately be managed within weeks. Consensus as to which tests and which results fall into these different categories should be established within practices. Patients' expectations and anxiety are important factors in determining the appropriate time latency from test performance to notification. Perhaps the most important definitions to establish first are those results that require same-day notification. A working definition for these might be "without same-day management, unnecessary harm might come to the patient." The following list defines some results of tests commonly ordered by the Ob/Gyn that require same-day management. These are results that may not be treated as critical values by a testing-performing site.

- Positive urine culture (when treatment had not been initiated; or when the bug is resistant to the prescribed antimicrobial)
- Positive chlamydia or gonorrhea
- Positive group A Sitreptococcus throat culture

- Quantitative beta-hCG, ordered to follow an abnormal pregnancy
- 24-hour urine protein 300 mg/24 hours
- Spot urine protein/creatinine ratio(U P/C) > 0.3
- SGOT or SGPT above normal
- Platelets < 100,000/dl

These are merely examples and are not meant to be an inclusive list.

Whether an electronic medical record is used or paper charts, a system must be built for alerting the ordering provider – or a clearly identified designee or covering provider – that same-day action may be necessary. The patient's condition may not warrant same-day intervention, but a provider should triage the result on the same day, instead of visiting the result when time allows. If tests are not sent to an electronic record which assigns priorities to result values, then accountability for result prioritizing should not rest only the ordering provider. Offices should set up guidelines for extenders to review results and assist in managing them in the appropriate timeframe. A fail-safe process should also be developed that defines responsibility for result management when the ordering provider is unavailable. The reliable system will be:

- Designed by all of the stakeholders
- Standard and consistent for all providers
- Accessible by the entire team
- Designed with enough redundancy to reduce errors of omission or delay

Documentation

Results are reviewed and managed most effectively in the context of the medical record. Test ordering, tracking, resulting, and management which is embedded within an electronic record offers a lot in the way of error reduction and good documentation. However, paper charts can effectively accomplish the same thing. Results should be:

- Presented attached to the chart
- Date stamped with arrival time
- Date stamped with review and notification time
- Management plan and follow-up plan documented either on the lab result or in medical record progress notes

Documenting these steps is important for many reasons. Describing the care episode thoroughly is important to good communication. Other reasons include supporting the level of service billed, and risk

management. Redundant and inefficient work can be avoided when any member of the care team can discern from the record which steps of the testing process have been completed.

Patient Notification

Case #9 describes a common office scenario. This patient had a normal Pap test and was not measurably harmed by the failure to notify, but such a patient certainly experiences needless worry over the possibility of an abnormal result. These experiences can lead to an erosion of confidence in the provider, and negatively impact perception of care quality.

The Institute of Medicine report "Crossing the Quality Chasm" suggests that increasing information exchange between patients and providers might help reduce errors [24]. The mantra "nothing about me, without me" has been advocated to empower the patient to become an active part of her healthcare management [25]. Patients want to be notified about all of their test results, not just abnormal ones [26]. The adage that "no news is good news" no longer has a place in healthcare. Practices should make a policy for the timeframe of result notification. They should post it for patients, and stick to it. A patient should be invited to contact the office about a result about which she did not get notified in the prescribed timeframe. Timely notification of all test results helps allay fears, helps reduce phone calls inquiring about normal results, and gives the patient a role in reducing the risk for errors in returning, responding, or notifying about abnormal results.

Follow-up

ACOG recommends that practices use a reminder system to increase patient compliance with the interventions providers prescribe [21]. Such a system would "close the loop" by tracking whether the patient in Case #7 shows up to her clinic visit consultation with a gynecologic oncologist after the cancer was detected on endometrial biopsy. These systems can also remind patients about missed appointments in the office. They can remind patients that expected lab or radiology tests were not received. They can remind patients to follow through with ordered procedures and consultations. The ideal system would be embedded in an electronic medical record and be initiated at initial encounters. However, paper-based systems can accomplish the same goal. ACOG suggests that reminder systems should have certain characteristics:

- Policies and procedures. The office's team members should decide on what should be tracked and should spell out all of the steps from beginning to end.
- Health Insurance Portability and accountability Act (HIPAA). Patient's privacy must be protected.
- Specificity. The data in the reminder system should be defined. The expected timelines for receiving information, notifying patients of information, or recognizing deficiencies must be defined.
- Central location. The system must be accessible by all of the stakeholders in the office.
- Reliability. The system should be run by a team of staff, not just one person. Cross-training and cross-coverage is necessary for success.
- Red Flags Rule compliance. The Federal Trade Commission holds healthcare providers to this rule, which requires offices to develop identity theft prevention and detection measures. (AMA: Protest your patients, protect your practice: what you need to know about the Red Flags Rule [27].)

Strategies employed at the time of patient result notification can increase follow-up rates. Yabroff et al. showed that interactive telephone counseling for notifying patients about abnormal Pap tests increased compliance with recommended follow-up over controls. Telephone counseling increased follow-up rates more than educational brochures or simple telephone delivery of scripted educational material [28].

Quality Measurement

Practices should identify quality indicators they feel are important to track and improve. A number of quality measures have been proposed to evaluate outpatient healthcare. The Healthcare Effectiveness Data and Information Set (HEDIS), developed by the National Committee for Quality Assurance (NCQA), is widely used (Table 3.1). The Joint Commission's National Patient Safety Goals are posted annually, and include recommendations applicable to the outpatient

Table 3.1 HEDIS measures applicable to the Ob/Gyn.

Adult BMI assessment	HPV vaccination
Colorectal cancer screening	Breast cancer screening
Cervical cancer screening	Chlamydia screening
Medication reconciliation post-discharge	Postpartum visit completion

Table 3.2 Joint Commission Ambulatory Health Care National Patient Safety Goals 2018 [18].

Identify patients correctly	Use at least two identifiers
Use medicines safely	Before a procedure, label medicines
	Take extra care with patients on blood thinners
	Take an accurate medicine history; reconcile medications
Prevent infection	Improve hand hygiene
	Use proven guidelines to prevent surgical site infections
Prevent mistakes in surgery	Do correct surgery on correct patient and at correct place on patient's body
	Mark correct place on patient's body
	Pause before surgery to do Time Out

setting (Table 3.2). The authors suggest some additional options (Table 3.3).

Quality Improvement Process – PDCA

At the authors' institution, care improvement projects are implemented using Lean principles – a set of practices adopted and adapted from manufacturing that focuses on elimination of waste. Projects are constructed on the framework of the model for improvement, or PDCA cycle: Plan, Do, Check, Act [29]. Briefly, successful process improvement requires:

- **Plan**. Take the time to identify a problem, form team of stakeholders to analyze the problem, and propose a solution.
- **Do**. Implement a solution.
- **Check**. Measure the results and collect data.
- **Act**. Analyze the data. Celebrate improvement. If the solution has not helped, revise it and repeat the cycle.

Many offices function by relying on team members to over-compensate for poor processes. Although outcomes are usually satisfactory because of successful work-around practices, most such systems contain inherent waste and inefficiency. Although process improvement projects take time and may keep clinicians from direct patient care, the downstream benefits and positive return on investment should be enjoyed in the forms of improved patient care, fewer adverse outcomes, operational efficiency, and more satisfied care teams [30].

Table 3.3 Other quality indicators.

Office efficiency/access	Ob/Gyn primary care	Surgery quality indicators
No shows	Postpartum depression screening	Consent forms completed
Wait time during office visits	Tdap administration	Transfer to hospital
Time from request to appointment	Influenza vaccination in OB	Surgical complications
Abandoned telephone calls rates		Surgical site infection
		Re-visit prior to scheduled post-op check appointment

Selecting a Quality Indicator

Whatever the process or outcome that is chosen for quality tracking, it should be evaluated to make sure it is the right one. At the authors' institution, the following criteria are applied to determine whether an indicator is suitable for tracking:

1. The indicator is measurable. The numerator and denominator can be determined.
2. Data elements are defined and clearly understandable.
3. The data are accessible.
4. The variables outside of my department's control are reduced.
5. A threshold or benchmark exists for comparison.
6. The indicator measures important aspects of care or service. Care may be compromised if performance is not optimal.
7. The results which are tracked will reflect an element of my department's quality of service.
8. There is consensus from the various providers that the indicators are important measures of care.

Summary

The need for a structured safety program in the office is important, in part, because the majority of patient contact occurs in that setting. Systematic and proven techniques should be employed to assure that diagnostic testing results are always seen, patients are notified appropriately, including appropriate follow-up tests or visits. Office procedures have become increasingly routine, including procedures that were previously performed in a formal operating room. Before procedures of this type are attempted in the office, the procedure rooms should have the appropriate equipment, personnel training, emergency resuscitation equipment (including training on proper use). Formal safety checklists should be put in place similar to what would occur in a formal operating room setting.

References

1 Kohn LT, Corrigan JM, Donaldson MS, eds; Committee on Quality of Health Care in America, Institute of Medicine. *To Err is Human: Building a Safer Health System*. Washington, DC: National Academy Press; 1999.

2 *Report of the Presidential Task Force on Patient Safety in the Office Setting*. Washington, DC: ACOG; 2010.

3 Wynia MK, Classen DC. Improving ambulatory patient safety learning from the last decade, moving ahead in the next. *JAMA*. 2011;306(22):2504–2505.

4 www.acog.org/About_ACOG/News_Room/News_Releases/2011/New_SCOPE_Program_Makes_Patient_Safety_a_Priority_No_Matter_the_Setting (downloaded April, 2012).

5 Psuhkar M. Lidocaine toxicity. *Anesth Prog*. 1998;45:38–41.

6 Campbell JR. Allergic response to metabisulfite in lidocaine anesthetic solution. *Anesth Prog*. 2001;48:21–26.

7 Fader DJ, Johnson TM. Medical issues and emergencies in the dermatology office. *J Am Acad Dermatol*. 1997;36:1–16.

8 Eisenberg MS. Cardiac resuscitation in the community: importance of rapid provision and implications for program planning. *JAMA*. 1979;241:1905–1907.

9 Kruskal JF. Lean approach to improving performance and efficiency in the radiology department. *RadioGraphics*. 2012;21:573–587.

10 Hirano H. *Putting 5S to Work*. Tokyo: PHP Institute, Inc.; 1993.

11 Haynes AB. A surgical safety checklist to reduce morbidity and mortality in a global population. *N Engl J Med*. 2009;360:491–499.

12 www.who.int/patientsafety/safesurgery/ss_checklist/en/index.html (downloaded April, 2012).

13 2012 Ambulatory Care National Patient Safety Goals (from www.jointcommission.org).

14 Leape LL, Brennan TA, Laird N, et al. The nature of adverse events in hospitalized patients. *N Engl J Med.* 1991;324:377–384.

15 Friedman AL. Medication errors in the outpatient setting. *Arch Surg.* 2007;142:278–283.

16 Elliot M. The nine rights of medication administration: an overview. *Brit J Nurs.* 2010;19:300–305.

17 Gleason KM. *Medications at Transitions and Clinical Handoffs (MATCH) Toolkit for Medication Reconciliation AHRQ Pub No. 11 (12)-0059.* Rockville, MD: AHRQ; 2011.

18 www.jointcommission.org/assets/1/6/2018_AHC_NPSG_goals_final.pdf (downloaded January, 2018).

19 Hickner JM, Fernald DH, Harris DM, Poon EG, Elder NC, Mold JW. Issues and initiatives in the testing process in primary care physician offices. *J Qual Patient Saf.* 2005;31(2):81–89.

20 Lapworth R, Teal TK. Laboratory blunders revisited. *Ann Clin Biochem.* 1994;31:78–84.

21 ACOG Committee Opinion 461. Tracking and Reminder Systems. Aug 2010.

22 Shojania KG. The effects of on-screen, point of care computer reminders on the processes and outcomes of care. *Cochrane Database Syst Rev.* July 8, 2009;(3).

23 Hanna D, Griswold P, Leape LL, Bates DW. Communicating critical test results: safe practice recommendations. *J Qual Patient Saf.* 2005;31(2):68–77.

24 Institute of Medicine. *Crossing the Quality Chasm; A New Health System for the 21st Century.* Washington, DC: National Academy Press; 2001.

25 Delbanco MD, Berwick DM, Boufford JI, et al. Healthcare in a land called PeoplePower: nothing about me without me. *Health Expect.* 2001;4(3):144–150.

26 Meza JP. Patient preferences for laboratory test result notification. *Am J Manag Care.* 2000;6:1297–1300.

27 Chicago, IL: AMA; 2009. www.ama-assn.org/ama1/pub/upload/mm/368/red-flags-rule-edu.pdf

28 Yabroff K, Kerner JF, Mandelblatt JS. Effectiveness of interventions to improve follow up after abnormal cancer screening. *Prev Med.* 2000;31:429–430.

29 Kim CS, Spahlinger DA, Kin JM, Billi JE. Lean health care: what can hospitals learn from a world-class automaker? *J Hosp Med.* 2006; 1(3):191–199.

30 *Going Lean in Health Care.* IHI Innovation Series white paper. Cambridge, MA: Institute for Healthcare Improvement; 2005 (downloaded April 2012 from www.IHI.org).

Principles for the Safe Use of Electrosurgery

Fidel A. Valea

History

The basic principle of using heat to cauterize bleeding tissue and destroy disease can be traced back to 3000 BC in ancient Egypt when a probe was heated and applied to bleeding tissue to achieve coagulation, hemostasis, and necrosis [1]. The history of electrosurgery dates back to the 1880s when William J. Morton first described the biological effects of a static induced current oscillating at approximately 100 kHz [2]. These effects were further studied by d'Arsonval, who found that high-frequency currents could be passed through living tissue without pain or muscular contractions if the oscillations exceeded 10,000 per second, with the only physiologic effect being an elevation of temperature associated with the absorption of oxygen and release of carbon dioxide [3]. Several other modifications ensued that led to the birth of "medical electrosurgery."

Joseph Riviere demonstrated that by using a small electrode, the density of the current was increased and led to destructive effects. He sprayed the spark from d'Arsonval's apparatus on the back of a musician's hand to treat an indolent ulcer. When the ulcer healed he expanded its use and attracted the attention of the medical community. In 1908 Beer was the first to adapt "fulguration," as it was called by Pozzi, to destroy bladder tumors through a cystoscope [4]. Independent of these discoveries, in 1906, Cook was accidently burned by a spark from a static machine and started using it to treat and eradicate small skin tumors, tonsils, and even hemorrhoids. Subsequent modifications led to the creation of what is the current-day "grounding pad" allowing for the production of much higher temperatures, 500–600°C, with more powerful effects.

The progress of this technology in the United States is in part due to the work of Clark who, by increasing the amperage, was able to treat larger and more "deep-seated" malignant tumors and was the first to study the biological effects of diathermy under

the microscope [5,6]. In 1908, De Forrest used a "cutting" current to make clean incisions in dogs that had little bleeding. At this point in the development of what would turn out to be modern-day electrosurgery, there were three separate and distinct forms of energy that had different tissue alterations: (1) electrodissection, (2) electrocoagulation, and (3) electrocutting.

In 1920, Bovie is credited with the development of the first commercially available electrosurgical device that on October 1, 1926, at Peter Bent Brigham Hospital, was used by Cushing to successfully excise an intracranial mass [7]. The basic principle – passing high-frequency alternating current into the body allowing the current to cut or coagulate – is still in use today and remains a fundamental tool in modern-day surgery [8].

Definitions

Electrosurgery is the use of high-frequency alternating electrical current (AC) passing through living tissues to achieve coagulation, dessication, or fulguration. *Electrocautery* uses electricity to heat a probe and uses heat conduction as the means to achieve coagulation, similar to a soldering iron. The electric current is not actually passing through the tissue but is used to generate heat at the tip of the instrument. *Diathermy* uses a high-frequency alternating electric field, as is used in a microwave oven, to produce heat in the tissue as opposed to electrocautery where heat is applied externally.

Basic Principles

There are three basic principles of electricity that govern this process: (1) electricity always seeks the path of least resistance, (2) electricity always seeks ground, and (3) there must be a complete circuit for electricity to flow. An understanding of how electrosurgery works and its associated complications is based on these three principles.

To understand the concept of electrosurgery, one must first understand the physical principles of electricity. When voltage is applied across a tissue it produces a "flow" of electrons in a circuit and an electrical current is generated. Voltage is the necessary force that drives this movement of electrons. As the electrons pass through the tissue, they encounter resistance, which converts electrical energy into thermal energy. In the operating room, this heat dissipates into the tissues, achieving the desired tissue effect [9]. After dissipating heat, the electrons return to the electrosurgical generator through either the grounding pad (monopolar) or the conducting instrument itself (bipolar) to complete the circuit.

Tissue Effects from Different Waveforms

In modern-day electrosurgery, an alternating current, near the radiofrequency range, is passed from the generator through a conductive element (hand piece) to the target tissue where it is converted to heat as the tissue resists the flow of current. This can lead to one of three distinct tissue effects that depend on the wave form: cutting, desiccation, or fulguration.

Cutting can be achieved by using a "cutting" current, which is no more than a pure sinusoidal wave pattern with low-amplitude (voltage) spikes. The waves are constant with no "down time" leading to a higher current density causing the target tissue to rapidly heat up to the boiling point and vaporize the intracellular fluid. This results in rupture of the cell membrane, thus dividing the tissue and dissipating heat in the form of vapor into the air. Although some heat is absorbed, the thermal effect on the target tissue is small and the desired cutting effect on the tissue is achieved.

Coagulation current is a modulated current that produced short burst of high-amplitude (voltage) waves that also heat up the target tissue but because these waves are delivered in very short bursts with lots of "down time" the tissue is not vaporized. Instead the intracellular fluid is evaporated, which is a slower heating process, and the cells have a chance to cool down in between each burst, producing less heat overall. Because the cells are not vaporized, the heat is not dissipated into vapor. Instead, the heat is absorbed by the target tissue, causing denaturation of protein that forms a coagulum [10]. Although the current density with coagulation current is low, the heat that is generated is absorbed and not dissipated; thus, the thermal injury to the tissue is greater than with cutting current.

With modern-day electrosurgical units one can also obtain a *blended waveform* that is commonly used to achieve some hemostasis while still trying to obtain the cutting effect. A blended waveform is a modification of the cutting waveform in which the continuous sinusoidal pattern is interrupted by varying degrees to allow for some cooling and hemostasis to occur while keeping the total energy density constant. To achieve this, the amplitude (voltage) of the cutting waveform is increased in return for some breaks in continuity to allow for cooling. As one goes from blend 1 to blend 3 the amount of time off in between wave spikes is increased, as is the amplitude of the waves (voltage). This allows for more of a coagulation effect that is "blended" into the cutting current. However, to achieve this effect the unit must be turned on to blend and the surgeon must press the cutting current button, as pressing the coagulation button will only produce a coagulation waveform (Figure 4.1).

Tissue Effects

In addition to the power settings and the waveform selected, there are several other factors that control the desired tissue effects. Perhaps the most important factor is how the surgeon manipulates the active electrode. Whether the surgeon chooses to place the electrode near or in direct contact with the tissue will have profoundly different effects.

Desiccation occurs when the coagulation current is in use and the electrode is in direct contact with the target tissue. Clinically, this manifests itself as a large eschar that will not divide despite increasing the power on the unit because the tissue has no water and hence no longer conducts electricity. Increasing the power in this setting leads to a greater area of destruction with no division of tissue.

Fulguration occurs when the electrode is in close proximity to the target tissue without touching it, creating an arc of electrons that produce a "spray" effect resulting in only superficial destruction of the tissue. In order to achieve this effect one must use high-voltage (coagulation) current and arc the electrons to the tissue. It is mostly used for superficial destruction of skin lesions or a broad area of oozing.

Activation time (how long the electrode is active) is yet another variable that can influence the tissue effects of electrosurgery. Too short an activation time will limit the amount of thermal injury, but will do so at the expense of not achieving the desired tissue

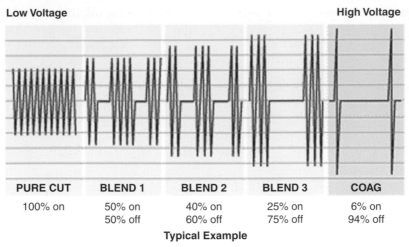

Figure 4.1 The relationship of instrument settings to voltage and current interruption.

effect. Conversely, too long an activation time will lead to more pronounced thermal injury to the surrounding tissue. Activation time is the result of two independent variables – (1) electrical current at the instrument tip, and (2) speed that the surgeon moves the electrode through the tissue. The slower the movement, the more thermal injury; the quicker the movement, the less the desired tissue effects [11].

The size of the electrode is yet another variable to consider when performing electrosurgery. A smaller, more pinpoint electrode tip will provide a much higher current density originating from the tip compared to a wider electrode tip such as a ball electrode for the same power settings on the same tissue type. The use of a needle-point electrode may allow use of lower power settings to achieve the same effects.

Finally, one must consider the target tissue when performing electrosurgery. Fat and bone have much higher resistance and are poor conductors of electricity. Conversely, skin, muscle, and fascia have high water contents and are excellent conductors of electricity as they have lower resistance than fat and bone. Hence it is not uncommon to turn up the power when going through fat and turn down the power when working on skin and fascia.

Electrosurgical Units

Electrosurgical units in use today are almost exclusively isolated solid-state generators in which the electrons are returned through the grounding pad to complete the circuit.

Monopolar Electrosurgery

This is the most commonly employed energy delivery system in the United States. It allows for the use of the various electrosurgical principles described above producing a variety of different effects. In this system the active electrode can be activated by hand or foot and delivers the energy through an "active electrode" at the surgical site. The grounding pad or return electrode is attached to the patient at a separate site that minimizes the potential for stray currents. The large size of the grounding pad allows safe passage of current from the patient back to the electrosurgical generator.

Bipolar Electrosurgery

With bipolar electrosurgery the active and return electrodes are in very close proximity at the surgical site and typically within the tip of the instruments. In this case the current does not flow through the patient and there is no need for a grounding pad. The electrical current only passes through the tissue between the two electrodes. As a result, much lower power settings are required and the potential for thermal injury is less than in monopolar electrosurgery. Unfortunately, the time needed to coagulate tissue is longer because of the lower power settings. In addition the potential for charring and tissue adherence with subsequent "tearing" of tissue is greater [12]. This modality is commonly used in neurosurgery where tissue destruction and the potential for stray currents must be minimized.

Feedback-controlled Bipolar Electrosurgery

Newer technologies have further enhanced the advantages and safety of electrosurgery, especially with laparoscopic use [13]. There are several instruments that use new bipolar technology "seal" and divide vessels with less energy and achieve more reliable results than traditional bipolar electrosurgery. One such device applies a precise amount of bipolar energy and pressure to fuse collagen and elastin within the vessel walls. This results in a permanent seal that can withstand three times the normal systolic pressure, and seals vessels up to 7 mm in size. This instrument must be used with a dedicated generator that senses the resistance of the tissue in the jaws of the instrument through feedback via the return electrode and turns off the electrical flow when the seal is optimal [14]. The jaws of this instrument have a larger surface area than traditional bipolar forceps and lead to a more reliable seal.

Another device uses pulsed bipolar energy delivered through the instrument to the tissue within the jaws, allowing for intermittent tissue cooling, which limits lateral thermal spread. The system automatically detects the optimal settings for the specific instrument, as well as a visual and audible impedance monitor to indicate when the coagulation is optimal. The system has two different modes: the vapor-pulse coagulation mode, and a tissue-cutting mode. In the vapor-pulse mode, high energy is delivered to grasped tissue, creating vapor zones. The current then travels around the high-impedance vapor zones, following the path of least resistance. The vapor zones subsequently collapse, and with each new energy pulse more and more tissue between the instrument jaws is coagulated, ultimately resulting in uniform coagulation of tissue. The tissue-cutting mode allows the surgeon to cut tissue using bipolar energy, thereby achieving simultaneous cutting and coagulation of tissue [15].

A third system provides vessel sealing by combining a compression mechanism that applies uniform pressure along the full length of the instrument jaw, achieving compression forces similar to those of a linear stapler but with thermal energy for sealing. The device also has a cutting mechanism to allow one-step sealing and transection of vessels and soft tissues [16].

Complications

Although electrosurgery is relatively safe, there are still complications that can occur.

Operating Room Fires

It is estimated that operating room fires occur about 550–600 times per year in the United States [17]. Most of these are associated with the use of electrosurgery and the greatest risk is around the time of induction of anesthesia. Electrosurgery can ignite flammable anesthetics, preps (chlorhexadine and iodophor), cleaning agents, benzoin, alcohol, certain ointments (petroleum jelly), and even combustible material such as drapes and clothes, especially when in proximity to an oxygen-rich environment. Key steps in reducing risk include limiting electrosurgery activation during induction of anesthesia, limiting free-flowing oxygen, assuring operating surfaces are dry of cleaning agents, avoiding use of electrosurgery after ointments have been placed, and avoiding pooling of prep agents around the patient.

Burns

The most common injury related to the use of monopolar cautery is a burn at the grounding pad, which is the return electrode site. Although most return electrodes in use today have "smart" technology where the generator actually senses if it is not applied properly and will not allow activation of the unit, a burn can still occur, especially if the return electrode is not large enough to disperse the energy. Sometimes improper contact is due to fluids or lotion at the site, too much hair, too much adipose tissue, scar tissue, bony prominences or surgical hardware in close proximity to the site. It is best to place the return electrode as close as possible to the operative site in an area that has well vascularized muscle under the skin with no nearby hardware.

Burns can also occur on the skin because of accidental activation of the electrode when it is not in its insulated container. In addition, alternative burn sites can occur when the skin is in contact with other conductive materials such as metal.

By following proper perioperative care, skin burns can be minimized although not completely eliminated. These principles include proper ground electrode placement, removal of all metal objects and avoidance of contact with any metal objects.

In minimally invasive surgery burns are potentially due to stray currents most often seen with the use of monopolar electrosurgery. With minimally invasive surgery the instruments are longer and, with the exception of the most distal tip, are not in the operative field of vision. Hence, they are more susceptible to stray currents due to insulation failures and coupling of the shaft to nearby tissue.

Direct coupling occurs when the monopolar electrosurgical unit is activated when the tip is either touching or in close proximity to another conducting metal instrument. The current would then flow from the active electrode through the other conducting instrument and can potentially damage structures in contact with that instrument. This injury can be minimized by visualizing the tip of the active electrode at all times and making sure it is clear of the surrounding instruments before activation.

Capacitance coupling is a rare event. Capacitance is the property of an electrical circuit that allows it to transfer an electrical charge from one conductor to another despite being separated by insulation. As the electrosurgical generator is activated, potential energy builds up along the active electrode. When that potential energy exceeds the insulator's capacity, it can be transferred to a nearby conductive element even if it too is insulated. It is directly related to the amount of energy used, the activation time, and the length of the instruments. The transfer can be between instruments or even from one instrument to skin or any intraabdominal organ if it is in close enough proximity. Laparoscopic instruments are long and frequently out of direct view during an operation, thereby putting this type of surgery at risk for a capacitance coupling event. Limiting activation times and using the lowest power setting necessary to achieve the desired effect can minimize the risk of capacitance coupling.

Insulation failures are not uncommon. In one series, 19% of reusable and 3% of disposable instruments had insulation breaks when tested [18]. In randomly selected surgical sets 71% had at least one instrument with a break in insulation. When there is a break in the insulation covering the active electrode, stray currents can develop which may go unnoticed by the surgeon and lead to significant surgical morbidity. This occurs predominantly when using coagulation current because of its high-voltage output. Another common cause is frequent resterilization of instruments, which can weaken, and possibly break, the insulation. Instruments should be checked periodically for insulation failures. Burns from insulation breaks can be minimized by: (1) limiting the amount of power used to the minimum necessary to achieve the desired effect; (2) using more cutting current; and (3) using an active electrode monitoring system.

Key Steps to Safe Electrosurgery

1. Train/certify OR technicians in equipment and technique
2. Provide surgeons formal didactic and hands-on training
3. Inspect unit regularly (by certified technician)
4. Inspect accessories prior to EVERY case (by OR technician and surgeon) in order to:
   a. Identify insulation defects
   b. Confirm that alarms are functional and audible
5. Allow dispersion of anesthetics, oxygen, OR gases, and vapors from cleaning agents before activating unit
6. Avoid use of flammable agents
7. Follow instructions meticulously for placement of dispersive electrode
8. Avoid accumulating pools of fluids
9. Place towels under patient; remove after prep is complete
10. Minimize buildup of N_2O under drapes
11. Use the lowest effective output settings
12. Always place electrode in safety holster
13. Always visualize tip when operating

Conclusion

Electrosurgery is a continuously evolving field and provides many benefits over other techniques including less blood loss, shorter operative times, and even less pain. It does have unique complications that can be minimized with a thorough understanding of the principles of electricity. Knowledge of these principles will allow surgeons across all disciplines to address more complex cases safely.

References

1 Breasted JH. *The Edwin Smith Surgical Papyrus*. Chicago, IL: Chicago University Press; 1930: 54.

2 Ward GE. Electrosurgery. *Am J Surg.* 1932;17(1):86–93.

3 d'Arsonval A. Action physiologique des courants alternatifs. *Comptes Rendus Societe de Biologie.* 1891;43:283–286.

4 Beer E. Removal of neoplasms of the urinary bladder. *JAMA*. 1910;54:1768–1769.

5 Clark WL, Asnis EJ, Morgan JD. *Atlantic Med J.* 1923;27.

6   Clark W. The desiccation treatment of congenital and new growths of the skin and mucous membranes. *JAMA*. 1914;63:925–928.

7   Cushing H. Electrosurgery as an aid to the removal of intracranial tumors with a preliminary note on a new surgical-current generator by W.T. Bovie. *Surg Gynecol Obstet*. 1928;47:751–784.

8   Jones CM, Pierre KB, Nicoud IB, Stain SC, Melvin WV. Electrosurgery. *Curr Surg*. 2006;63(6):458–463.

9   Wang K, Advincula AP. "Current thoughts" in electrosurgery. *Int J of Gynecol Obstet*. 2007;97:245–250.

10 Gallagher K, Dhinsa B, Miles J. Electrosurgery. *Surgery*. 2010;29(2):70–72.

11 Van Way III CW, Hinrichs CS. Electrosurgery 201: basic electrical principles. *Curr Surg*. 2000; 57(3):261–264.

12 Tucker RD, Voyles CR. Laparoscopic electrosurgical complications and their prevention. *AORN*. 1995;62:51–59.

13 Hay DJ. Electrosurgery. *Surgery*. 2007;26(2):66–69.

14 Kennedy JS, Stranahan PL, Taylor KD, Chandler JG. High-burst-strength, feedback-controlled bipolar vessel sealing. *Surg Endosc*. 1998; 12:876–878.

15 Presthus JB, Brooks PG, Kirchof N. Vessel sealing using a pulsed bipolar system and open forceps. *J Am Assoc Gynecol Laparosc*. 2003;10(4):528–533.

16 Newcomb WL, Hope WW, Schmelzer TM, et al. Comparison of blood vessel sealing among new electrosurgical and ultrasonic devices. *Surg Endosc*. 2009;23(1):90–96.

17 Hart SR, Yajnik A, Ashford J, Springer R, Harvey S. Operating room fire safety. *Ochsner J*. 2011;11(1):37–42.

18 Montero P, Robinson T, Weaver J, Stiegmann G. Insulation failure in laparoscopic instruments. *Surg Endosc*. 2010;24:462–465.

The Obstetric-Gynecologic Hospitalist

An Illustrative Study of the Development of an Obstetric-Gynecologic Hospitalist Program

Christopher C. Swain and Alan M. Dulit

Illustrative Case

A 28-year-old woman, G2P1001 at 34 2/7 weeks gestation, presented to labor and delivery at 2230 hours following a fall down a small flight of stairs. The patient reported that she slipped, landed on her buttocks, and slid down three stairs. She denied any direct abdominal trauma. She complained of mild low back pain but denied any abdominal pain, vaginal bleeding, or symptoms consistent with rupture of membranes. She further denied any additional trauma, pain, or contractions, and she reported good fetal movement. The patient reported that her pregnancy had been uncomplicated prior to her fall, and her previous pregnancy with term vaginal delivery was without complication.

Upon arrival, the patient was placed on external fetal monitoring in the Obstetrics Triage Unit. The nurse documented a normal fetal heart tracing showing a baseline heart rate of 130 bpm with moderate variability and accelerations. No decelerations were present and no contractions were noted on external tocometry. A nurse examined the patient, noting a mildly obese female in no apparent distress. The patient was ambulatory and showed no limitations of mobility. Vital signs were normal with a blood pressure of 130/72. The patient had no visible contusions, abrasions, or lacerations. A pelvic exam revealed no evidence of vaginal bleeding, and the cervix was noted to be closed and thick. This report was telephoned to the patient's obstetrician at 2315 hours. The physician requested that the patient remain on continuous fetal monitoring, and ordered initial laboratory tests which included a complete blood count, type and screen, prothrombin and partial thromboplastin times, fibrinogen, urine analysis, and Kleihauer–Betke test. The patient was moved to an observation bed for overnight assessment.

At 0045 hours, the nurse telephoned the physician to report normal initial lab results which included a hemoglobin and hematocrit of 12.8/38.6, respectively, and normal coagulation studies. The Kleihaeur–Betke test was still pending. The nurse also reported that the patient had some mild abdominal cramping and one episode of vaginal spotting. The fetal monitoring was reported as continuing to be normal with heart rate of 130–140 bpm with the presence of accelerations and moderate variability; decelerations were absent. No contractions were noted on external tocometry. To further evaluate the spotting, the physician ordered a fetal ultrasound and requested that the patient remain on continuous fetal monitoring.

At 0220 hours, the nurse telephoned the physician to report a prolonged fetal heart rate deceleration with a fetal heart rate in the 80s for the past two minutes. The nurse stated that the patient was writhing in the bed and complaining of severe abdominal pain. Further, she reported that the patient had begun to experience profuse vaginal bleeding and had passed a clot of approximate 150 cm³. The physician ordered preparations for urgent cesarean delivery to commence as soon as he could arrive at the hospital, which was located approximately 20 minutes from his home.

At 0246 hours, the physician arrived to the operating theater to initiate the emergent cesarean delivery which was performed under general anesthesia, delivering a 5 lb, 1 oz male at 0248 hours. Surgery revealed a large volume of intrauterine blood, with an estimated 80% placental abruption. The infant received Apgar scores of 0, 2, and 5 at 1, 5, and 10 minutes, respectively, and was transferred to a tertiary neonatal intensive care unit where he developed seizures within 12 hours. The neonate's clinical course and radiologic studies while in the NICU were consistent with hypoxic ischemic encephalopathy. At one year of age the infant was noted to have severe, permanent cognitive and developmental delays.

Aftermath

A lawsuit naming the obstetrician, the Labor and Delivery nurse, and the hospital was brought on behalf of the infant. This suit alleged that the delay in treatment of fetal distress resulted in severe and permanent neurological injury.

Following this event, a root-cause analysis was undertaken by a hospital safety committee to identify potential areas of improvement. The study found that, although surgery was initiated within 30 minutes of the sentinel event, the delay in response time due to the lack of immediate obstetrician availability was a key factor contributing to the outcome in this case. The committee strongly recommended that continuous in-house Ob/Gyn physician coverage should be considered for the hospital.

Analysis

The 375-bed full-service hospital had 2,200 births per year and a Level II Neonatal Intensive Care Unit. To further determine the cost-effectiveness and associated benefits of the proposed program of continuous coverage, a comprehensive needs analysis was performed to evaluate the hospital's entire obstetric and gynecologic service line. The goal of this analysis was to identify areas where patient safety might be improved by the immediate availability of an obstetric and gynecologic provider. Additionally, they sought to determine other benefits that would be provided to the hospital and to the medical staff if continuous

Ob/Gyn coverage were instituted within the facility. The results of the analysis are listed in Figure 5.1.

Analytical Details

Expedite delivery of emergency obstetric care: The hospital recognized that *Delay of Care* is a significant issue that threatens patient safety. A 2000–2009 retrospective study by The Doctors Company showed that in half of neonatal brain damage and death cases, delay in treatment of fetal distress was the major allegation [1]. Although the hospital had a policy mandating a maximum 30-minute response time to attend in-house emergencies, the hospital recognized that this response time is often insufficient to effectively manage catastrophic obstetric emergencies.

Improve the management of Obstetric Triage patients: Unscheduled patients frequently presented to the hospital with pregnancy-related complaints. Hospital policy required that patients of less than 20 weeks gestation be seen in the main Emergency Department, while patients greater than 20 weeks gestation were sent to the Labor and Delivery Triage Unit for evaluation. Patients arriving to this Triage Unit were often evaluated only by a nurse, followed by a telephone consultation with a physician. The hospital recognized that the Labor and Delivery Triage Unit was the only unit in the entire hospital where patients presented with unscheduled problem visits and were subsequently discharged without having been evaluated by a physician. This process was seen as a safety

- Lack of immediately available obstetric emergency care
- RNs designated as "qualified medical personnel" for the evaluation of Obstetric Triage patients with subsequent routine discharge of patients without a physician evaluation resulting in a potential safety risk and a source of patient dissatisfaction
- Need improved process to manage unassigned obstetric patients
- Need improved process to manage unassigned gynecological patients
- No emergency preparedness drills
- Lack of surgical assistants for cesarean deliveries
- No immediate physician support for the midwife service
- Insufficient proctoring of family practice residents
- Family practitioners need additional support
- Unable to perform VBACs
- Inability to perform timely Ob/Gyn consults
- Need to develop a high-risk service
- Difficulties recruiting and retaining new obstetricians
- Obstetric nursing dissatisfaction and turnover
- Diminished productivity of staff Ob/Gyn physicians

Figure 5.1 The benefits provided to the hospital and the medical staff if continuous Ob/Gyn coverage were instituted within the facility.

and quality issue, a medico-legal risk, and a source of patient dissatisfaction. The 24/7 presence of a physician on the Labor and Delivery Triage Unit would allow all of these unscheduled patients to be evaluated by a physician prior to admission or discharge.

Improve the process for managing unassigned obstetric patients: Hospital policy required that unassigned obstetric patients with no local obstetrics provider be evaluated by the on-call Ob/Gyn physician. These unassigned patients were frequently high-risk due to lack of consistent prenatal care and health risks associated with low socioeconomic status. This policy required a local physician to leave his home or office to commute to the hospital and physically evaluate these patients. The physicians were dissatisfied with this process, which was viewed as an increased liability risk as well as a costly disruption to their practice and quality of life.

Improve the process for managing unassigned gynecology patients: Unassigned gynecologic emergency patients were evaluated in the Emergency Department by emergency physicians. After the determination that a patient required admission or surgery, the patient was then assigned to the on-call Ob/Gyn physician. These gynecologic emergency patients were often uninsured and frequently had problems that necessitated immediate surgical intervention. The management of these patients required a significant time commitment and was disruptive to the scheduled activities of staff Ob/Gyn physicians.

Develop emergency preparedness drills: The Joint Commission advocates using mock obstetrical emergency training drills as a risk reduction strategy [2]. The hospital's analysis revealed that there was sporadic performance of these drills in the unit due to limited availability of the medical staff for participation. Increased physician availability on the Labor Unit would facilitate regular performance of clinical drills to help nurses and physicians prepare for obstetric emergencies such as emergent cesarean section, shoulder dystocia, and postpartum hemorrhage.

Provide surgical assists for cesarean deliveries: Hospital policy required the presence of two surgeons for cesarean delivery, therefore community physicians were being called upon to assist on unscheduled cesarean deliveries. The analysis proposed that an in-house physician would be readily available to provide this service.

Improve midwife support: Midwife practitioners, limited by their scope of practice, are unable to perform surgical procedures or manage high-risk or complicated obstetric patients. Midwives require a readily available physician support system. The analysis further noted that in-house physician availability could provide ready access to obstetric consultation for high-risk patients and co-management of complicated labors, thereby reducing unnecessary delays of care.

Improve proctoring of Family Practice residents: The hospital had Family Practice residents managing obstetric patients under the guidance of experienced Family Practice attending physicians. These attending physicians did not have surgical privileges, relying on local obstetricians to provide surgical back-up. It was determined that an in-house obstetrician could improve this process by reducing the burden of interruptions to private obstetricians and could enhance the overall learning experience of the Family Practice residents.

Provide additional obstetric support for Family Practitioners: The hospital had several community Family Practice physicians providing obstetric services. These community physicians were unable to perform cesarean deliveries, requiring the back-up support of local obstetricians. The analysis recommended that an in-house obstetrician could potentially alleviate delays in care and improve this process while placing fewer burdens on the staff obstetrician.

Increase ability to offer vaginal birth after cesarean (VBAC): Hospital policy required immediate physician availability for any patient attempting to undergo vaginal birth after cesarean delivery. For this reason, many local physicians were not offering VBAC because they could not safely fulfill this requirement. Consequently, patients desiring VBAC were delivering at a competitor hospital. Twenty-four hour, dedicated in-house physician coverage would satisfy the requirement for immediate physician availability for VBAC and could help reduce the hospital's cesarean delivery rate [3].

Expedite Ob/Gyn consultations: Obstetric and gynecologic consultations are time-consuming and further increase the workload of staff Ob/Gyn physicians. The hospital determined that in-house Ob/Gyn physicians could manage most of these consultations, allowing staff physicians more time to focus on other duties.

Develop a high-risk perinatal service: The hospital's Maternal–Fetal Medicine (MFM) service was focused primarily on outpatient duties. The office workload of the perinatal service made it very difficult for the MFM team to manage an inpatient population. Some patients were being transferred to nearby tertiary facilities to be managed by a more comprehensive high-risk perinatal service. An in-house obstetric team could co-manage these high-risk patients in partnership with the MFM team, allowing the MFM specialists to focus more on consultative services. This could improve the productivity of the MFM service, improve the hospital's ability to manage high-risk patients, and improve the Neonatal Intensive Care Unit census.

Improve recruitment and retention of Ob/Gyn physicians: The hospital determined that additional support of in-house Ob/Gyn physicians could enable improved lifestyles and provide enhanced support for newer physicians. To meet the growing needs of the community, the hospital must strive to retain current providers and recruit additional Ob/Gyn physicians. Recruiting and retaining physicians has become more difficult, in part, due to the greater emphasis on lifestyle and personal time by physicians of generations X and Y [4]. Physicians coming out of training today increasingly seek employment; they want a job with a steady paycheck and predictable hours [5]. An improved work environment could increase physician retention and improve recruiting success.

Improve obstetric nursing satisfaction and reduce turnover: Low levels of nursing satisfaction and a high degree of nursing turnover were observed on the labor and delivery unit. The nurses were reportedly uncomfortable with being required to render clinical opinions and manage emergencies, often single-handedly, while awaiting the attendance of a physician. Having a physician present and readily available would potentially lead to improved teamwork, communication, and cohesiveness, resulting in an increased level of nursing satisfaction [6].

Diminished productivity of staff physicians: Staff physicians were making multiple trips to the hospital each day to manage routine patient care needs. Additionally, these physicians were being called to the hospital to perform consultations and manage unassigned obstetric and gynecologic patients. A 2002 study of medical hospitalists by Wachter and

Goldman reported that "the average primary care physician would realize a yearly net gain of about $40,000 by forgoing hospital care, simply by replacing wasted commute time with increased ambulatory productivity" [7]. An in-house Ob/Gyn physician can function in a manner similar to a partner *in absentia*, allowing the staff physician more time to complete office hours, perform surgery, or get a few more hours of sleep [8].

Post-analysis Decision

Following the analysis of the hospital's obstetrics and gynecology services as related to the provision of in-house Ob/Gyn staffing, the hospital resolved to implement a comprehensive obstetric-gynecologic hospitalist program. This analysis helped to identify and focus the goals and parameters of the new program.

Program Structure

The Obstetric-Gynecologic Hospitalist Program was staffed by seasoned, board-certified Ob/Gyn physicians who did not have private practice affiliations within the community. Thus, the hospitalists could focus their efforts solely on assigned responsibilities within the hospital while providing assistance to all community physicians without being viewed as competitors. In addition to board certification, the hospitalists were required to complete recent training in Advanced Cardiac Life Support, Neonatal Resuscitation, Advanced Fetal Monitoring, Operative Delivery, Postpartum Hemorrhage, and Shoulder Dystocia Management.

The core duties of the hospitalists were defined as: (1) management of obstetric emergencies, (2) management of unassigned gynecological emergencies; and (3) evaluation of unscheduled Obstetric Triage patients. Utilizing the Obstetric Triage Unit as a "home base," the hospitalists were readily available to respond to emergencies within the Labor and Delivery Unit. Additionally, the hospitalists had sufficient availability to engage in educational programs and drills for nurses and residents, provide surgical assists for unscheduled cesareans, perform consultations, and provide assistance and support for the Maternal–Fetal Medicine Service and other local obstetric providers.

Recognizing that the hospitalist on duty might occasionally be involved in a surgical case and unable to respond immediately to a simultaneous emergency, the hospital maintained an emergency back-up call Schedule composed of the Ob/Gyn staff physicians on a rotating schedule. The back-up system served two purposes: (1) it identified a second physician to be called in the rare event of a dual emergency situation; and (2) it provided a rotating physician referral list for those patients seen in the Emergency Department requiring outpatient follow-up.

In an effort to address the above-described concerns and to achieve an overall enhancement of the Women's Service line, the hospital implemented an Obstetric Gynecologic Hospitalist program.

Cost Considerations

Cost is the principal factor restricting implementation of obstetric-gynecologic hospitalist programs. Obstetric-gynecologic hospitalists capture professional fees primarily from obstetric triage visits, surgical assists, unassigned deliveries, consults, and emergency gynecologic cases. It is unlikely that professional fee revenue will sufficiently offset the expense of a program; so other revenue sources must be considered when evaluating the cost-effectiveness of an obstetric-gynecologic hospitalist program.

One source of revenue that can be realized from an obstetric-gynecologic hospitalist program involves utilizing the hospitalists, rather than a nurse, to consistently evaluate patients in the Obstetrics Triage Unit. In many hospitals it is common practice for a nurse to triage an OB patient, communicate with the doctor by telephone, and discharge the patient – all without generating an appropriate hospital charge for the visit. Evaluation of obstetric triage patients by obstetric hospitalists improves patient safety and enhances patient flow, while enabling hospitals to capture significant new revenue.

Having an obstetric-gynecologic hospitalist program often allows hospitals to eliminate a daily physician-on-call expense, as the hospitalists will assume primary responsibility for unassigned patients. Also, many hospitals realize savings related to the proctoring of residents and medical students, utilizing the Ob/Gyn hospitalists to provide this supervision. Subsidies that are routinely paid for this service to private physicians can be discontinued when the resident and student teaching responsibilities are transferred to the hospitalist service. Generally, the hospitalists can provide this without incurring additional expense to the hospital.

The ongoing support that Ob/Gyn hospitalists provide to community obstetric providers will eliminate many unnecessary commutes to the hospital, potentially allowing these providers to be more productive in the office, resulting in increased service volume for the hospital. This physician support could help decrease nightly calls, allow more flexible schedules, increase personal time, and enhance the lifestyle of the community Ob/Gyn physicians. Structuring this more favorable work environment could help recruit new physician practices to the hospital, and reduce "burn-out" of the existing physicians.

Upon request, hospitalists may also provide call coverage services for private practices. The hospitalists can charge the practice a fair and reasonable fee for the delivery of private patients during the coverage period and the private physician is often able to bill the global fee for the pregnancy management. These delivery fees offer additional revenue for a hospitalist program.

Ob/Gyn hospitalists often work closely with MFM specialists to co-manage a high-risk obstetric service. This collaboration allows MFM physicians to increase outpatient productivity by reducing their clinical load in the hospital. A continuously staffed high-risk service can readily accept and manage high-risk transports and could help reduce unnecessary transports out of the hospital. A high-risk service could lead to an increased NICU census.

Delivery in a facility with 24-hour in-house obstetric coverage has been identified as a practice that reduces obstetric litigation [9]. Hospitals with 24/7 Ob/Gyn hospitalist programs have expanded physician availability that can improve emergency outcomes and reduce overall hospital malpractice exposure. Some hospitals have found the implementation of an Ob/Gyn hospitalist program allows them to reduce their insurance reserves or premium requirements.

As may be seen by the above discussion, an obstetric-gynecologic hospitalist program has many potential mechanisms to generate the revenue necessary to justify and sustain its existence. A 2013 study by Allen et al. demonstrated the implementation of 24-hour in-house obstetric coverage to be a cost-effective strategy for most medium to large size hospitals, and can produce better fetal outcomes in hospitals where obstetricians cannot respond to obstetric emergencies within 30 minutes [10]. These mechanisms will vary greatly from hospital to hospital, and a true cost analysis must consider the impact of multiple revenue variables.

When viewed in totality, these revenue sources and cost savings can often reveal a cost-effective, and even profitable, hospitalist program.

Discussion

The obstetric-gynecologic hospitalist care model is a rapidly growing phenomenon within the specialty of obstetrics and gynecology, mirroring the popularity of the original hospitalist model introduced in a 1996 *New England Journal of Medicine* article by Wachter and Goldman, describing a "hospitalist" as a physician specializing in the care of hospitalized patients [11]. The concept of obstetric-gynecologic hospitalists first began to take shape in 2002–2003. An article by Frigoletto and Greene in 2002 suggested a role for future obstetrician-gynecologic hospitalists [12]. In 2003, Weinstein coined the term "laborist" to describe a physician whose sole focus of practice is treating a patient in labor [13].

Today the titles "Ob/Gyn Hospitalist," "OB Hospitalist," or "Laborist" are often used interchangeably to describe any hospital-based physician specialized in providing care to obstetrics and gynecologic patients within the hospital. However, a laborist is generally defined as an individual who cares for obstetric patients on labor and delivery *only*, whereas the Ob/Gyn hospitalist, or OB hospitalist, provides a broader level of service encompassing both obstetric and gynecologic patients within the hospital and emergency department.

The obstetric-gynecologic hospitalist model takes into consideration the fact that patients want and expect to be delivered by the physician whom they chose to provide their prenatal care; and private physicians want and need to deliver these patients to sustain their practices. The Ob/Gyn hospitalist is not intended to be a replacement for the private Ob/Gyn physician, but rather can serve as an extension of the private Ob/Gyn practice that can be utilized in times of need.

First and foremost, the obstetric-gynecologic hospitalist is an emergency responder who will react to any obstetric or gynecologic emergency within the hospital. Additionally, there are other core functions that are commonplace in most Ob/Gyn hospitalist programs, including the management of the obstetrics triage unit, evaluation and management of unassigned obstetric patients, and the management of any unassigned gynecology patient requiring urgent care from an Ob/Gyn specialist.

In California, around-the-clock labor and delivery (L&D) coverage was noted to be associated with

decreased odds of cesarean delivery and increased likelihood of trial of labor after cesarean and achieving vaginal birth after previous caesarean [14]. Full-time laborist programs have also been shown to decrease cesarean section rates in term primiparous patients [15]. And in a 2013 study, Srinivas et al. demonstrated that the implementation of laborists improved obstetric outcomes including decreased term NICU admissions, reduced preterm deliveries and fewer babies born at < 2500 g [16].

The continuous presence of an Ob/Gyn hospitalist on the Labor Unit creates ongoing opportunities for education and support. This ready availability allows for improved emergency preparedness by enhancing the timely ability to respond to emergencies. The hospitalists will have availability to participate in mock drills, educational seminars, and assist with the training of nurses, medical students, and residents. Also, ready availability assures that non-Ob/Gyn obstetric providers will have continuous access to an Ob/Gyn specialist.

Most Ob/Gyn hospitalist programs provide additional support services for local physicians to assist with the management of patients in labor. Such services often include VBAC management, supervising oxytocin augmentation, ordering epidurals, amniotomy, placement of fetal scalp electrode, evaluation of bleeding, and review of questionable tracings. In this scenario, the private physician at home or in the office, continues to be the "captain of the ship" regarding the management of the laboring patient, with the Ob/Gyn hospitalist playing a supporting role. Some programs provide a more extensive level of physician support that includes call coverage and rounding assistance. This level of support allows private physicians to periodically sign-out their inpatient service to the Ob/Gyn hospitalist team, permitting the Ob/Gyn hospitalists to take over as the "captain of the ship," managing all patient care decisions. The provision of more extensive physician support services is dependent upon the volume of the hospitalist service and the safe availability of the Ob/Gyn hospitalist.

To facilitate an effective patient care team, it is important that patients be educated to anticipate the potential involvement of the Ob/Gyn hospitalist in their hospital care. The Ob/Gyn hospitalists may be introduced as practice "associates" who are continuously at the hospital to enhance patient safety. Some practitioners introduce the hospitalist concept by assuring the patient that "I, or one of my associates, will be at the hospital 24 hours a day, seven days a week, to assist you." The American College of Obstetricians and Gynecologists recognizes the obstetric-gynecologic hospitalist model as a potential solution to achieving increased patient satisfaction [8]. Hospitalist experience has shown that patients appear to be willing to trade familiarity (of their primary doctor) for availability (of the hospitalist) when it comes to hospital care [7].

Effective communication is a necessary component of any successful Ob/Gyn hospitalist program. Patient handoffs occur regularly between hospitalists and primary physicians; appropriate management of transition of care is essential to patient safety and is conducive to a healthy partnership. The Joint Commission estimates that 80% of serious medical errors involve miscommunication between caregivers when responsibility for patients is transferred or handed-off [17]. A successful Ob/Gyn hospitalist program should have a defined protocol outlining physician-to-physician communication surrounding patient handoffs and a reliable mechanism for obtaining prenatal records.

The current environment for obstetrician-gynecologists and for hospitals providing Ob/Gyn services is a challenging one. Decreasing reimbursements, heavy call burden, high patient volume and the need to juggle busy office practices together with hospital duties, have all contributed to decreased quality of life for Ob/Gyns.

Hospitals and physicians alike must operate within a medico-legal environment that places increasing demands on physician time and hospital resources. This case was presented to be illustrative of the many challenges facing Ob/Gyns and hospitals in trying to provide excellent obstetric and gynecologic care. The obstetric-gynecologic hospitalist model has been proposed as a solution to many of these challenges. While not all hospitals will have all of the problems attributed to the facility in the case study, few institutions have none.

As noted in the ACOG Committee Opinion No. 459, the Ob/Gyn hospitalist model has the potential to provide benefits to practicing Obstetrician-Gynecologists, to hospitals, and to patients and their families. "The American College of Obstetricians and Gynecologists supports the continued development of the obstetric-gynecologic hospitalist model as one potential approach to achieving increased professional and patient satisfaction while maintaining safe and effective care across delivery settings" [8]. While it is obvious that the immediate availability of emergency obstetric services translates into improved patient safety in the face of catastrophic emergencies, there are many opportunities to investigate other benefits that may be provided by an Ob/Gyn hospitalist program.

Summary

The thoughtful development of a comprehensive obstetric-gynecologic hospitalist program can result in a cost-effective model that provides increased value through a wide variety of services. The continuous on-site availability of an Ob/Gyn specialist affords many benefits to patients, hospitals, and practicing physicians. Such programs increase patient safety, promote risk reduction, and improve clinical outcomes, while enriching the quality of life of obstetricians and gynecologists. The Ob/Gyn hospitalist model is a trend that is likely to see increasingly wide adoption in the coming years.

References

1 Ranum, D. (September 24, 2011). A Study of OB Claims. Seminar/PowerPoint presented to The Society of OB/GYN Hospitalists. Denver, Colorado.

2 Joint Commission on Accreditation of Healthcare Organizations: Sentinel event alert. Issue 30, July 21, 2004. Available at: www.jointcommission.org/assets/1/18/SEA_30.PDF

3 Klasko SK, Cummings RV, Balducci J, DeFulvio JD, Reed JF 3rd. The impact of mandated in-hospital coverage on primary cesarean delivery rates in a large non-university teaching hospital. *Am J Obstet Gynecol.* 1995;172:637–642 (II-2).

4 Weinstein L, Wolfe H. The downward spiral of physician satisfaction: an attempt to avert a crisis within the medical profession. *Obstet Gynecol.* 2007;109:1181–1183.

5 Cors WK, Rohr R. The 'ist' explosion: driving forces, current trends and future directions for hospitalists. *Physician Exec.* 2010;36(3):12–14.

6 Wolfe S. Hospitalists: good or bad news for nurses? *RN.* 2000;63(3):31–33.

7 Wachter RM, Goldman, L. The hospitalist movement 5 Years Later. *JAMA.* 2002;287:487–494.

8 The American College of Obstetricians and Gynecologists. Committee opinion no. 459: The Obstetric-Gynecologic Hospitalist. *Obstet Gynecol.* 2010;116(1):237–239.

9 Clark SL, Belfort MA, Dildy GA, Meyers JA. Reducing obstetric litigation through alterations in practice patterns. *Obstet Gynecol.* 2008;112(6):1279–1283.

10 Allen A, Page J, Cahill A, et al. The cost effectiveness of 24 hr in-house obstetric coverage. *AJOG*. 2013;S48. Supplement to January 2013.

11 Wachter R, Goldman L. The emerging role of "hospitalists" in the American healthcare system. *N Engl J Med*. 1996;335(7):514–517.

12 Frigoletto FD, Greene MF. Is there a sea change ahead for obstetrics and gynecology? *Obstet Gynecol*. 2002; 100(6):1342–1343.

13 Weinstein L. The laborist: a new focus of practice for the obstetrician. *Am J Obstet Gynecol*. 2003;188:310–312.

14 Cheng Y, Cassidy A, Darney BG, et al. Labor and delivery coverage: around-the-clock or as-needed? *AJOG*. 2013;S48. Supplement to January 2013.

15 Iriye B, Huang WH, Condon J, et al. Implementation of a full-time laborist program is associated with a substantial reduction in cesarean section rate. *AJOG*. 2013;S58. Supplement to January 2013.

16 Srinivas S, Macheras M, Small DS, Lorch S. Does the laborist model improve obstetric outcomes? *AJOG*. 2013;S48. Supplement to January 2013.

17 Zhani E. Joint Commission Center for Transforming Healthcare Tackles Miscommunication Among Caregivers. 2010. www.centerfortransforming healthcare.org/news/detail.aspx?ArticleId=294153 (accessed April 29, 2012).

Transparency and Disclosure

Sandra Koch

Disclosure of Adverse Events

Disclosure of adverse events is difficult for clinicians. It's especially difficult in obstetrics and gynecology as any adverse event related to an unborn or newborn baby increases the degree of emotional stress already present in these challenging conversations. This chapter will review general information about disclosure and transparency and further review evidence that disclosure is beneficial to patients, clinicians, and the healthcare system. At the end of the chapter there is a discussion based on three adverse events used to illustrate different disclosure styles and to discuss the impact they might have.

In 2000, the Institute of Medicine released the report "To Err is Human" that documented the large number of medical errors that occurred in hospitals. [1]. Suddenly, addressing patient safety and medical errors had become part of the healthcare discourse. All stake holders in healthcare – consumers, providers, administrators, insurers, federal and state governments – have a vested interest in insuring patient safety by reducing errors and avoiding patient harm. Despite the best intentions, errors will still happen. When an adverse event happens how one discloses the event is essential to the well being of the patient, the clinician and the institution. The Joint Commission released the following standard (R1.1.2.2 in 2001) [2]: "The responsible licensed independent practitioner or his or her designee clearly explains the outcome of any treatment or procedure to the patient and, when appropriate, the family, whenever those outcomes differ significantly from the anticipated outcomes." The American Medical Association followed with this strong statement: "a patient suffers significant medical complications that may have resulted from a physician's mistake … the physician is ethically required to inform the patient of all the facts necessary to ensure understanding of what has occurred" [3]. Many patient safety organizations around the world made statements strongly recommending disclosure of unexpected outcomes, adverse events, and medical errors [4].

Eighty percent of physicians studied by Iezzoni et al. [5] stated that fear of being sued would not dissuade them from full disclosure to a patient when a medical error was made. There was a difference noted between physicians practicing in small private settings as compared with those in university or medical center practices. The survey revealed that more physicians in universities and medical centers (78%) completely agreed with the need to report all serious medical errors as compared to physicians in one- or two-person practices (61%). One in five physicians reported that fear of being sued was a barrier to fully disclosing errors to patients.

Patients and Families

Unexpected outcomes, adverse events, and medical errors happen. It's important to understand what effect they have on the various parties involved.

Patients and families suffer consequences from adverse events. Patients are vulnerable when they receive health care. Even when the treatment plan is clear and the outcome is as expected, some patients will experience emotional distress. When an adverse event occurs, patients may experience both physical and psychological difficulties. Injury from a medical error is different from other injuries due to the trust inherent in the physician–patient relationship. Adding to this, they may need additional medical treatment to recover from the mishap, again requiring that they entrust themselves to a healthcare professional – perhaps the same professional that was involved in the mishap in the first place. There may be long-term consequences for the patient, including chronic pain, disability, and secondary depression. All of these may have an impact on the patient's finances and on personal and work relationships.

Families are also at risk for negative effects, especially if the adverse outcome involves death or disability. Financial, physical, and psychological stress can all be increased. Family members often are unable to move on and ruminate endlessly about the details of the adverse event [6].

Clinicians

Despite knowing and recognizing that medical mistakes and errors do occur, the impact on clinicians can be devastating. Clinicians can experience feelings of being singled out, depression, anxiety, guilt, and humiliation [7]. This can then affect their ability to concentrate, which in turn may further affect their work performance. Clinicians often do not recognize the emotional impact on themselves. Further complicating the situation is that institutions, healthcare organizations, and departments often lack the systems to identify and offer help to clinicians involved in medical error [8]. The term "The Second Victim" was first introduced by Dr. Albert Wu to describe the impact on clinicians involved in medical errors. By using the term, we formally recognize the consequences experienced by clinicians when they are involved in a medical error, especially one that results in patient harm. Recognition by the clinician, their colleagues, and the institution can help all involved in medical errors to successfully cope and learn from the error. It also can help prevent the development of dysfunctional behavior, the clinician leaving medicine, or suicide [7].

Barriers to Disclosure

Many clinicians have difficulty with disclosure. The most common barriers include a lack of training in how to disclose, a fear of being sued, and a culture of blame [9,10]. David Marx, author of the Just Culture Physician Algorithm, emphasizes the importance of creating a blame-free culture in which staff is comfortable reporting and exploring adverse events in order to reduce their recurrence. Because many adverse events are the culmination of an unfortunate sequence of events, every opportunity to analyze the pathway leading to the event has the potential to reduce the risk of recurrence [11].

Medical Liability

How does disclosure of medical errors impact future litigation? The University of Michigan published its litigation experience before and after instituting a policy of complete disclosure and early resolution

of adverse events. After adopting the policy, they saw the rate of new medical malpractice claims fall from 7.03 to 4.52 per 100,000 patient encounters. The number of lawsuits fell from 2.13 to 0.75 per 100,000 patient encounters. The time for resolution of claims fell from 1.36 years to 0.95 years and the total costs for liability, including patient compensation and non-compensation-related legal expenses, also fell. This information suggests that full disclosure of adverse outcomes may lead to a reduction in liability claims and a decrease in total liability expenditure [12].

Liability carriers are also supporting full disclosure. The Doctor's Company actively supports full disclosure and offers guidelines and best practices to providers [13]. COPIC, a Colorado-based medical liability carrier, developed an early offer program started in 2000. The program is known as the 3Rs – Recognize, Respond, and Resolve. Under this program the patient does not give up the right to sue. This program has received excellent physician and patient feedback and demonstrated reduced liability costs for those involved.

As fear of being sued is often listed as a barrier to disclosure, it is important to understand why patients file lawsuits. Only 2% of patients harmed by medical error file a claim. Lawsuits by patients without a valid claim significantly outnumber patients who sue with a valid claim.

Poor communication clearly plays an important role in determining which patients file lawsuits. A total of 44% sued either because they "Believed there was a cover up" or "Suing to obtain more information". Some physicians are more likely to be sued due to their lack of empathy and communication skills, not their clinical skills. A number of studies have specifically looked at the factors that determine which clinicians are sued. Mothers of infants who were permanently injured or

Table 6.1 Reasons why parents sued after an adverse event involving a newborn [14].

32%	To sue by an influential other (often another healthcare provider)
24%	Needed money
24%	Believed there was a cover up
23%	The suit was over a child with no future
20%	Reported suing to obtain more information
19%	Sued for revenge/license (to punish the physician)

who had died were significantly more likely to sue if they felt their physician did not listen, was unwilling to discuss the events openly, or to review the long-term outcome for their infant [14]. Mothers interviewed after having recently delivered a healthy newborn were significantly more likely to complain of poor communication when their clinician had a history of multiple prior suits [14]. These studies underscore the importance of communication and suggest that effective post event management of adverse events, errors, and poor outcomes could significantly impact the desire for patients to seek legal action.

Apology Laws

Apology laws prohibit certain statements and expressions of sorry from being used as an admission of guilt in a court of law during malpractice litigation. There is variation between states as to exactly which statements are restricted from use. There has been some preliminary evidence that states where apology laws have been passed have seen lower liability payments and faster resolutions for claims with serious adverse events [15]. It is not necessary to live in a state that has an apology law in order to disclose. Disclosure is now the standard of care in every state.

Benefits of Disclosure

Disclosure has been demonstrated to benefit both parties through a strengthened physician–patient relationship. There is evidence to support that patients recover more quickly, both emotionally and physically, when full disclosure has been made [16]. The sense of trust created is a very powerful tool. Chapman and Thomas have studied the language of apology in detail and describes the importance of apology in this way: "When one's sense of right is violated, that person will experience anger. He or she will feel wronged and resentful at the person who has violated their trust. The wrongful act stands as a barrier between the two people, and the relationship is fractured. They cannot, even if they desired, live as though the wrong had not been committed. Something inside the offended calls for justice. It is these human realties that serve as the basis of all judicial systems" [17]. They point out that humans, when it comes to apology, speak five different languages, as listed below:

1. Expressing Regret "I am sorry"
2. Accepting Responsibility "I was wrong"
3. Making Restitution "What can I do to make it right?"
4. Genuinely Repenting "Making an earnest effort not to repeat the same mistake"
5. Requesting Forgiveness "Will you forgive me?"

There is significant overlap between what patients want following a medical mishap and these languages. Patients want and expect a timely and full disclosure of the event, expressions of sympathy, an acknowledgment of responsibility, an understanding of what happened, and a discussion of what is being done to prevent recurrence [18,19]. By incorporating these languages in our interactions with patients, we can assist in the healing of all concerned.

How to Disclose?

Disclosure of an adverse event means communicating bad news. If done with adequate knowledge and preparation, it can be a compassionate, constructive dialogue that strengthens the clinician–patient relationship. It can be the first step in providing resolution and emotional healing for all parties involved.

Despite the emergence of evidence-based medicine, much of clinical care remains an art form and not an exact science. Things will go wrong, and when they do, it is the obligation of the clinician to examine carefully the events to understand better how they unfolded. Guessing, surmising, assuming are all very dangerous terms when communicating about adverse events. There are times when the cause will be straightforward, uncomplicated, and easily assessed. In other situations the cause may never be determined. It is the responsibility of the clinician to exercise due diligence in investigating the medical mishap. It is also the responsibility of the physician to communicate **only** what is known and the process that may be undertaken to gain more information to the patient and the family. When there is an adverse event it is extremely important not to publically speculate about the causes.

The decision of how much to disclose is unclear. Many experts teach the disclosure process as a balance beam approach [20]. This is a way to evaluate response strategies and their repercussion along a continuum. On the left side of the balance beam there is no disclosure. As you move to the right end the amount of disclosure increases. At the far right of the balance beam, complete disclosure is followed by the assignment of responsibility (Figure 6.1) [6].

Many clinicians have a hard time dealing with unanticipated adverse events; some may be unable to keep an intellectual distance from the patient's

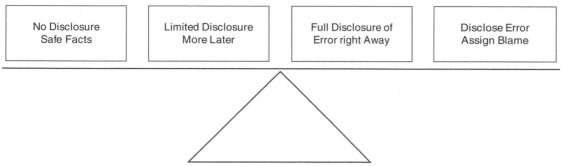

| No Disclosure Safe Facts | Limited Disclosure More Later | Full Disclosure of Error right Away | Disclose Error Assign Blame |

Figure 6.1 Disclosure continuum. Moving from under-disclosure to over-disclosure. Balanced communication is the goal.

situation and therefore may have a difficult time analyzing the facts to make the reasoned evaluation. Learning tools to assist in disclosure will help to bring this back in to focus and will lead to the best possible outcomes for patients, their families, and the providers involved. It is advisable to consider a team approach to the meeting; including another physician or a member of the nursing staff can be helpful to keep the conversation on track. There might also be specific hospital policy regarding the attendance of others such as the risk manager. Clinicians who expect themselves to be perfect will have a particularly difficult time with adverse events and will benefit greatly from structure and assistance. It will allow the clinician to maintain the focus on patient care.

Most clinicians will be apprehensive before a disclosure discussion. Dealing with their own fallibility, failed responsibility, or fear of an inability to respond to a reaction of grief from the patient are common concerns [21]. If disclosure of an adverse event is done well it leaves everyone with a shared understanding; if done poorly, it can leave a patient feeling abandoned, uncared for, and angry. It can leave the clinician emotionally distressed. The key to a successful meeting is careful planning.

Prior to the meeting the clinician must have a full understanding of the case. There should be no distractions. The meeting should take place in a private space where the conversation is unlikely to be interrupted. Cell phones and pagers should be turned off. Sitting down and making eye contact with the patient also helps to convey an important message.

Begin the conversation with a brief review of the entire case; discuss your understanding of the sequence of events – what is known and what is not yet determined. Make sure that the patient and their family do not encounter emotional distance, excuses,

or inappropriate body language as you explain the events. It is important to take your time and make sure that the patient and support people understand the information. Lead the discussion at a level appropriate for the patient and her family. Give them time to ask questions as the conversation proceeds. This should be a discussion and not a lecture. They should understand clearly what the initial assessment of the situation was, how and why the care plan was chosen, and what changed.

Move to expressing empathy to the patient and the family. One of the most powerful things a clinician can do to heal the patient emotionally – and him-/herself – is to apologize. The simple act of formally apologizing can do much to diffuse the hurt and anger that follows injury. Remember that there are five different languages that communicate an apology and be sure to take the opportunity to use each of them as appropriate. Try to avoid discussion of your own feelings. This discussion should focus entirely on the patient's situation.

Failure to communicate openly, take responsibility, and apologize can increase the patient's anger and the likelihood of litigation. In cases where mistakes were clearly made, being sincere, caring, and concerned may be your only defense.

It is crucial during this discussion to ask the patient about their feelings. It is your opportunity to truly understand what the patient/family thinks happened. If they are angry, find out why and to whom is their anger directed. Listening to the concerns of the patient and family may be difficult; however, it is your opportunity to fully understand their perspective. It can give you the information to meet their emotional needs most effectively.

At the close of the meeting with the patient and family, take the opportunity to assess their grasp of the events. Ask that they restate their understanding of the situation. Take the time to give additional explanation as needed and to correct any misunderstanding that becomes evident. With the patient's consent, include the family in this final discussion, ensuring that all issues and questions have been addressed. Often it is an extended family member that pushes the patient to seek legal action [6]. Make sure that the patient and family know that a full review will be taking place and that you will be meeting with them as often as needed.

Carefully document your conversation after the conclusion of the meeting. Make note of the names of those attending the meeting, the date and times, and an overview of the discussion, highlighting misunderstandings and sources of anger from the patient or family. Indicate the patient's level of understanding. Finally, document the plan for subsequent meeting(s) to review any additional information. Clinicians often underestimate the importance of follow-up and ongoing communication [6]. Part of taking responsibility means that you will work diligently to discover the causes of the event and keep the patient and their family informed.

Responsibility also means managing complications from the adverse event. If there are changes made following a full review, knowing this may prevent others from suffering the same problem will also help the patient and family to cope. It gives a positive meaning to their experience to know that their suffering helped improve the healthcare system.

Regardless of the cause of the adverse event, the attending physician is ultimately the one who must take responsibility for discussing it with the patient

Table 6.2 Breaking bad news.

Carefully review the case prior to meeting
Choose a private place to meet, cell phones/beepers off
Begin with a brief overview of the case – make sure the patient/family understand
Apologize/empathize
Ask about their emotions/who are they angry with, what are they angry about
Request that the patient/family review their understanding of the events with you – answer any additional questions or clarify points as needed
Arrange follow-up
Document the meeting, date/time who was there, sources of confusion or anger
Document any follow up that was arranged

(see [2]). Taking responsibility is one of the five languages of apology. Taking responsibility does not mean that you caused the adverse event. It means that you understand the responsibility you have accepted inherent in the doctor–patient relationship. It means that the adverse event took place under your care. Patients look to their physician as the leader of the team. By accepting the patient's trust you have a responsibility to provide their care before, during, and after an adverse event. The patient should understand that you or your designee are in charge and have control over their care. Distancing yourself from the patient at the time of an adverse event simply adds the feeling of abandonment to an already difficult situation. Being sincere, caring, and concerned is not only the best way to avoid legal action; it is ethically the right thing to do.

Following are three cases that illustrate the disclosure process. They do not attempt to outline a complete conversation, but rather to illustrate the balance beam approach to disclosure.

Cases

Case #1 – Unexpected Outcome – No Error Was Made

AB was a 19-year-old woman G1P0 who presented to the emergency room with RLQ pain. She was sexually active and using depoprovera injection for contraception. She received her last depo injection 6 wks ago. In the emergency room she was noted to have a positive bHCG of 1950 and a complex right adnexal mass with no evidence of an intrauterine pregnancy was seen on transvaginal ultrasound. She was counseled that both the viability and location of the pregnancy test were unknown. She was offered three treatment options: (1) re-evaluation in 48 hours with follow-up bHCG, (2) diagnostic laparoscopy, or (3) methotrexate for presumed ectopic pregnancy. Although this was an unplanned pregnancy, the patient was clear that she would continue the pregnancy if it was healthy. She wished to avoid surgery and to preserve her fertility. The physician advised her that the most likely location of the pregnancy was in the tube. After discussion with the physician, she opted to receive methotrexate. Over the following 2 weeks her bHCG level rose and she received an additional methotrexate injection following the standard protocol for treating ectopic pregnancy. Follow-up ultrasound revealed a gestational sac at 5 wks. Dr. Smith would like your advice on how this should be communicated to the patient.

Approach #1

AB, the ultrasound result shows some fluid in the uterus. We will need to continue to check your HCG levels and repeat the ultrasound in a week.

Approach #2

AB, the ultrasound result shows fluid in the uterus. This may indicate that the pregnancy was located in the uterus not in the tube. We will need to continue to check your HCG levels and repeat the ultrasound in a week.

Approach #3

AB, the ultrasound shows an early intrauterine pregnancy. The information we have lets us know that this is not a healthy pregnancy; however, this is good news as it means you have an increased chance of conceiving normally when you are ready. We will need to continue to check your HCG levels and repeat the ultrasound in one week.

Approach #4

AB, the ultrasound result shows an early intrauterine pregnancy. In our discussion I told you that I thought it was most likely an ectopic pregnancy. I see now that I was wrong. I would not have used methotrexate had I known this.

Discussion

In determining which approach is best, the clinician has to take into account their personal communication style. The difficulty with approach #1 is that it is dishonest. The patient sees a copy of the ultrasound report saying that an intrauterine pregnancy is evident and may feel deceived. Approaches #2 and #3 let the patient know that there is a possibility that an intrauterine pregnancy is present, but does not confirm this information. Either of these options meets the goals we established above. These options are safe and allow the patient's clinical course to progress with more conversation to follow. Approach #4: this disclosure exceeds what is actually known. This is an example of speculation. It potentially exposes the clinician to significant anger from a patient who may feel she was given poor treatment initially and it undermines the initial reasonable evaluation that took place in the emergency room.

Case #2 Straightforward Case with Medical Error

LR is a 38-year-old woman G2P2 with a history of menometrorrhagia. Ultrasound showed a leiomyoma within the endometrial cavity. She was scheduled for hysteroscopy with a planned resection of the leiomyoma. During surgery the leiomyoma was identified and resection performed. The circulating nurse was tracking the sorbitol medium being used. She was recording the total amount running in and the amount coming out and noted a discrepancy. She informed the physician of the discrepancy at 500, 800, 1,000, 1,200, and 1,500 cm^3. She also noted that there was a lot of fluid leaking onto the floor. The anesthesiologist was aware of the situation. Serum electrolyte levels were ordered in the recovery room and the results showed the patient to be severely hyponatremic. She was admitted to the ICU for treatment of acute water intoxication. Dr. Farnsworth would like your assistance in communicating this to the patient.

Approach #1

LR, your electrolyte levels became unbalanced during the surgery. We will need to admit you to the ICU while they normalize.

Approach #2

LR, during your surgery your electrolyte level became unbalanced. We need to admit you to the ICU while they normalize. It happened because too much of the fluid we were using for the hystcroscopic resection entered your bloodstream, diluting your electrolytes. I am not sure why this happened – we will look into this.

Approach #3

LR, during your surgery your electrolytes became unbalanced. We need to admit you to the ICU for acute treatment. It happened because too much of the fluid we were using for the hysteroscopic resection entered your bloodstream, diluting your electrolytes. We had some difficulty with the system we use for evaluating the fluid shifts in the operating room. We routinely measure the amount of fluid entering and returning to prevent this from happening. In your case the circulating nurse noticed a significant leakage of fluid on the floor and felt this accounted for the mismatch. We will be conducting a full review and will let you know what we find.

Approach #4

LR, during your surgery your electrolytes became unbalanced. We need to admit you to the ICU for acute treatment. It happened because too much of the fluid we were using for the hysteroscopic resection entered your bloodstream, diluting your electrolytes. We routinely measure the amount of fluid entering and returning to prevent this from happening. In your case the circulating nurse noticed a significant leakage of fluid on the floor and felt this accounted for the mismatch. I dismissed the discrepancy due to this and see now that that was a mistake. We will be conducting a full review and will let you know what we find.

Discussion

The difficulty with approach #1 is that the patient again may feel a lack of transparency is present given that the only reasonable cause for the electrolyte abnormality is the excessive absorption of the sorbitol solution. Not disclosing this is dishonest and may cause the patient to feel the physician was trying to hide something. Approaches #2 and #3 let the patient know that there is an explanation for the hyponatremia and that an evaluation is being done to determine if changes need to be made in order to prevent this from happening again. Either of these options meets the goals we established above. These approaches are safe and allow the patient to understand what happened without assigning blame; additional conversation will need to take place so that the patient is informed of the results of the review. Approach #4: this disclosure has full transparency and also assigns responsibility. It is honest. It seems to go beyond what is necessary and may lead the patient to doubt the clinician's ability. In fact, it may expose the clinician to litigation.

Case #3 Case with the Cause of an Unexpected Outcome Not Immediately Known

CG is a 24-year-old primigravida with an uncomplicated pregnancy. She was admitted to labor and delivery at term in early labor after an uncomplicated prenatal course. She progressed to 5 cm dilatation with Pitocin augmentation; the fetal monitor initially showed a category 1 tracing; however, the tracing had deteriorated and was now category 2. The anesthesiologist was notified of the possible need for a C-section. Over the next hour the fetal monitor deteriorated to a category

3 pattern. The obstetrician managing the patient made the decision that a C-section was indicated. The anesthesiologist was notified, she was involved in another patient's care and was unable to be present for an hour. The patient received position change, increased fluid, oxygen, and the pitocin was discontinued. The tracing returned to a category 2. The C-section was performed under epidural anesthesia with the father of the baby in the room to attend the birth. When the baby was delivered the initial APGAR was 1, the pediatrician attempted to resuscitate the baby for 30 minutes but was unsuccessful. The baby was pronounced dead. Dr. Smith would like your assistance in discussing the outcome with the parents.

Approach #1

CG, we are so sorry to tell you that your baby did not survive. Sometimes things happen, we may never know why.

Approach #2

CG, we are so sorry to tell you that your baby did not survive. Sometimes things happen, we may never know why. An autopsy may be able to give us some insight as to what happened.

Approach #3

CG, we are so sorry to tell you that your baby did not survive. Sometimes things happen, we may never know why. An autopsy may be able to give us some insight as to what happened. As you know, the C-section was performed because we were concerned about the baby's heart rate. This may have been a factor in the outcome. We will be conducting a full review and will let you know what we find.

Approach #4

CG, we are so sorry to tell you that your baby did not survive, sometimes things happen, we may never know why. An autopsy may be able to give us some insight as to what happened. As you know, the C-section was performed because we were concerned about the baby's heart rate. I am concerned that the delay caused by the lack of availability of the anesthesiologist may have been too much for the baby to tolerate. I had notified the anesthesiologist over an hour before the initial decision to move to a C-section and do not understand why anesthesia was not prepared. We will be conducting a full investigation.

Addendum

Autopsy showed that the baby had a lethal congenital anomaly of the GI tract not visible by ultrasound.

Discussion

The difficulty with approach #1 is that the patient knows there was a problem with the heart tracing. Not discussing this may cause the patient to feel the physician was trying to hide something. It certainly gives the impression that the physician is unwilling to discuss details of the events. Approaches #2 and #3 let the patient know that the physician is aware of the fetal heart rate abnormalities and that only an autopsy will be able to give the additional information needed to help understand the newborn's death. Either of these options meets the goals we established above. These options are safe and allow the patient to understand what happened; they don't assign blame. They leave room for the additional conversations that will need to take place as a review is performed and the autopsy is completed. Approach #4: the physician clearly implies that the abnormal fetal heart tracing is related to the death. This is an assumption that was later found to be incorrect. The physician goes further to express anger and blame the anesthesiologist for delaying the delivery of the baby and implies that this may have contributed to the outcome. After the autopsy findings are back and the cause of death becomes known, this patient will still remember that she was mishandled and her ability to trust the same facility in the future will be compromised. The information given was honest and yet still may have created unnecessary emotional harm.

Post-disclosure Care

It is important to have continued interaction with the patient after an adverse event and the initial disclosure discussion. It takes time for patients to process what they have experienced. New questions and emotions will emerge. During follow-up meetings it is important to again ask about how the patient is doing emotionally. Are they angry? If so, with whom and why? This is an appropriate time to offer counseling services to anyone perceived to be struggling. Medical mishaps can leave a patient constantly thinking about the incident, unable to let it go. Therapy may avert this reaction.

Discuss with them the result of any review that was performed and any changes that were made to prevent the same thing from happening again. Give them an opportunity to ask further questions regarding the event.

Giving the patient assistance in obtaining the medical, emotional, and financial support that they need in dealing with the consequences of the adverse event significantly impacts their attitudes toward the responsible clinicians. If we suffered an injury at the hands of another we would certainly appreciate compassion, care, and compensation.

Summary

The conversation that you have following an adverse event is critical to resolution for everyone involved. If you use an organized approach, it can be a compassionate, constructive dialogue. A careful assessment can also help identify systems issues that will improve care for future patients. This approach is the best way to show your patient and their family that you and the healthcare team want to assist them as they move forward.

References

1   Kohn LT, Corrigan JM, Donaldson MS, editors. *To Err is Human: Building a Safer Health System.* Washington, DC: National Academy Press, Institute of Medicine; 1999.

2   July 2001, the Joint Commission for Accreditation of Healthcare Organizations (JCAHO) Patient Safety Standards (R1.1.2.2 in 2001).

3   American Medical Association. Code of Medical Ethics Opinion 8.12 on "Patient Information"; 2003.

4   Australian Council for Safety and Quality in Health Care, Standard for Open Disclosure, 2003; United Kingdom, National Patient safety Agency, 2009; National Patient Safety Foundation, 2003; National Quality Forum 2009, Safe Practice #7, Disclosure; Canadian Medical Association, 2004 (Code of Ethics updated 2004, Item 14).

5   Iezzoni LI, Rao SR, DesRoches CM, Vogeli C, Campbell EG. Survey shows that at least some physicians are not always open or honest with patients. *Health Affairs.* 2012;31(2):383–391.

6   Pichert JW, Hickson GB, Pinto A, Vincent CA. Communicating about the unexpected outcomes, adverse events, and errors. In: Carayon P, ed., *Handbook of Human Factors and Ergonomics in Health Care and Patient Safety*, 2nd ed. Boca Raton, FL: CRC Press; 2011: 401–422.

7   Wu AW. Medical error: the second victim. The doctor who makes the mistake needs help too. *BMJ.* 2000;320(7237):726–727.

8 Weiss PM. Medical errors and the second victim. *The Female Patient*. 2011;36(2):29–32.

9 Finkelstein D, Wu AW, Holtzman NA, Smith MK. When a physician harms a patient by a medical error: ethical, legal, and risk-management considerations. *J Clin Ethics*.1997;8:330–335.

10 Goldberg RM, Kuhn G, Andrew LB, Thomas HA Jr. Coping with medical mistakes and errors in judgment. *Ann Emerg Med*.2002;39:287–292.

11 Marx D. *Whack-a-Mole: The Price We Pay For Expecting Perfection*. Eden Prairie, MN: By Your Side Studios; 2009.

12 Kachalia A, Kaufman SR, Boothman R, et al. Liability claims and costs before and after implementation of a medical error disclosure program. *Ann Int Med*. 2010;153(4):213–221.

13 Disclosure Resources. www.the doctors.com.

14 Hickson GB, Clayton EW, Githens PB, et al. Factors that prompted families to file medical malpractice claims following perinatal injuries. *JAMA*. 1992;267:1359–1363.

15 Does Sorry Work? The Impact of Apology Laws on Medical Malpractice. Ho, Benjamin and Liu, Elaine, Does Sorry Work? The Impact of Apology Laws on Medical Malpractice (December 1, 2010). Johnson School Research Paper Series No. 04-2011. Available at SSRN: http://ssrn.com/abstract=1744225 or http://dx.doi.org/10.2139/ssrn.1744225

16 Allan A, McKillop D. The health implications of apologizing after an adverse event. *Int J Qual Health Care*. 2010;22:126–131.

17 Chapman G, Thomas J. *The Five Languages of Apology*. Hyderabad: Jaico; 2006.

18 Gallagher, TH, Waterman AD, Ebers AG, et al. Patients' and physicians' attitudes regarding the disclosure of medical errors. *JAMA*. 2003;289:1001–1007.

19 Mazor KM, Simon SR, Yood RA, et al. Health plan members' views about the disclosure of medical errors. *Ann Intern Med*. 2004;140:409–418.

20 Hickson GB, Pichert JW. *Disclosure and Apology. National Patient Safety Foundation Stand Up for Patient Safety Resource Guide*. North Adams, MA: National Patient Safety Foundation; 2008.

21 Woods JR, Orzovsky FA. *What Do I Say? Communicating Intended or Unanticipated Outcomes in Obstetrics*. San Fransisco, CA: Jossey Bass; 2003.

Surgical Checklists

John S. Wachtel and Abraham Lichtmacher

Most medical organizations today advocate for the use of checklists as a way to standardize key processes and to help prevent the multitude of errors that can occur in modern medical therapy and in all health systems. While the proven effectiveness and use of checklists has been widespread for many years in high-reliability organizations, and particularly in the aviation industry, medicine has been slow to adopt this valuable technique to improve patient outcomes. There are now numerous examples throughout the medical literature, including the fields of Obstetrics and Gynecology, demonstrating the effectiveness of checklists and protocols to reduce errors and improve patient safety. The Institute of Medicine (IOM) has encouraged the use of checklists since 1999 [1] and beginning in 2011, the American College of Obstetricians and Gynecologists (ACOG) has published a series of checklists on numerous subjects.

One of the earliest success stories of the benefits of checklists in medicine was from the pioneering work of Pronovost and colleagues at Johns Hopkins. They decreased the number of catheter related bloodstream infections in ICUs in Michigan to zero by using a simple five-item checklist prior to each catheter insertion [2]. In the field of obstetrics, ground-breaking work has been done by Clark and colleagues at the Hospital Corporation of America (HCA) proving the clinical effectiveness of checklists and protocols in improving patient outcomes in some of the more common and critical areas of our specialty [3,4]. In gynecologic surgery as in the general surgical arena, the adoption of the World Health Organization (WHO) Safe Surgery Checklist has been shown to dramatically reduce surgical errors [5].

At its core, the checklist is essentially a tool that reduces reliance on memory for standardized processes, improves reproducibility, eliminates variability which can result in error, and ultimately is a communication tool that improves teamwork. In some cases variation is expected and indeed a desired outcome. A good example is a work of art that is unique and different every time. On the other hand, checklists are essential in those endeavors that require a consistent, non-variable result. Any time a process or an action is expected to produce the same result, standardization is essential. Examples of this principle are universal and are applied in everything from a manufacturing process to a basic cookbook recipe. Altering the process, as for example, leaving out an ingredient in a recipe, will produce a different result. In the case of a surgical process, leaving out a crucial step would also potentially produce a different result, one that could prove to be harmful to the patient. The checklist represents the steps that need to be taken in the correct sequence to produce the desired results.

WHO Surgical Checklists

In 2002, the World Health Assembly (WHA) in 2002 adopted a resolution which urged countries to focus on and improve patient safety in the world as it relates to healthcare delivery. In response to this resolution, the World Health Organization (WHO) brought together experts from around the world under its focused safety campaigns called Global Patient Safety Challenges. Initial focus was placed on reducing infection in a variety of healthcare settings. This was done through a campaign to improve hand hygiene. Continued efforts by the WHO in 2007 began to focus on the previously underappreciated worldwide problem of patient safety in the surgical arena. The effort and its recommendation is outlined in the monograph *WHO Guidelines for Safe Surgery 2009 Safe Surgery Saves Lives* [6]. Ten objectives were outlined as shown in Table 7.1. The primary tool detailed in this monograph was the use of a checklist to enhance communication among members of the surgical team and increase standardization thereby reducing errors. The surgical procedure is a process composed of three distinct phases. The initial phase occurs during the preparation for surgery and

Table 7.1 World Health Organization: ten essential objectives for safe surgery.

Objective 1: The team will operate on the correct patient at the correct site
Objective 2: The team will use methods known to prevent harm from administration of anesthetics, while protecting the patient from pain
Objective 3: The team will recognize and effectively prepare for life-threatening loss of airway or respiratory function
Objective 4: The team will recognize and effectively prepare for risk of high blood loss
Objective 5: The team will avoid inducing an allergic or adverse drug reaction for which the patient is known to be at significant risk
Objective 6: The team will consistently use methods known to minimize the risk for surgical site
Objective 7: The team will prevent inadvertent retention of instruments and sponges in surgical wounds
Objective 8: The team will secure and accurately identify all surgical specimens
Objective 9: The team will effectively communicate and exchange critical information for the safe conduct of the operation
Objective 10: Hospitals and public health systems will establish routine surveillance of surgical capacity, volume and results

WHO Guidelines for Safe Surgery 2009 [6].

before induction of anesthesia. Once anesthesia has been initiated but before the actual procedure starts would represent the second phase of the procedure. The final phase is after the surgery has been completed with the closure of the wound but before the patient is moved from the operating room.

By dividing the surgical procedure into phases, specific components of the process can be identified and incorporated as part of the checklist. Many of the processes followed during any surgical procedure are routine. The WHO recommendation for the implementation of the checklist is that individual hospitals and physicians develop their own checklist that is reflective of their local culture and processes. The modification of the checklist to meet the needs of the local hospital needs to be undertaken with a critical eye, and as recommended by the WHO it should follow seven specific principles.

1. The checklist should focus on most critical issues.
2. It should be brief, allowing it to be completed quickly without interfering with the surgical procedure.

3. Every part of the checklist must have an associated action.
4. The checklist should promote some verbal interaction among team members.
5. The development of the checklist needs to be a collaborative process that involves all individuals who will ultimately use it.
6. Any effort to modify the checklist should be in collaboration with representatives from groups who might be involved in using it.
7. Before a checklist is adopted it should be tested in a limited setting to be certain that it meets the needs of the facility.

Once the checklist is implemented, it should be integrated into processes that may already exist in the hospital. The WHO Surgical Safety Checklist (Figure 7.1) was presented as an example which may be modified to meet the needs of the local hospital [7].

Types of Checklists

Checklists that have been adopted in medicine and throughout other high-reliability organizations fall into four principal categories [8]. These depend upon the number of people involved and how the correct actions are verified.

1. Static Parallel Checklists: These are completed by a single person. Typical oxytocin checklists or those used for anesthesia machine checklist are examples.
2. Static Sequential with Verification: These require two individuals, with one person reading the list and the second person verifying that the elements have been completed. Typical examples of this type would include the five-element checklist to prevent catheter-associated bloodstream infection [2] or the administration of blood products.
3. Static Sequential Checklists with Verification and Confirmation: These checklists are used by larger teams of care providers, with one individual reading the list and other team members verifying and confirming the tasks. The best examples are the time-out checklists now routinely used in most operating rooms or the use of shoulder dystocia checklists.
4. Dynamic Checklists: These checklists utilize a flow chart to guide more complex decision-making. Recent examples would include checklists for management of hypertensive crises in obstetrics or for the management of Category 2 fetal heart rate monitor tracings.

Surgical Safety Checklist

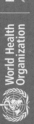 **World Health Organization** | **Patient Safety**
A World Alliance for Safer Health Care

Before induction of anaesthesia

(with at least nurse and anaesthetist)

Has the patient confirmed his/her identity, site, procedure, and consent?
☐ Yes

Is the site marked?
☐ Yes
☐ Not applicable

Is the anaesthesia machine and medication check complete?
☐ Yes

Is the pulse oximeter on the patient and functioning?
☐ Yes

Does the patient have a:

Known allergy?
☐ No
☐ Yes

Difficult airway or aspiration risk?
☐ No
☐ Yes, and equipment/assistance available

Risk of >500ml blood loss (7ml/kg in children)?
☐ No
☐ Yes, and two IVs/central access and fluids planned

Before skin incision

(with nurse, anaesthetist and surgeon)

☐ **Confirm all team members have introduced themselves by name and role.**

☐ **Confirm the patient's name, procedure, and where the incision will be made.**

Has antibiotic prophylaxis been given within the last 60 minutes?
☐ Yes
☐ Not applicable

Anticipated Critical Events

To Surgeon:
☐ What are the critical or non-routine steps?
☐ How long will the case take?
☐ What is the anticipated blood loss?

To Anaesthetist:
☐ Are there any patient-specific concerns?

To Nursing Team:
☐ Has sterility (including indicator results) been confirmed?
☐ Are there equipment issues or any concerns?

Is essential imaging displayed?
☐ Yes
☐ Not applicable

Before patient leaves operating room

(with nurse, anaesthetist and surgeon)

Nurse Verbally Confirms:
☐ The name of the procedure
☐ Completion of instrument, sponge and needle counts
☐ Specimen labelling (read specimen labels aloud, including patient name)
☐ Whether there are any equipment problems to be addressed

To Surgeon, Anaesthetist and Nurse:
☐ What are the key concerns for recovery and management of this patient?

This checklist is not intended to be comprehensive. Additions and modifications to fit local practice are encouraged.

Revised 1 / 2009 © WHO, 2009

Figure 7.1 World Health Organization Surgical Safety checklist.

Clinical Scenario

We would like to examine a clinical example of the use of a static sequential checklist with verification and confirmation. The following clinical example occurred at one of the authors' institutions. This demonstrates a failure of the time-out process in gynecologic surgery.

A very experienced and prominent gynecologic surgeon had two cases scheduled in the operating room to follow each other on the same day. Patient A was a 42-year-old woman with large symptomatic uterine fibroids who requested and was scheduled for a total abdominal hysterectomy (TAH). Patient B was a 46-year-old woman, also with large symptomatic uterine fibroids, who requested that a total abdominal hysterectomy AND bilateral salpingo-oophorectomy (TAH-BSO) be performed. According to the surgeon, surgical resident, anesthesiologist, and the group of circulating and scrub nurses, both cases were completed uneventfully and without complication. On postoperative day #5, the surgeon received the final pathology reports on both patients. At this time, she recognized that, unfortunately, Patient A had undergone a TAH-BSO and Patient B only a TAH.

A root-cause analysis was performed to help determine how this error had occurred, dramatically affecting two patients. Some of the problems uncovered in the review included the following.

1. Hierarchal problems. Both patients were evaluated at the surgeon's private office and not seen by the junior gynecologic resident until the time of surgery. The resident was concerned that the proper procedure was not being done on Patient A. However, she was reluctant to inquire or challenge the experienced surgeon, who was more familiar with the patients.

2. Multitasking and distraction. The anesthesiologist who participated in the time-out, and by hospital guidelines was to be responsible for ensuring the correct procedure was performed, was covering two operating rooms simultaneously. He left the OR to deal with some problems in the other room he was covering and did not recognize the wrong procedures were being performed.

3. Communication issues. In the middle of both the first and the second cases, both the scrub nurse and the circulating nurse who participated in the time-out were relieved by back-up nurses. In both cases, the precise surgery planned was not shared with the relief nurses, who were unaware that the incorrect surgeries were being performed.

4. Physician fatigue. While it was difficult to assess the contribution of fatigue to this medical error, the primary surgeon had an emergency surgery during the night prior to these scheduled hysterectomies. This was probably not the only reason for the surgeon performing the wrong procedures, but she felt this did affect her recall of the patients' preferences for the type of surgery.

This unusual case of "wrong site surgery" was a failure of the time-out procedure and the use of a preoperative checklist. It required the failure of numerous individuals who could have taken the responsibility to ensure that the correct patient received the correct surgery. While the primary surgeon had the greatest responsibility to ensure this event did not occur, an appropriate system had been designed by the hospital to prevent such occurrences. The case emphasizes the importance of every member of the surgical team taking responsibility for all aspects of the procedure, including that the planned surgery was accomplished.

Barriers to Implementation

Why has the correct use of checklists been so slow to be integrated into the medical culture? While there are numerous contributing factors, the most common problem has been physician resistance. Many doctors consider checklists to be an affront to their intelligence and to be a challenge to their autonomy. Unlike aviation pilots, who recognize the enormous benefits of checklists and embrace the concept, many surgeons who should be role models dismiss the use of these tools as an intrusion on their ability to provide the best care for their patients. This ignores the reality of the increasing complexity of modern medicine that can no longer rely solely on the primary doctor's memory and knowledge base. Modern medicine has become much more of a "team sport," incorporating shift work and numerous handoffs which can lead to communication errors. A properly designed checklist may help to mitigate some of these problems and help to deal with the inherent fallibility of all humans, including surgeons.

Medicine has been frequently described as an art, as in the "art of medicine." The implication is that creative interpretation should be accepted as part of the practice of medicine. In 1951, T. L. Fisher, MD Secretary-Treasurer for the Canadian Medical

Protective Association, discussed that 50 years after the introduction of the surgical sponge count, it was still felt by many surgeons and hospitals that it, "was an unnecessary refinement of the surgical Art" [9]. The point is underscored with the observation that "responsibility for error in the absence of a count will rest on their [the surgeons'] shoulders," which reinforced the long-held approach of assigning fault for an error to an individual. With the increasing focus on systems and a team approach to the care of the patient, this lingering sentiment has begun to shift.

Despite the evidence that the use of a checklist reduces potential of error, there has been resistance to the acceptance for the use of checklists in medicine until recently. The often-used refrain against practicing cookbook medicine still describes the lingering attitude that resists the introduction of standardization in medicine. This attitude, however, does underscore the fact that the diagnosis and treatment of diseases is filled with a significant amount of variation that cannot be completely eliminated by the use of standardized processes. Yet in those areas where the use of a uniform process clearly demonstrates a better outcome, the implementation of that process must be supported. The use of a well-designed process or checklist should be viewed as a "safe harbor" that has the potential of not only protecting the patient from harm, but also the physician from inappropriate assignment of fault for an error.

Another barrier to acceptance of checklists may be the absence of definitive scientific evidence to show that a particular protocol represents the "best" care. Do not let perfection be the enemy of good. In fact, there are relatively few instances where unequivocal scientific data exist to show that a single management strategy is ideal. This should not prevent a checklist from being created, as simply the act of standardizing care, even if the checklist is not perfect, will lead to improved outcomes. The best example of this in our specialty is the use of an oxytocin protocol. While no single method of administering oxytocin has been proven to be ideal (low dose versus high dose, timing of dosage changes, etc.), there are robust data to show improved outcomes even if the checklist may be imperfect or flawed. "A successful checklist does not have to be based on a proven best practice (such as multiple randomized clinical trials) when the existence of such a proven best practice is not present" [10].

Yet another barrier to acceptance of the checklist is the concern that it may not apply to all patients.

Because of specific circumstances, the checklist may not be the best way to manage a particular patient. No protocol or checklist is perfect and a disclaimer should always be included that the checklist can be altered or ignored to manage the individual needs of the patient. However, the critical thinking involved in modifying a protocol for a specific patient must be documented in the medical records to explain the rationale for nonstandard treatment.

Medical knowledge is constantly changing. It must also be recognized that any checklist must be a living document, subject to scheduled review and either reaffirmation or revision as necessary. Dates of review and revision should be prominently displayed on each document. The more controversial the checklist may be, the sooner it should be re-evaluated for its effectiveness. If possible, data should be collected before and after any intervention to show the actual effectiveness. If the desired outcome is not achieved with improved patient care, then the checklist should be amended or eliminated. This should help to allay the fears of outliers who have difficulty accepting these concepts.

Clinical Scenario

Let's examine another clinical example where a checklist failure has occurred in the OR. This problem happened in the Labor and Delivery suite and again is an uncommon occurrence. Because Cesarean section is usually the only surgical procedure performed in the delivery room, the time-out procedure is often taken lightly by the surgical team.

A 42-year-old patient was undergoing her third Cesarean section scheduled at term. The time-out procedure was done, which confirmed that the patient's signed operative consent form was for a "repeat Cesarean section." All surgical team members concurred with the planned operation. After safely delivering the baby and closing the uterine incision, the surgeon looked over the drapes and asked the patient if she still wanted to have her tubal ligation performed. She confirmed her desire to have a permanent sterilization procedure completed. The circulating nurse correctly noted that the surgical consent form did not include a tubal ligation procedure, and objected to allowing this to occur. A lengthy discussion ensued between the surgical team, the circulating and scrub nurses as well as the anesthesiologist, all of whom had been involved in the preoperative time-out. Fortunately, in the state where this occurred, there was a requirement for a separate sterilization form to be signed by the patient at least 3 days in advance of the surgery. As this document was in the chart and both the surgeon and surgical assistant stated the patient had reiterated her desire for a sterilization procedure prior to the operation, the nurse relented and allowed the desired surgery to occur. The patient's husband, who was also present in the OR, confirmed the patient's request for a tubal ligation and was a strong advocate for ensuring that this surgery was completed.

Careful attention to the correct surgical procedure during the time-out is essential, especially when multiple procedures are planned and especially if multiple surgeons are involved. The cavalier attitude of the obstetrical team was inappropriate as second procedures such as a cerclage removal or tubal ligation are not uncommon in Labor and Delivery. This example reflects the attitude and culture in many operating rooms around the country about the importance and effectiveness of checklists. Until the entire medical community recognizes the inherent value of checklists and embraces the concept, unfortunate medical errors will occur. "While the science of checklists, much like the science of safety and quality, is rapidly evolving, many believe that medical checklists can help prevent errors, mitigate harm and reduce the costs associated with them" [11].

How to Produce a Checklist

The World Health Organization in its WHO Surgical Safety Checklist 2009 Implementation Manual discusses the process for the acceptance and implementation of a surgical checklist [6]. An initial step in this process is the formation of a multidisciplinary team (i.e., surgeons, anesthesiologists, operating room nurses, operating room administration, nurse anesthetists, and others) that is responsible for the development and implementation of the checklist. The focus has clearly been shifted from the individual to the team for the responsibility of ensuring the safety of the patient. Patients and families now have the expectation that every member of the team is responsible for their safe care [12]. The organization of the team approach to the delivery of care to the patient is highly dependent on effective communication among all members of the healthcare team. Many strategies have been developed for improvement of such communication. AHRQ's TeamSTEPPS [13] has received much attention and acceptance as a strategy for improving

communication among healthcare teams. The use of a checklist helps improve such communication and its development and acceptance within an organization is best achieved as a team effort.

The perioperative process is well-defined. Many procedures have been developed in response to a variety of regulatory and patient safety initiatives, such as The Joint Commission's Universal Protocol for Preventing Wrong Site, Wrong Procedure and Wrong Person Surgery™ which became effective July 1, 2004. Although these do not specifically require the use of a checklist, they do clearly delineate specific steps and verification processes that need to be carried out during this perioperative timeframe. These requirements can serve as a starting point in identifying the focus of the checklist as well as the elements, which should be included in a given checklist. Atul Gawande, the lead physician in the WHO Safe Surgery Saves Lives project, in The Checklist Manifesto described his trial and error process of developing a checklist [14]. He then listed the routine steps that should be followed in developing a surgical checklist. These steps are further elaborated in the Implementation Manual of the WHO Surgical Safety Checklist 2009.

An important consideration in the development of a checklist is to keep it simple. As the practice of medicine has taken on an increasing complexity, there is often a desire to make the checklist all encompassing. The WHO Implementation Manual notes that the checklist should be brief and focused. It usually should be possible to complete the checklist in under 1 minute, so that it does not interfere with the process of the surgery [6]. As acceptance of the checklist develops, it may be expanded based on the needs of the organization. Despite the best efforts of those involved in the development of a checklist, this process must be considered an ongoing one. Modifications should be made in response to changes in regulatory and local requirements for perioperative patient safety as well as the effectives of the initial checklist. In order to evaluate the effectiveness of the checklist, its use needs to be continuously monitored. Does it do what it is meant to do? Has it improved the process and patient outcomes? Continued reliance on an ineffective and unworkable process as outlined in a checklist will reduce its acceptance and will eventually make it ineffective.

An example of a comprehensive checklist composed of elements recommended by various organizations is presented in Figure 7.2. Although it contains most of

COMPREHENSIVE SURGICAL CHECKLIST

Blue = World Health Organization (WHO) Green = The Joint Commission – Universal Protocol (JC) 2010 National Patient Safety Goals Orange = JC and WHO

PREPROCEDURE CHECK-IN	SIGN-IN	TIME-OUT	SIGN-OUT
In Holding Area	**Before Induction of Anesthesia**	**Before Skin Incision**	**Before the Patient Leaves the Operating Room**
Patient/patient representative actively confirms with Registered Nurse (RN):	**RN and anesthesia care provider confirm:**	**Initiated by designated team member** All other activities to be suspended (unless a life-threatening emergency)	**RN confirms:**
Identity □ Yes Procedure and procedure site □ Yes Consent(s) □ Yes Site marked □ Yes □ N/A by person performing the procedure	Confirmation of: identity, procedure, procedure site and consent(s) □ Yes Site marked □ Yes □ N/A by person performing the procedure	**Introduction of team members** □ Yes **All:** Confirmation of the following: identity, procedure, incision site, consent(s) □ Yes Site is marked and visible □ Yes □ N/A	Name of operative procedure Completion of sponge, sharp, and instrument counts □ Yes □ N/A Specimens identified and labeled □ Yes □ N/A Any equipment problems to be addressed? □ Yes □ N/A
RN confirms presence of: History and physical □ Yes Preanesthesia assessment □ Yes	Patient allergies □ Yes □ N/A Difficult airway or aspiration risk? □ No □ Yes (preparation confirmed)	Relevant images properly labeled and displayed □ Yes □ N/A Any equipment concerns? **Anticipated Critical Events**	**To all team members:** What are the key concerns for recovery and management of this patient?
Diagnostic and radiologic test results □ Yes □ N/A Blood products □ Yes □ N/A Any special equipment, devices, implants □ Yes □ N/A	Risk of blood loss (> 500 ml) □ Yes □ N/A # of units available _____ Anesthesia safety check completed □ Yes	**Surgeon:** States the following: □ critical or nonroutine steps □ case duration □ anticipated blood loss **Anesthesia Provider:** □ Antibiotic prophylaxis within one hour before incision □ Yes □ N/A □ Additional concerns?	
Include in Preprocedure check-in as per institutional custom: Beta blocker medication given (SCIP) □ Yes □ N/A Venous thromboembolism prophylaxis ordered (SCIP) □Yes □ N/A Normothermia measures (SCIP) □ Yes □ N/A	**Briefing:** All members of the team have discussed care plan and addressed concerns □ Yes	**Scrub and circulating nurse:** □ Sterilization indicators have been confirmed □ Additional concerns?	April 2010

The JC does not stipulate which team member initiates any section of the checklist except for site marking.
The Joint Commission also does not stipulate where these activities occur. See the Universal Protocol for details on the Joint Commission requirements.

AORN

Figure 7.2 Association of Peri-Operating Registered Nurses Surgical Checklist.

Perioperative Checklist - Rochester General Hospital

L&D OR

Date: _____

Patient Name: _____ DOB: _____

Pre-Op Diagnosis: _____

Post-Op Diagnosis: _____
(If Different)

Procedure: _____

Confirmed Not Confirmed

Notes/Concerns:

1. Patient Identification with 2 identifiers

2. Allergies

3. Consent signed

4. H&P updated today

5. Antibiotics given

6. DVT Compression Sleeves On

7. Surgical Time Out

8. Specimens _____

9. Placenta Sent

10. Pathology Sheet Signed

Only use WorldWide Medical markers. Order at 866-997-0576 or www.checklistboards.com

Figure 7.3 Rochester General Hospital Perioperative Checklist Board.

Produced by: Checklist Boards Corporation 11 Schoen Place, Pittsford NY 14534.

the elements currently recommended and required for review and verification prior to surgery, it may be difficult to implement initially and too time-consuming.

In developing the checklist, it is important to consider the form that it will take. It must be remembered that the checklist is designed to stimulate communication between all members of the team. As such it needs to be interactive and verbal. There are various formats to the checklist that can achieve this interaction. Figure 7.3 shows an example of a perioperative checklist in use at Rochester General Hospital that requires the input of information that is specific to the intended surgery and patient, as well as the use of a standardized list of items that require verification in every surgery. Although the checklist is carried out as an interactive process, the additional use of a color-coded response verification assists in visual confirmation of the completion of the checklist. This laminated checklist is displayed prominently in every operating room and is visible to every participant in the surgical procedure. Although the checklist appears in black and white for this chapter, we encourage the use of red/green color coding. The presence of any non-verified response as evidenced on the list as coded in black, prevents the procedure from being initiated.

Implementation of the Checklist

We would like to present an example of the implementation of a checklist at one of the authors' hospitals. As a result of a "near miss" during a surgical procedure it was determined that the time-out process had become less effective. Although it was routinely carried out before the surgery, many of the participants involved had become inattentive. This was often the result of an individual focusing on their specific tasks rather than being an active participant in the process. Because the process did not require an interactive response from every participant in the surgical procedure, the benefit of a team-based approach to the surgical procedure was lost. The perioperative time-out became the focus of a checklist process. The champions of this perioperative checklist process were the chiefs of their respective surgical departments. Every member of the operating team including the surgeons, nurses, resident physicians, and surgical techs was required to participate in an interactive training process that reviewed the need for participating in a perioperative time-out process and how it would be carried out. Individuals were not allowed to participate in a

surgical procedure until they completed the training process. The process involved the use of a specific basic checklist. The surgeon is required to take the lead in initiating the process before the surgery can start as well as carrying out the second portion of the time-out at conclusion of the surgery before the procedure can be completed and the patient moved out of the operating suite. Every surgeon was given a small laminated pocket card (Figure 7.4) which served as a checklist template for the interactive process to be initiated by the attending surgeon and then participated in by the entire team at the beginning and end of a surgical procedure. It was kept very simple to start, and additional items may be added that are department-specific, but the basic requirements are preserved. A necessary component of the new process is that all work stops when the time-out is performed. There must be verbal interaction and agreement between all members of the surgical team. Any member of the team can prevent the procedure from beginning if there are discrepancies in the process.

The purpose of this approach was to create a verbal participatory team interaction around the time-out process that had been previously employed but had become simply another step in the operative procedure. In many instances the time-out process had simply become another step in a larger perioperative process and often became reduced to "was the time-out observed, yes or no." Employing this simple checklist requires all participants to stop what they are doing and verbally follow and respond to a simple checklist. An ongoing evaluation of this new process is being performed. Some of the criteria that are being monitored by the respective chiefs of the surgical departments are how many times a procedure is stopped because some element of the checklist is not verified correctly. Additionally, the time-out at the end of the procedure is being monitored for concordance

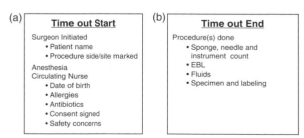

Figure 7.4 Rochester General Hospital Surgeon's Time-out template.

of documentation between the nursing, anesthesia, and operative notes as to the actual procedure performed, level of blood loss, and proper documentation of surgical specimens.

The example presented underscores the process in producing a checklist. Although every checklist will be different based on the procedure or treatment being described, the principles remain the same. It must be noted that medical care remains a complex process with many variables and potential outcomes. Despite evidence that standardizing a process to reduce variation and thereby reduce errors that could impact patient safety, there needs to be initial consensus on the evidence that supports a particular process. Lacking such evidence or consensus makes the development of a checklist problematic. The American Congress of Obstetricians and Gynecologists has increased interest for the development of checklists in a variety of clinical settings through its publications. These publications can serve as the building blocks for checklists that can be developed and find acceptance at the local hospital.

Conclusion

Obstetrical and surgical care in the twenty-first century has become far too complex with more information than one individual can possibly manage. Without the use of validated tools such as team training, standardized communication techniques, simulation training, and the widespread use of checklists and protocols, we will not be able to reduce the frequent preventable errors that occur in our increasingly complicated hospitals. "Checklists are an integral part of a safer medical system advocated by the Institute of Medicine in which reliance on memory and vigilance are to be avoided" [1]. We look forward to the time when checklists become ingrained into the culture of medicine just as they have been adopted in other high-reliability industries.

Appendix 1: Stanford Hospital Surgical Checklist (based on [15]).

SURGICAL SAFETY CHECKLIST

STANFORD
HOSPITAL & CLINICS
Stanford University Medical Center

SURGEON WHO MAKES THE INCISION CONDUCTS THE TIME OUT

Before Induction of Anesthesia → **Before Skin Incision/Procedure** → **Before Patient Leaves Room**

O.R. BOARDING CHECKLIST

IN PRE-OP AREA

CIRCULATOR VERIFIES:

- Equipment/Instrument status
- Patient ID
- Site Marking by Surgeon
- Consent complete and accurate
- Current H&P (within 30 days/update 24hrs prior to scheduled procedure)
- Confirmation of Allergies
- Allergy band on
- Latex allergy
- Attending Surgeon/Proceduralist Contacted

IN OPERATING ROOM

If patient bypassed pre-op verification Boarding Checklist to be completed in OR

ANESTHESIOLOGIST AND CIRCULATOR VERIFY:

- Correct patient, procedure, and site
- Anesthesia Safety Check completed
- ASA Class recorded
- Oximeter on and functioning
- Airway status assessed
- Blood available (if applicable)
- ABO blood group verified (if applicable)
- UNOS ID # (if applicable)

TIME OUT

SURGEON / PROCEDURALIST TO LEAD THIS PROCESS

ALL TEAM MEMBERS PARTICIPATE

STOP!

TIME OUT PAUSE

- ■ TEAM MEMBER INTRODUCTION
  (First case and any subsequent personnel changes)
- Correct patient, procedure, and position
- Correct operative site/side
- Consent is complete, accurate, and signed
- Surgical site marked by surgeon, mark visible after prep/after drape
- Confirmation of Allergies
- Images/implants available (if needed)
- Prophylactic antibiotics given /time/ re-dose time
- DVT Prophylaxis
- Procedure duration
- Anticipated blood loss
- Are we all in agreement/any special patient concerns?

POST EVALUATION / TEAM DEBRIEFING

(COMPLETED IN OR/PROCEDURE ROOM)

ALL TEAM MEMBERS PARTICIPATE

- Name of procedure recorded
- Wound class recorded
- Counts are correct (or NA)
- ID and Allergy Bands in place
- Read back specimen labeling & Path form completed per protocol
- Equipment/Instrument problems to address
- Key concerns for recovery and management of patient
- Recovery destination notified

Based on the WHO Surgical Safety Checklist

04/13/09; 11/15/10; 2/21/11; 3/4/11; 3/14/11 rev 18

References

1   The Institute of Medicine. *To Err is Human: Building a Safer Health System*. Washington, DC: National Academy of Sciences, National Academic Press; 1999.

2   Pronovost P, Needham D, Berenholtz S, et al. An intervention to decrease catheter-related bloodstream infections in the ICU. *New Engl J Med*. 2006;355: 2725–2732.

3   Clark SL, Belfort MA, Meyers JA, et al. Improved outcomes, fewer cesarean deliveries and reduced litigation. results of a new paradigm in patient safety. *Am J Obstet Gynecol*. 2008;199:105.e1–7.

4   Clark SL, Belfort MA, Saade GA, et al. Implementation of a conservative checklist based protocol for oxytocin administration: maternal and fetal outcomes. *Am J Obstet Gynecol*. 2007;197:480.e1–5.

5   Hayees AB, Weiser TG, Berry WR, et al. A surgical safety checklist to reduce morbidity and mortality in a global population. *N Engl J Med*. 2009;360:491–499.

6   WHO. *WHO Guidelines for Safe Surgery: 2009: Safe Surgery Saves Lives*. Geneva: WHO.

7   DeVries EN, Prins HA, Crolla RMPH, et al. Effect of a comprehensive surgical safety system on patient outcomes. *N Engl J Med*. 2010;363:1928–1937.

8   Peleg M, Boxwala AA, Ogunyemi O, et al. GLIF3: the evolution of a guideline representation format. *Proceedings of the AMIA Symposium*; 2000:645–649.

9   Fisher TL. The counting of sponges. *Can Med Ass J*. 1951; 64:165–166.

10 Fausett MB, Propst A, Van Doren K, Clark BT. How to develop an effective obstetric checklist. *Am J Obstet Gynecol*. 2011;205:165–170.

11 Winters BD, Gurses AP, Lehmann H, Sexton JB, Rampersad CJ, Pronovost PJ. Clinical Review: Checklists – translating evidence into practice. *Crit Care*. 2009; 13(210): 1–9.

12 Leonard M, Graham S, Bonacum D. The human factor: the critical importance of effective teamwork and communication in providing safe care. *Qual Safety Health Care*. 2004; 13(Suppl 1): 85–90.

13 Agency for Healthcare Research and Quality (AHRQ). Team Strategies and Tools to Enhance Performance and Patient Safety. http://teamstepps.AHRQ.gov/ (accessed March 25, 2012).

14 Gawande A. *The Checklist Manifesto. How to Get Things Done Right*. New York, NY: Metropolitan Books; 2009.

15 WHO. *Implementation Manual: WHO Surgical Safety Checklist 2009*. Geneva: WHO.

Chapter

8

What is a High-reliability Organization?

Joseph C. Gambone and John P. Keats

You are the chair of the Department of Obstetrics and Gynecology at a highly regarded local hospital, Community General, where you and your 30 colleagues perform almost 400 deliveries a month in addition to a large number of gynecologic surgeries. An important part of your role as department chair is to sit on the medical executive committee (MEC) of the medical staff. You have been called to a special meeting of the MEC one evening. Upon arrival, you are greeted by the chief of the medical staff. As you enter the room you are surprised to find not only the hospital CEO and CMO present, but the entire Quality Committee as well as the chair of the hospital board. Clearly there is something important to be discussed!

As everyone is seated, the chief of the medical staff announces that he will show a 10-minute video clip to set the stage for the upcoming discussion. The video clip is a portion of a speech given in 1999 by a well-known national expert on patient safety and quality improvement, describing his wife's experience during 60 days of hospitalization in several highly regarded institutions in the north-east for a serious neurological illness. He then reviews a litany of significant problems they experienced. These problems included numerous medication errors, incorrectly performed diagnostic procedures, disorganized laboratory results, a loss of continuity of care with every provider handoff, and an inability to get consistent information relating to his wife's care and prognosis. This ordeal was all set against a backdrop of a lack of respect for their time and privacy. He concludes with these sobering remarks – "We are doing harm and we need to stop it. We could be a lot better than we are." (The video is available for viewing on YouTube at www.youtube.com/watch?v=00aa6xc0xf4. It is highly recommended that the reader view the entire 10-minute video.)

As the video clip concludes and the lights are raised, the chief of staff announces that an influential patient safety organization has just released the results of a large national survey of safety structure, processes, and outcomes for hospitals around the country. Your facility has earned an undistinguished and disappointing "D" grade, while several nearby competitor hospitals have all earned "A"s or "B"s. The results will be published in the local newspaper in the morning, and reporters are already calling the hospital asking for comments about this poor performance and what plans the hospital is making to improve the safety of care. This MEC meeting was called to formulate a plan and a response to the survey. As the chief of staff reviews the various components of the analysis, you are thinking that surely your department has not contributed to this low safety score — everyone in your department does such a conscientious job. However, as the chief of staff lists category after category of performance measures, your impression begins to change. Teamwork training? Sure, you recall that this was offered a year or so ago, but all the doctors in your department thought that was something only nurses should attend. Medication reconciliation? That form was such a bother! Hand hygiene? Of course everyone scrubbed for surgery, but did it really matter on routine rounds when you were in such a hurry to get to the office? Retained foreign objects? Well, there was that retained surgical sponge in the cesarean delivery patient, but that was an emergency after all and represented an isolated event. Thromboembolism prophylaxis? We did have two cases of postoperative deep vein thrombosis after major surgeries last month, but at least they didn't have pulmonary emboli. As you think more about these past events you soon realize, to your surprise, that your department had contributed significantly to the hospital's poor safety record. How did such a "highly regarded" department come to this sad state, and what could be done about it?

Once the chief of staff has reviewed the entire report, he introduces a consultant who addresses the sobered and silent audience. She describes the urgent need to turn the hospital as a whole, and the Ob/Gyn department in particular (ouch, you are thinking) into an integrated high-reliability organization (HRO). By this she explains that she means establishing work environments that are able to accomplish complex and potentially dangerous tasks successfully and without error repetitively over extended periods of time. You listen with increasingly rapt attention as she lays out the components that will be required for you and your colleagues to make the journey from your current unsafe environment to one of high reliability. She explains what organizations of high reliability are and emphasizes that they are appropriate for modern healthcare. She gives reasons why healthcare has lagged behind as an industry in the area of error prevention and how strong, innovative leadership will be needed to catch up. She then lays out a plan for consideration by the leadership of Community General Hospital. Her plan includes Seven Steps to High Reliability, where Step One is:

> Step One: Acknowledge the need and the intent to become highly reliable.

What is a High-reliability Organization?

A high-reliability organization (HRO) is an organization that operates in a complex environment or system, manages high-risk activities, and successfully avoids catastrophes despite complexity and significant risk factors. The classic examples of HROs are nuclear power plants and aircraft carriers. Any errors, no matter how small, can have catastrophic outcomes in and on these facilities – a core meltdown or the loss of an aircraft and pilot. The complexity of the machines and technology used to operate a nuclear power plant or an aircraft carrier require teams of individuals who have been specially and carefully trained to run them. These teams must exist within a culture that accepts the need to recognize and react to the early signs (weak danger signals) of error and prevent the error before it happens.

Modern healthcare is clearly a high-risk, high-impact activity and health care institutions that are now transforming themselves into HROs are planning to deliver the best health outcomes, even while dealing with unexpected events. Many of these organizations train everyone involved in patient care to be aware of the five components of *mindfulness*,

where failure is recognized as always possible, expertise is recognized regardless of rank, the unexpected is met with resilience, smaller tasks are performed in the context of the bigger picture, and hierarchy can be flattened depending on the situation [1]. (See components in the context of health care in Table 8.1.) Caregivers in some of these institutions are able to avoid error effectively, partly because they have become expert at the process of *thin slicing* – making instant decisions, *in the blink of an eye*, despite an overload of variables [2]. Healthcare organizations that are moving toward transformation into an HRO are particularly able to do so because of strong and focused leadership committed to the education and training necessary to transform.

It has been clear for some time that there is too much preventable error in healthcare [3] and that we are not moving fast enough to correct this situation [4]. So why is it taking so long to adopt the techniques of *complexity science* [5] and high reliability and incorporate them into the healthcare setting? Part of the problem is due to the belief by many that healthcare is distinct from other industries. It would thus be improper to treat it like other activities that use statistical tools and teamwork to improve. Frequently, a lack of enlightened and effective leadership is the underlying problem.

Are HROs Appropriate for Healthcare?

Healthcare organizations are indeed somewhat different from the typical HRO. Rather than dealing with carefully designed, highly predictable mechanical processes, they must address the unique challenges of individual patients and their inherent unpredictability. Yet many processes within healthcare are coming to more closely resemble those of other industries through application of the tools of complexity science and high reliability. The art of medicine that has been traditionally characterized qualitatively for so many years has evolved to include highly complex and risky activities. The *art* parts, including effective communication and compassion, are still essential for quality care, but the complexity parts must be subjected to scientific techniques and tools that can improve performance and reduce error.

There are over 10,000 diagnoses listed by the World Health Organization as ICD-9 and now ICD-10 diagnostic codes. There are over 4,000 procedures

Table 8.1 Components of mindfullness () and strategies and tools for healthcare based upon them.

1. Constant concern about the possibility of failure – even when it is highly unlikely.

   Healthcare team members are trained to notice and record near-misses and even not-so-near ones (weak signs of failure) when performing procedures that have become routine. Facilitated by:

   Periodic "cause and effect" analysis of near-misses to improve the process.

2. Deference to expertise and experience – regardless of rank or status.

   Everyone on the healthcare team respects and values the opinions of other members without "grading" them based purely on position or title. Facilitated by:

   Team resource management and leadership that fosters a safe environment (fair and just culture) for open communication.

3. Commitment to resilience – adapting to the unexpected.

   Healthcare team reacts appropriately to an unexpected event during a procedure. Facilitated by:

   Drills and simulations designed to test "what if?"

4. Sensitivity to operations – performing a specific task while mindful of big picture.

   Each member of the healthcare team is capable of performing their specific part of a procedure while also being focused on the overall goals and desired outcomes. Facilitated by:

   Leadership that fosters team accountability for health outcomes.

5. Ability to alter and flatten hierarchy as best fits the situation.

   Healthcare team members able to make instant decisions "in the blink of an eye" that alter the usual routine to prevent error. Facilitated by:

   Leadership that fosters team training, open communication and innovative thinking.

with current procedural terminology (CPT) codes, many of which are complex and risky. And there are 6,000 drugs that can be prescribed, many dangerous and unforgiving of error [6–8]. Two of the 10 "High Alert" medications published by the Institute for Safe Medication Practice are magnesium sulfate and oxytocin, both used in obstetrical care (www.ismp.org/, accessed March 9, 2013).

Just as the aviation industry had to recognize that flying modern aircraft was too complicated for one or even a few individuals to manage, healthcare providers should recognize the need for a team approach to healthcare delivery. Strong leadership is critical to inform and guide the way to high reliability in the current complex and "error-prone" healthcare system.

The Need for Transformational Change in Healthcare

Unlike nuclear power plants and aircraft carriers, early medical practice started out with far less complexity and much less machinery and testing. For centuries, individual providers, physicians and nurses, applied relatively simple and uncomplicated procedures to *sometimes* cure disease but *mostly* to relieve suffering and provide comfort to individual patients. Error was common and often accepted due to the uncertainty of diagnoses and the application of unreliable treatments. As the noted British physician Cyril Chantler has stated, "Medicine [the practice of] used to be simple, ineffective and relatively safe. Now it is complex, effective and potentially dangerous" [9].

Furthermore, the traditions of the practice of medicine were deeply rooted in the predominance of *individual* analysis and decision-making. This long-standing "solo" or individualistic culture is very resistant to change or questioning. The "captain of the ship" mentality remains pervasive in healthcare, yet it is incompatible with HROs.

As organizations or facilities, nuclear power plants and aircraft carriers were never in a situation where mistakes were acceptable even though they occurred on occasion. Because error could not be tolerated, however, a culture of strict prevention and high reliability was always necessary from the very beginning. When organizations that must be highly reliable drift from a strong culture of error prevention, catastrophic events can occur. This was seen recently in Japan during an earthquake and the tidal wave that followed.

In the latter part of the twentieth century, the nature of healthcare processes began to change. Surgical procedures requiring teams of highly trained individuals with complex machinery, including robotic technology, is now commonplace. Modern testing procedures, using radioactive isotopes and magnetic imaging machines, are performed, often on a daily basis. These changes often seem to have occurred overnight. The fact is that they have been evolving over many years, yet the necessary "cultural changes" for safe and reliable execution have lagged behind the dramatic evolution in technology and processes. A cautionary lesson is seen through the experience of Eastman Kodak. Kodak *invented* digital photography but failed as a business because they could not *adapt and change* from a culture that was committed to film. They failed to make the necessary transformational change.

Unlike industries that have been designed from their inception with processes and culture of high reliability, healthcare organizations must now transform. Powerful people at Kodak were able to block necessary change. They were in a position to reject, often for selfish reasons, the innovation that was needed to survive. Today's healthcare leaders are encountering similar obstructive behavior as they try to lead this process of transformation. Organizations like Kodak and modern healthcare institutions can do all of the strategic planning to recognize that change is needed, and even why, where, and how to change, but without strong leadership that recognizes and acts to transform an inappropriate culture into one that adapts, little will change. Informed leaders in all industries know all too well that "culture eats strategy for lunch every day."

> Step Two: Establish leadership that makes patient safety the top priority.

Why Has Healthcare Lagged So Far Behind?

There are a number of reasons why healthcare has been slow to recognize the problem of medical error and adopt proven methods to reduce it. The recognition and acceptance of the problem of medical error in medical practice took many decades. In the early part of the last century (1914) Ernest Codman identified, measured, and researched medical error and tried to make improvements in patient safety at a prominent hospital in Boston [10]. He lost hospital privileges and was expelled from the medical society and from the Harvard faculty for his efforts. It was not until the early part of this century (2000) when the Institute of Medicine (IOM) published their seminal article on patient safety, *To Err is Human* [3] that a concerted and sustained effort has begun to identify and reduce error.

The prevailing culture at many healthcare facilities promotes the idea that healthcare is *so* different from other industries that proven techniques in industrial error reduction, such as checklists and crew resource management, are somehow inappropriate and ineffective for healthcare. However, recent experience with these *reliability-increasing* tools in healthcare settings has shown that they are not just effective, but also acceptable [11,12].

Despite assertions to the contrary, the medical–legal climate in the US likely sustains some barriers to identifying and reducing errors in healthcare. Keeping information about errors quiet and working within a culture that will not effectively investigate actual errors or near-misses in care processes is an important barrier. And not disclosing an error when it happens frequently leads to an inability to properly investigate the causes of mistakes so that they may be prevented in the future. In the past, many risk managers and legal advisors have counseled "silence" above all else when mistakes happened and this behavior is not conducive to the prevention of error.

The lack of effective leadership may be the most important barrier to the transformational change necessary to make healthcare organizations safe and highly reliable. Without the proper leadership, caregivers in healthcare organizations may not feel safe to report and explore the causes of errors. Strong leadership can make individuals who expose error feel valued for their efforts and opinions on how to improve patient safety.

Leadership for Transformational Change

Leading an organization that has always been highly reliable is challenging enough, but an even greater task is to lead organizations, like those in modern healthcare, including Community General, that have evolved over time. Transforming a culture of low expectation [13] that has been "error-tolerant" and somewhat "error-concealing" into one that has the goal of reducing error to the lowest possible level is a daunting task. What characteristics and styles of leadership are needed, and what must the leader do to transform such an organization?

According to Kotter [14], both leadership and management are necessary for transformational change. Leadership entails establishing direction, aligning people, and then motivating and inspiring them. A good leader must be a teacher, a coach and an attentive and active listener. The style of leadership must be committed to change but open to suggestion and skilled at selecting and working with day-to-day management. Managing an organization involves planning and budgeting, organizing and staffing, and controlling and problem-solving [15]. Without competent management, even the best leaders may fail.

Listed in Table 8.2 are the eight basic errors that can undermine a successful effort for transformational change. Having an understanding of the concepts of

Table 8.2 Kotter's eight basic errors that undermine successful change.

1. Failure to establish a sufficient sense of urgency for change
2. Failure to build a powerful enough guiding coalition for change
3. Failure to establish a clear vision for change
4. Failure to adequately communicate the vision for change
5. Failure to identify and remove obstacles to the new vision for change
6. Failure to plan and create short-term wins
7. Failure to avoid a premature declaration of victory
8. Failure to anchor all changes in the organizational culture

leadership, vision, and culture are the main deterrents to committing these errors [15]. Selection of a strong leader for Community General as it moves to become highly reliable at delivering healthcare will be key to successful change.

Transformational Change at Community General Hospital

The special MEC meeting at Community General hospital provided an eye-opening learning opportunity for you as the chair of Ob/Gyn and for all of the clinical leadership. After the presentation by the special consultant on patient safety, the hospital board directed the CEO of the hospital to supervise the formulation and implementation of a plan to identify and reduce medical error. This will represent the beginning of the transformation of Community General into a highly reliable organization (HRO).

As chair of the department of Ob/Gyn, you were surprised and honored to be put in charge of a task force that will lead this change. You are thinking – we are a significant part of the problem, so we should be a significant part of any improvement effort. The chief of the medical staff knows that you are highly regarded within your department and that you have a national reputation for quality, both in your specialty and in other specialties.

Among your stronger qualities is your ability to listen to the feelings and opinions of everyone involved in an activity. Members of your department recall your comment to them at a staff meeting that "we are all born with two ears and one mouth, and we should use them in that proportion." You know that it is important to value expertise regardless of the level of authority of the individual giving advice. You also

know that even if you are only performing a part of a bigger task that you must be aware of the big picture. And, most importantly, you know that modifying the beliefs about the way things should be done, the *unwritten rules* in any organization, referred to as its *culture*, will be essential to improve. Transforming Community General into an HRO will require that a leader change the attitude that "patients are ill and mistakes will happen" to one that is committed to reducing error to the lowest level possible. With the help of the special consultant that was hired to advise on the transformation to an HRO you lay out the elements of the program for improvement.

> Step Three: Lead the organization into a "fair and just" culture: one that encourages and rewards the identification of system changes to prevent human errors from harming patients.

Building a Culture of Safety

For centuries, medical practice was regarded as following the dictum of *primum non nocere*, or *first, do no harm*. Changing this fundamental rule from a verbally celebrated "slogan" to a working commitment is paramount. Building a culture of safety, by first keeping the patient safe, must be the initial element of the program of improvement at Community General. As the head of the special task force, you know that your leadership and the leadership of many others in the organization will be crucial to establishing this culture of patient safety. First, you will have to promote, by example and some cajoling, a "fair and just culture" [16] for guiding the way things are done at Community General. A fair and just culture is one that models and fosters behavior that promotes learning and improvement by openly identifying and examining the weaknesses of the organization [17]. Open exposure and discussion about areas of weakness at Community General will need to become just as important as pointing out areas of excellence. All caregivers must feel that they are safe and secure when voicing concerns about medical error [16]. A newer added dictum for medical practice should be *primum non tacere* or *first, be not silent* [18].

This element of the plan for improvement at Community General helps to define the essence of reliability, consistent effectiveness with the smallest amount of error possible. During the process of promoting transformation to an HRO, it will be important for everyone at Community General to realize that it is "*high* reliability" and not "*complete, total or absolute* reliability." Mistakes may still happen but at exceedingly lower rates. Perfection, no matter how laudable, will not be attainable. In fact, *trying* to be perfect is fine, but *expecting* to be perfect can make it more difficult to be extremely good or the best. The six-sigma initiatives (referring to six standard deviations on the normal curve of one million events) in other industries [19] strive for zero errors but expect no more than 3.4 defects (errors) out of one million events – extremely good, but not perfect. Currently, medical error (as high as 34% of patient encounters in one international study) is at about the level of baggage handling! (see Chapter 4 for more on Building a Culture for Safety).

> Step Four: Establish team-based care processes that make all team members accountable for outcomes.

Moving from Solo Decision-making to Teamwork

When the complexity of any activity exceeds the ability of one or just a few individuals to carry out the activity in a consistently error-free way (reliability), teamwork and the use of tools like checklists have been shown to result in better outcomes [11,20]. Years ago, the aviation industry learned that the complexity of their activity would not allow high reliability unless they changed how they managed flight operations. They learned that they needed to transform from a culture of solo decision-making to one of crew resource management and checklists.

The initial test flight of the celebrated B-17 bomber in 1936 resulted in a fiery crash soon after takeoff, with the loss of several lives. On this initial test flight, the B-17 was guided by a single decision-making test pilot. Checklists, now standard in aviation, had not yet been "invented." The test pilot forgot to do something essential that caused the B-17 to crash. Flying the modern aircraft had become too complicated for one (even very experienced and intelligent) individual to do reliably. Checklists were devised for this remarkable aircraft and operating the B-17 became highly reliable. *Crew* resource management, referred to as *medical team* management in healthcare, promotes a system of shared decision-making that improves safety in aviation and now in healthcare.

> Step Five: Apply both the science and the art of communication to care processes.

Communication

The *art* of communication in healthcare, such as a good bedside manner, is not adequate for creating and maintaining an HRO. The *science* of communication must also be appreciated and applied. Casual and informal communication about patient issues and management must be replaced by more formal and standardized methods. Many medical mistakes are directly connected to poor communication between and among healthcare providers [21]. Handwriting that cannot be read by others should be replaced by readable printed communication. Paper charts that are lost or cannot be easily transported from one facility to another will need to be converted to electronic health records that can be accessed easily from different sites. Written prescriptions, hand-carried by patients to pharmacies, will be replaced by electronic prescriptions, now mandated by the Centers for Medicare and Medicaid (CMS).

Verbal communication should be improved so that a surgical team can accurately and safely start, perform, and complete a potentially dangerous procedure. Are we about to surgically remove the correct limb? The transfer of patient care from one provider to another or from one team of providers to another team should be formalized so that any misunderstanding about the correct diagnosis and treatment is prevented. And the patient and their family members need to know and be told (in common, understandable language) all aspects of the care that is being given. Quality research actually shows that clinical outcomes are better when patients and their loved ones are better informed about the care process. Healthcare then simultaneously becomes more reliable and more humane (see Chapter 5 for more on Communication).

> Step Six: Use proven tools and techniques that increase reliability.

Adopting Tools for Performance Improvement

Once effective leadership at Community General has begun the process of creating a just and fair culture (one that looks for, admits to, and finds ways to correct errors) based on a priority of patient safety, the implementation of proven performance-improving tools should take place. These powerful tools and techniques are covered in Chapter 6 of this section in more detail and with examples. They include "The Voice of the Customer," where patients and providers are surveyed to determine quality issues. Run charts and control charts are used to differentiate between common (random) cause variation and special cause variation that could represent a need for improvement. SMART (Specific, Motivational, Accountable, Responsible, and Touchable) goals are established to set realistic expectations about *how* and *how soon* Community General can become an HRO. Other statistical tools such as "Cause and Effect," "Pareto," and "Force Field" diagrams should be used to guide improvement efforts. Better communication and respect for the opinion of all caregivers occurs when "Nominal Group Technique" is used to identify improvement opportunities.

And finally, the PDCA, or Plan, Do, Check, Act system (also known as PDSA, where "S" is Study) to guide the improvement process is a very powerful tool (see Figure 8.1). All of these efforts must be continued and sustained by strong effective leadership. Continuous improvement [22] should be the goal of these efforts at Community General and without the use of effective tools for improvement and others that will be available in the future it will be difficult to transform into an HRO.

> Step Seven: Continuously measure performance and feedback results for improvement.

Looking back on the special MEC meeting that the chief of the medical staff called for along with the presentation that happened, you realize that your work as the special task force leader will need to be accepted, effective, and ongoing. Improving and becoming highly reliable will be a journey and not just a goal!

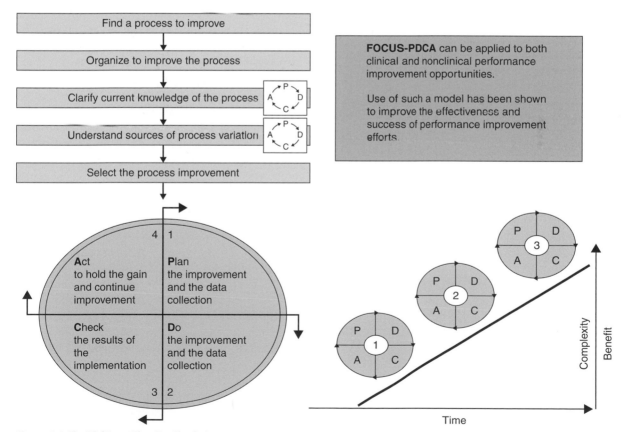

Figure 8.1 The PDCA – or Plan, Do, Check, Act system.

References

1   Weick KE, Sutcliffe KM. *Managing the Unexpected: Assuring High Performance in an Age of Complexity*. San Francisco, CA:Jossey-Bass; 2001.

2   Gladwell M. *Blink*. New York, NY: Little, Brown, and Co; 2005.

3   Kohn LT, Corrigan J, Donaldson MS. *To Err is Human: Building a Safer Health System*. Washington, DC: National Academy Press; 1999.

4   Leape LL, Berwick BM. Five years after *To Err is Human*: what have we learned? *JAMA*. 2005;293(19):2384–2390.

5   Zimmerman B, Lindberg C, Plsek P. *Edgeware: Insights from Complexity Science for Health Care Leaders*. Iriving, TX: VHS; 2001.

6   Gawande A. *Cowboys and Pit Crews*. New York, NY: The New Yorker; 2011. Available at www.newyorker.com/online/blogs/newsdesk/2011/05/atul-gqwand-harvard-medical-school-commencement-address.html (accessed June 15, 2012).

7   Beyea SC. High reliability theory and highly reliable organizations. *AORN J*. 2005;81:1319–1322.

8   Breeden JT. Challenges,change, and relevance. Presidential address. *Obstet Gynecol*. 2012; 120(1): 1–4.

9   Chantler, C. The role and education of doctors in the delivery of health care. *The Lancet*. 1999;353:1178–1181.

10 Gambone JC, Reiter RC. Elements of a successful quality improvement program in obstetrics and gynecology. *Obstet Gynecol Clin N Am*. 2008;35:129–145.

11 Haynes AB, Weiser TG, Berry WR, et al. A surgical safety checklist to reduce morbidity and mortality in a global population. *N Engl J Med*. 2009;360:491–499.

12 Neily J, Mills PD, Yinong Young-Yu, et al. Association between implementation of a medical team training program and surgical mortality. *JAMA*. 2010;304(15):1693–1700.

13 Chassin M, Beecher E. The wrong patient. *Ann Intern Med*. 2002;136:826–833.

14 Kotter JP. Leading change: why transformation efforts fail. *Harvard Bus Rev*. 2007;73(2):660–668.

15 Kotter JP. *A Force for Change: How Leadership Differs from Management*. New York, NY: The Free Press; 1990.

16 Marx D. *Patient Safety and the 'Just Culture': A Primer for Health Care Executives*. New York, NY: Trustees of Columbia University in the City of New York, Columbia University; 2001.

17 Frankel A, Graydon-Baker E, Neppl C, et al. Patient safety leadership walkrounds. *Joint Comm J Qual*. 2003;29(1):16–26.

18 Dwyer J. *Primum non tacere* – an ethics of speaking up. *Hastings Center Report*. 1994;24:13–18.

19 Chassin MR. Is health care ready for sigma six quality. *Milbank Q*. 1998;76(4):565–591.

20 Pronovost P, Needham D, Berenholtz S, et al. An intervention to decrease catheter-related blood stream infections in the ICU. *N Engl J Med*. 2006;355:2725–2732.

21 Muphy JG, Dunn WF. Medical errors and poor communication. *Chest*. 2010;138:1292–1293.

22 Berwick DM. Continuous improvement as an ideal in health care. *N Engl J Med*. 1989;310:53–56.

Powerful Tools for Quality Improvement

John P. Keats

The quest for improvement in the processes of care should be a permanent part of any clinical setting for the delivery of women's healthcare, whether in the hospital, an ambulatory surgery center, or physician office. To effectively embark on a journey to improve the delivery of care requires an initial understanding of the use of several powerful tools that will enable an organization to analyze an existing process as well as determine the best method to correct deficiencies or improve performance. The goal of the use of these tools is illustrated in Figure 9.1. Many healthcare facilities are very adept at generating data – i.e., raw numbers that describe a clinical parameter over a discrete period of time, usually as a percentage per month. Many quality improvement committees in hospital departments look at raw data in table form, month after month, describing clinical processes or outcomes such as cesarean section rate, postoperative wound infection rate, etc. Data such as this are not useful in determining whether there is a problem with your processes of care, and even less useful in determining what to do if there is a problem. The use of quality improvement tools will take these raw data and present them in a way that conveys information [1] – i.e., an awareness of how these data reflect the appropriateness of the processes of care and whether they are functioning as they should to produce the best outcomes for our patients. Furthermore, the use of more sophisticated tools will transform this information into knowledge. This implies a deeper understanding of the processes of care to the point that one can diagnose where and why they are malfunctioning and pose hypotheses as to what might be done to fix the problem. This will lead one lastly to wise actions; the development and testing of a possible solution to the problem, seeing if it is effective, and then further refining the solution to lead to sustained improvement over the long-term.

Data ⟹ Information ⟹ Knowledge ⟹ Wise Actions

Figure 9.1 Steps in process improvement.

Before embarking on an explanation of these tools, it will be helpful to pick a specific scenario as an example. We can then show how each tool could be applied to this case. Let's take as an example a common source of dissatisfaction among obstetrician/gynecologists – the operating room runs chronically late, with start times for surgery getting further and further behind schedule the later in the day a case is planned. Like many processes in a complex place like an operating room, there are certain to be many factors that play into this. As the person responsible for quality improvement in your department, you would like to improve this process. From your personal experience, you suspect that this problem begins at the start of each day because the 7:30 AM case often has a skin incision time of 8:00 AM or later. However, being an experienced quality improvement expert, you know that you should first gather data, apply your QI tools to it, and determine if this is really a place to begin to solve your operating room problem.

Voice of the Customer

First you should establish if this is truly a problem for the Ob/Gyn physicians in your hospital and how pervasive or difficult this problem really is. A tool to do this would be to devise a short survey on operating room times and ask all the physicians who use the operating rooms to complete it. This is called using the "Voice of the Customer" [2]. It will establish whether this is a serious enough issue for you to devote time to it. Equally important, it will establish a baseline against which to judge the future success of any quality improvement efforts you choose to make. Let us assume that your survey reveals that late surgery start times are indeed a source of extreme dissatisfaction amongst your surgeons. Some have even considered not admitting their surgical patients to your hospital. You now know that this is a quality-of-care issue that should be addressed. You continue your efforts at data collection to further analyze the issue.

Run Charts and Control Charts

You ask the operating room manager to begin to track surgery start times for the first scheduled case in each room and aggregate them on a weekly basis as percentage of cases where the skin incision occurs within 15 minutes of the scheduled start time of 7:30 AM. If you are fortunate, there will be records of surgery start times going back several months so that you can recreate some historical data. You can then apply the first of our tools, the run chart, to display these data in a way that conveys information. A run chart is a depiction of the results of a process over time (Figure 9.2). In this case we would plot out the weekly percentage of cases that start on time, which we have defined as the skin incision occurring no later than 7:45 AM, with weekly intervals along the x-axis and percentage "on time" on the y-axis. Once you have sufficient data to plot 10 or more points, you draw a median line such that an equal number of points lie above and below this line. You can then continue to add data points as time goes by. One should typically see data points arrange themselves randomly on either side of this median line. This is what is referred to as "common-cause variation." This is the random variation inherent in any process. You would not expect to see precisely the same rate of on-time OR starts, deliveries in an Ob unit, or the outcomes of any process each and every week or month. There will be variation, but this random or common-cause variation should result in measured values arranging themselves on both sides of a median line over time. When we see this pattern we speak of the process in question as being "in control," and we can predict that over time we will

not see very wide variations away from this established median value. However, should you start to see seven or more points on one side of the median line, or five or more points that steadily increase or decrease, that would indicate "special-cause variation." This is a term that indicates that something has changed about the process itself, which should be investigated. The process is now referred to as being "out of control." Perhaps a certain surgeon or anesthesiologist has gone on an extended vacation! Then you would know that they were a direct contributing cause to your problem of late starts in the OR. But how many people take five to seven weeks off? By just using a run chart, you might miss the crucial knowledge that a single person or event over a short period of time is causing most of your problems. Identifying this type of situation requires the next tool described below.

A more sophisticated tool that you could use instead is a control chart. This is a special type of run chart that includes upper and lower control limits (Figure 9.3). It is similar to a run chart and is initially constructed in the same way, except the initial line drawn through the first 10 data points is the arithmetic mean of those results. The upper and lower control limits are then added to the chart, and are calculated to correspond to three standard deviations above and below that arithmetic mean. On a control chart, even a single data point above or below the control limits indicates special-cause variation. Using this tool, you'll recognize a change in your OR process when that problem surgeon or anesthesiologist is gone even for just a week!

SMART Goals

So, you have followed your OR start times for several months using a control chart, and have determined

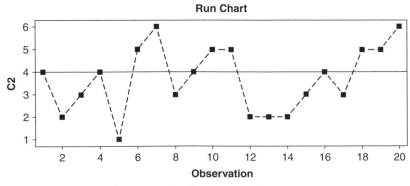

Figure 9.2 A run chart depicting results of a process over time.

that there is no special-cause variation. The percentage of on-time cases varies randomly around your mean line, but you are unhappy to learn that what you suspected is in fact the case. The percentage of on-time cases first thing in the morning is very low, with a mean result of 20%. You want to improve this, and believe that it will be the first of possibly many steps to make the OR more efficient. The next step in any quality improvement process after a problem has been identified is to set a goal. Appropriate goals in quality improvement should conform to the acronym SMART (Figure 9.4). Your goal should be *specific*. To say that your goal is to improve OR start times is too vague. More appropriate would be to say that your goal is to increase the percentage of on-time OR cases to 60%, with on-time defined as skin incision within 15 minutes of scheduled start time. Your goal should be

measureable. We have already established in the previous section how you will continue to plot OR on-time percentages on your control chart. Your goal should be *attainable*. Setting your goal at 100% on-time starts would be unrealistic and counterproductive. Given the unpredictable nature of patient problems that could be discovered in the pre-op area, you would never be able to attain a 100% goal. Setting a goal at an unattainable level simply works to discourage anyone involved in implementation of your plan. They know the goal will never be reached, so why try at all? Make sure your specific goal is ambitious enough to inspire people to work to achieve it without being impossible to fulfill. Your goal should be *relevant*. This means it is something that is worth expending time and energy over, and will clearly improve the safety or well-being of patients or satisfaction of other relevant constituents, in this case gynecologic surgeons. Lastly, the goal should be *time-bound*. Setting open-ended goals invites the attitude that "we will achieve this goal some day, but what's the rush." In these cases "some day" never comes and the goal is never achieved. Decide on a timeframe for your goal that is reasonable. In this case your complete goal might be to increase the percentage of on-time OR starts to 60% within 6 months.

Cause and Effect Diagrams

You have identified a problem and set a SMART goal. Now you need to begin a search for solutions. To do that you have to first identify all the possible causes for the problem, and decide which one(s) are the right ones to address. A useful tool for this is the cause and

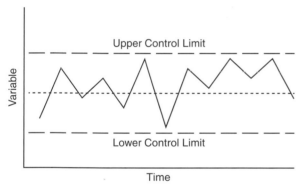

Figure 9.3 A control chart – a special type of run chart that includes upper and lower control limits.

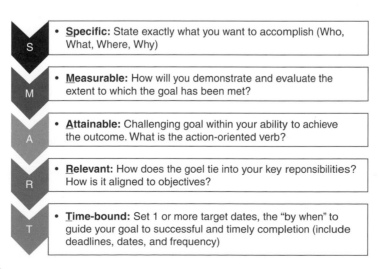

Figure 9.4 SMART goals.

effect diagram, also called an Ishikawa diagram after the Japanese industrial improvement expert who first devised it. This is a powerful way to frame and illustrate a root-cause analysis. Another common name is the fishbone diagram, because its shape is reminiscent of a fish skeleton (Figure 9.5). To construct a fishbone diagram, you place a statement of the problem to be analyzed in a box to the extreme right, which represents the fish's head. You then draw a "spine" extending horizontally to the left and connect it to several angled ribs. The ribs can vary in number, but four to six is common. These ribs are then labeled with major categories of factors that might contribute to the effect seen in the fish's head. The identity of these categories will depend on what type of problem is being considered. In healthcare, common categories would include People, Methods, Equipment, Materials, Machinery, and Environment. Branching off from each major category, depicted as horizontal lines, would be potential causes of the problem or possible subcategories that would be further subdivided. In our example, the People category could include major subdivisions of patient, surgeon, anesthesiologist, pre-op nurse, and circulating nurse. Under each subdivision would be listed causes that pertain to that person, such as patient forgot to fast, or surgeon arrived in OR late. Materials could include things like surgical consent is not on chart, or pre-op labs were not drawn. Machinery might include the CO_2 canister on the anesthesia machine needing to be changed. The important thing is to gather a group of people who actually work in that area who can brainstorm all the possible causes of

delay that contribute to late OR starts first thing in the morning. Capture on the diagram all possible causes without regard to how much you might believe that they contribute to the problem. A completed cause-and-effect diagram will often be very extensive, listing dozens of possible contributing factors. If the diagram becomes too large or unwieldy, it is possible to subdivide the topic by making each major category into its own separate fishbone. For example, create a diagram whose head reads "Patient not ready for transport from pre-op by 7:15" and go from there in delineating possible causes.

Pareto Diagram

Once you have completed your cause-and-effect diagram, you may be somewhat dismayed by the number of possible causes for late OR starts. It will become readily apparent that you cannot correct all the possible causes, so how do you decide where to focus your efforts? The answer lies in our next tool, the Pareto Diagram (Figure 9.6). Vilfredo Pareto was a nineteenth-century Italian economist. His studies of the economy of his native country led him to conclude that at the time 80% of the wealth of Italy was controlled by only 20% of the population. From his work was derived the Pareto Principle, which is more widely known as the 80/20 rule. In general, for any observed effect, 20% of the contributing causes account for 80% of the effect. We can confidently predict that while you cannot correct all the possible causes of late OR starts, if you can correctly identify and correct the 20% that

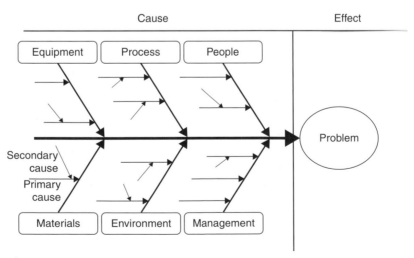

Figure 9.5 A fishbone diagram.

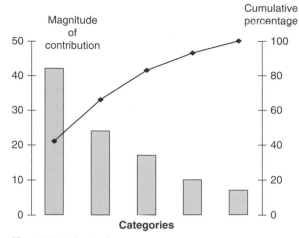

Figure 9.6 A Pareto diagram.

contribute most to the problem you can improve by 80%.

To identify those 20% will require construction of a Pareto diagram. To do this you will need to take all the causes identified on the cause-and-effect diagram and list them, by groups, on a checklist. This checklist can be distributed in the operating room, and completed with the help of the OR personnel or others that you enlist to aid in this project. Every time a first-of-the day OR case starts late, the checklist is completed, indicating which one or more factors contributed to the late start for that particular case. The checklists are collected daily and the results compiled over a period of a week, a month, or longer. The longer the data collection period the more accurate your results are likely to be. For each possible cause you determine a percentage of contribution, with the numerator being the number of times that box was checked and the denominator being the total number of check marks in the entire sample. The Pareto diagram is then constructed with each cause represented as a bar in a bar graph. The height of the bar corresponds to the absolute magnitude of contribution which is the number of times that box was checked during your observation period. The bars are listed in size order, with the tallest (highest contribution) to the left of the graph. Another set of dots is placed, on or over each bar, that represents the cumulative percentage contribution of the bars as you read from left to right and these are connected with a curved line. Typically, the slope of the cumulative percentage line will be fairly steep to the left of the diagram and then flatten out to the

right as there are smaller and smaller contributions by those factors.

Often, it is possible to visually identify an "inflection point" where the slope rapidly switches from steep to flat. True to the Pareto Principle, this is often at around 80% of the effect and will encompass only about 20% of your listed causes. You will then know to focus your efforts on correcting those 20% – what the process improvement expert Joseph Juran called the "Vital Few" as opposed to the "Trivial Many." If you started out with many possible causes, you may still find that even 20% of your causes are too many to address. You may choose to focus on the 10% that cause 70% of the effect, or the 5% that cause 50%, etc. Whatever you decide is the appropriate cut-off, the Pareto Diagram will show you which of the many possible causes should be addressed to most efficiently solve your problem.

Nominal Group Technique

Now you have identified the single or small group of causes that are most responsible for delays in the start time of the first cases in your operating room. You next need to come up with a way to eliminate that cause to the extent possible. You may be confident that you know how to fix it, given that you are a quality improvement expert. It is best to resist the urge to craft a solution yourself and impose it on the people working in the operating room for a number of reasons. First is the so-called "NIH" effect, which stands for "Not Invented Here." When people working in a complex environment are confronted with the need to change behaviors or ways of getting work done, they are much more likely to be cooperative if they feel that they, or at least their representatives, have had a hand in crafting the new work flow. If they feel that the change was "not invented here," the result is often a passive–aggressive approach to the implementation process that delays the entire effort or sometimes sabotages it completely. A second reason for not imposing solutions unilaterally is that often there are simpler or better solutions known to people working in the "front line" that may not be apparent to you.

A tool to avoid the NIH effect and increase the chance of crafting an optimal solution is the Nominal Group Technique. To do this, for each cause that you want to address you will need to assemble one or more representatives of each possible stakeholder group involved in this process. In this case there may be quite a number of groups that need to be represented – surgeons, anesthesiologists, pre-op nurses, circulating nurses, scrub techs, admitting clerks, nursing leadership, hospital administration, medical staff leadership, etc. The group is gathered in an appropriate-sized room with a commitment to eliminate possible sources of distraction such as cell phones or call responsibilities. Note paper and writing implements are provided. Possible causes to be addressed are taken one by one. For each cause, the process is the same and consists of several steps. First, after the cause is stated, each participant takes several minutes to individually and silently record all possible solutions to the problem they can think of. Participants are encouraged to list literally every solution they can think of, no matter how implausible or unlikely. Once everyone has finished writing down their ideas, a "round robin" is conducted where each participant in turn is asked to read off one solution from their list. All solutions are recorded on a flip chart, with no discussion of any kind at this time. You keep going around the room for as many rounds as it takes to have everyone read off every item on their list of solutions. Duplications should be recorded only once, even if several people thought of the same solution. Once all solutions are listed, participants can now ask clarifying questions about any solution of the person who made the suggestion. After all clarifying questions have been asked, similar solutions can be combined into a single one and the list rewritten on a flip chart for all to see. Each participant is then given an opportunity to express what they see as the pros and cons of each proposed solution. Once this has been done, the final step is for the group to vote to establish the group's preferred solution. Each participant picks the five solutions that they believe are most important and silently votes on the solutions in rank order, giving their preferred solution a "5," second favorite a "4," etc. The coordinator then reads out each solution and every participant indicates the number score they gave to that one. Once all votes have been tallied, the solution with the highest point total is recognized as the group's choice.

The Nominal Group Technique has several advantages. As previously stated, it involves all stakeholders from the beginning of the procedure to determine the optimal or most highly favored consensus solution to the identified cause. It gives everyone at the table an opportunity to express their ideas as to what a best solution would be. Often in healthcare, perceived hierarchies prevent some people from speaking in open meetings, with doctors or administrators dominating the conversation at the expense of nurses or clerks. Yet it is sometimes these latter individuals who have the clearest concepts of how to fix a problem that they deal with on a regular basis. The silent recording of ideas guarantees that all possible solutions are brought out and considered. Sometimes even wild or implausible ideas, after clarification and discussion, lead to new insights on possible solutions that no one had previously considered. Use of this technique will lead you to devise a solution or set of solutions that will be most likely to solve your problem and can be implemented with buy-in from all stakeholder groups.

Force Field Diagram

Now you have crafted a solution to each of the top causes you have chosen to address. These solutions must now be implemented, and our next tool will make successful implementation more likely. Whenever you are trying to change behaviors in an organization, you will meet resistance at some point. That is because change of any kind is nearly always perceived as a loss by someone – whether it is physicians who will now be asked to show up to the OR earlier in the morning, or pre-op nurses who will be tasked with checking lab results at the end of their day for the next day's patients. Whatever the solution you've decided on, it is best to anticipate where this resistance will come from and give some thought as to how to counter it even before you are confronted by it. A force field diagram is a way to organize your strategy around this issue (Figure 9.7). For each solution, a force field diagram requires you to list possible driving forces and restraining forces for that particular solution in the categories of patient influences, personal influences, educational influences, economic influences, and administrative influences. Additional categories can be added if desired. For each category, you and your colleagues or advisors should consider what forces exist in your organization that will either help to drive the change you're seeking or hinder it. You can then develop strategies to enhance the driving forces and diminish the restraining forces. Putting these strategies in place to the extent possible before starting the actual implementation of your change solution will make it much more likely that the solution will be implemented successfully.

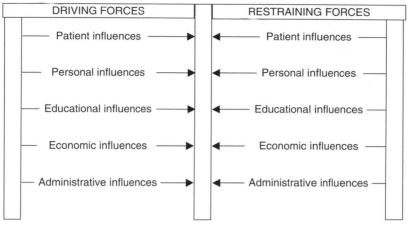

DRIVING FORCES	RESTRAINING FORCES
Patient influences ⟶	⟵ Patient influences
Personal influences ⟶	⟵ Personal influences
Educational influences ⟶	⟵ Educational influences
Economic influences ⟶	⟵ Economic influences
Administrative influences ⟶	⟵ Administrative influences

Figure 9.7 A force field diagram.

A corollary to this is to consider a pilot program to implement your solution rather than rolling it out across the organization as a whole at the start. Perhaps yours is a large institution with several OR areas. Start your change process in only one area, or perhaps with just one service. It is especially helpful, and often critical, to identify one or more "champions" – people who are particularly invested in seeing your program be successful. Having a physician as one of the champions would be particularly valuable. By being the first to embrace a change, they can inspire by example those that might otherwise be reluctant. These individuals are frequently those that can be identified as "innovators" under the paradigm described by Everett Rogers in his classic book *Diffusion of Innovations* [3]. These are the 2%–3% of individuals in a population who embrace change and adapt readily to new situations and environments. Enlisting these individuals as allies in your change process has the added benefit that they will help you co-create. As a new process is instituted, innovators will tend to examine it with a critical eye and give you feedback on how the process can be further refined and improved. Incorporating these recommended changes early in the process improvement program will make it easier for the other people involved to follow suit as the program is gradually incorporated by individuals in the other populations defined by Rogers as the early adopters, early majority, late majority, and finally the laggards.

PDSA Cycles

Once the process improvement program is underway, you can anticipate that there will be multiple changes identified (by innovators and others as described above) that will need to be incorporated to allow you to reach your stated goal. The tool that describes the iterative process that will best accomplish this is referred to as PDSA cycles [4]. The acronym stands for Plan–Do–Study–Act (sometimes PDCA, or Plan–Do–Check–Act), and is a well-recognized part of any attempt to change the way a task is accomplished in a complex work environment. These words represent the phases of installing a new or re-tooled work process.

The first phase is *Plan*. This is when an opportunity for improvement is recognized and a plan formulated for its correction. This also includes all of the necessary "who, what, where, when" of the project, as well as designing an appropriate measurement strategy. This phase encompasses many or all of the tools discussed in this chapter. Once your problem is identified and you have devised a solution, with buy-in from all participants, it is time to implement or test your solution. This is the *Do* phase. As stated above, it is best to accomplish this initially with the innovators and champions amongst your stakeholders and to pilot it on a small scale if feasible. Next is the *Study* phase. This is where you review the results of your small pilot or the results obtained with a limited number of participants. Huddle with your innovators and process stakeholders to review what worked, what didn't work, and what should be done differently. Unfortunately, this is where many well-intended improvement projects fall short – they simply didn't put enough effort into devising a meaningful strategy for measurement. However, change ideas that are driven and informed by data are typically the most potent and most sustainable.

Then you enter the *Act* phase, where you incorporate the suggested improvements into your change efforts. Others suggest the "A" includes act, adapt, or abandon. You then enter the cycle again, planning the next round of implementation of your improved process, and expanding the scope of sites and individuals involved. Look at what you've learned, what your data are telling you. Do you need to adapt or change the approach? Did you uncover negative effects or no change? Should you abandon and begin with an entirely new plan? Use the cycle to inform and drive your process. Repeated turns of this PDSA "wheel" will eventually yield the best method for improving the process you are targeting, the engagement of the broadest number of people involved in the process itself, and the best possible outcomes for your efforts.

Sustaining Quality Improvement

Just because you have made changes in a care process does not guarantee that improved outcomes will be the result. A perennial question in the field of quality improvement is how do we know that a change is an improvement [5]? The answer lies in continuous monitoring of a process after changes are made. Using one of the tools already discussed, the run or control chart, you will need to follow the process along after you have made changes. In this case you would continue to monitor OR start times and the percentage of on-time surgeries on a regular basis. If your implemented changes have indeed improved the process, you should have clear evidence of this in your charting. You should see a steady progression of data points above the previously established mean or median, with the likelihood that the line connecting the data points will show a steady rise and establishment of a new plateau well above the previous rate. Once you see this pattern and have several data points to confirm this, you should then establish a new mean around the newer data points.

Once this new mean is established you will have two remaining challenges. The first is to decide if you are satisfied with the results as depicted in the new mean percentage of on-time OR starts. Has your SMART goal been met? If not, you will need to consider a new round of process improvement by asking some questions. Has the new process been fully implemented and is everyone following the process correctly? Is there still resistance predicted by your force field analysis that needs to be addressed? It is possible

that the new process is being diligently adhered to, and what you are observing is simply the maximum improvement that can be expected from the changes you have put in place. In that case you will need to go back to your Pareto diagram and select another series of changes to implement in exactly the same fashion as described above. Because most hospital processes are extremely complex, and the causes of poor outcomes are usually multifactorial, it is often the case that several iterations of the quality improvement process will be required to reach the consistent high-performing outcome that you are seeking.

If you have chosen your targeted changes with care, you will reach the point that your results are now at the level that your SMART goal has been fulfilled. Congratulations! You have successfully made the QI journey by converting data to information, using that information to derive knowledge about your processes of care, and letting that knowledge guide you in the choice of wise actions. That, however, brings us to the second challenge mentioned at the start of this section. The second challenge is to *sustain* this improvement in outcomes over the long-term. This will require ongoing, intermittent monitoring of the results for an extended period using your now familiar tools. Without this monitoring, there is all too frequently the tendency for people to slip back into old habits and ways of accomplishing tasks. You will see a degradation of results back to the old baseline, but a vigilant quality improvement expert like yourself will see early warning signs of this displayed in your run charts. At that point action can be taken to assess what is occurring and reinforce the appropriate methods that have been instituted. One technique to delay or better yet avoid this problem is to celebrate success. It is very reinforcing of new behaviors to reward people in some overt way when the goal is initially reached and when it is periodically sustained. These celebrations need not involve anything tangible, although that is a frequently used option. Often simple verbal recognition by leaders in an appropriate forum of a team's efforts and success will energize everyone to continue on the path that has been set. At some point, typically after 12–18 months, the new process will have become ingrained and part of the culture of work in the unit under observation. At that point surveillance can be relaxed, but typically revisited at least annually with appropriate recognition conveyed to all involved if the improved outcomes are sustained.

Lastly, once the SMART goal has been reached in the required timeframe and you are ready to enter the surveillance phase, it would be appropriate to check back in with those customers who started this entire process. Your surgeons have played a role in the solution to this problem as stakeholders. They likely have had to change some of their own behaviors, and hopefully have been recognized for their contribution to the improved outcomes. At this point it would be time to reissue your original "Voice of the Customer" survey, and compare the current results with the previous ones. Hopefully you will see that overall satisfaction with the performance of the operating room has increased, and maybe those physicians threatening to go elsewhere have changed their minds. It is likely that an added benefit would be reduced stress on the nursing staff and other OR personnel now that late OR start times have been reduced as a source of friction with the physicians. Good work!!

References

1   Kelley L. *How to Use Control Charts for Healthcare*. Milwaukee, WI: ASQ Quality Press; 1999.

2   Carey R, Lloyd R. *Measuring Quality Improvement in Healthcare*. Milwaukee, WI: ASQ Quality Press; 2001.

3   Rogers EM. *Diffusion of Innovations,* 5th ed. New York, NY: Free Press; 2003.

4   Lighter D, Fair D. *Quality Management in Healthcare*, 2nd ed. Burlington, MA: Jones and Bartlett; 2004.

5   Ransom S, Joshi M, Nash D. *The Healthcare Quality Book*. Chicago, IL: Health Administration Press; 2004.

Simulation and Drills

Shad Deering

Introduction and Background

The old adage of "see one, do one, teach one," once the mainstay of medical education, has fallen under scrutiny and ultimately been deemed an ineffective way to maintain patient safety in the complex system of modern healthcare. The practice of simulation in the field of obstetrics and gynecology has evolved into an essential element of education and training as well as a critical component of team training as a strategy to improve care and patient outcomes. Simulation training allows individuals and teams to learn and practice basic and advanced procedural tasks as well as the opportunity to manage life-threatening emergencies in a controlled environment using mannequins. It also provides an opportunity for personnel to perfect effective communication skills during "practice runs" of chaotic and uncommon events that are part of the specialty. This method of training breathes new life into the aforementioned educational process and allows the "see one" to provide controlled exposure so that the "do one" may be purposely executed without the need to "learn" on actual patients.

In the past several years, these efforts have been endorsed by several national organization across the spectrum of medicine involved in women's health care including the American Academy of Family Physicians, the American Academy of Pediatrics, the Association of Women's Health, the American College of Nurse Midwives, the American College of Osteopathic Obstetricians and Gynecologists, the American College of Obstetricians and Gynecologists (ACOG), and the Society for Maternal–Fetal Medicine (SMFM) [1].

Case Presentation

A young woman at 39 weeks' gestation presented to triage in July with the complaint of regular uterine contractions for the last several hours. Her prenatal course was unremarkable. Her past obstetrical history was pertinent for a significant postpartum hemorrhage.

Her uterine contractions were every 2–3 minutes and her cervix was 6 cm dilated. She was admitted to labor and delivery. She had several severe-range blood pressure readings that were written on the fetal heart tracing and not entered into the electronic medical record and the information was not communicated during the transfer from the triage nurse to the labor nurse. During labor, she had mildly elevated blood pressure readings. She progressed to C/C/+2 and had a strong desire to push. A viable female infant was delivered vaginally without complications by a new intern resident. The placenta was delivered intact. No vaginal lacerations were noted on exam. Subsequently the patient had profuse vaginal bleeding and a boggy uterus was palpated. Oxytocin was administered, but the bleeding persisted. The attending staff was called and uterotonics were requested. Methergine was administered with resultant severe blood pressure elevations requiring intravenous labetalol. There was no improvement in the patient's vaginal bleeding. The team asked for the release of two units of packed red blood cells, but the new nurse on the floor tasked with calling did not know the phone number and had difficulty finding it, resulting in a delay of approximately 10 minutes. The patient was given a single dose of misoprostol rectally with improvement in her bleeding, but she continued to be mildly hypotensive and tachycardic. After two units packed red blood cells were transfused, her vital signs improved and the remainder of her postpartum was uneventful.

Obstetric and Gynecologic Simulation: Background and Current Evidence

Background

The driving force for the use of simulation in obstetrics and gynecology has been the recognition that it may improve patient safety and outcomes. In the past, training was often focused on individual skills, with the assumption that a technically proficient provider is the key to good outcomes. What has become clear, however, is that this is only a part of the solution and that other factors, such as communication, teamwork, and systems issues play a huge part in patient care and are often the areas where mistakes occur. In fact, it has been shown that the root cause of more than 60% of sentinel events is a breakdown in communication or teamwork [2]. Simulation is unique in that it can address all of these areas and teach and improve the technical and knowledge skills as well as provide the opportunity to practice communication and teamwork in ways that conventional lectures and instruction cannot (Figure 10.1).

The need for simulation training in obstetrics and gynecology is now widely recognized, especially in the climate of reduced work hours and more emphasis on demonstrating competency through direct assessment rather than just case numbers recorded. ACOG and the SMFM have created dedicated simulation committees to facilitate the incorporation of simulation into resident education as well as at the staff level and in the hospital systems. ACOG promotes the importance of drills and simulation that allows for team review of protocols and management of common emergencies [3]. ACOG also encourages the reinforcement of these protocols through the use of posters, pocket cards, or other aids [3].

Many institutions across the country are now developing and opening simulation centers to assist in the training of their medical students, residents, nursing staff, and physician staff. Simulation training may focus on individual tasks, such as fundamental laparoscopic skills or episiotomy repair, or on emergency clinical situations where knowledge, communication, and teamwork are all required and allow for both individual and team training. Examples include obstetric scenarios for shoulder dystocia and maternal cardiac arrest and gynecologic surgical simulations for operative hemorrhage.

Residency programs are also incorporating dedicated training time at these centers, or with stand-alone task trainers or mannequins if centers are not readily accessible, as mandatory portions of their curriculum to encourage exposure and education. Although it cannot always be avoided, learning and "practice" by residents and junior staff on live patients does pose an interesting ethical dilemma on the topic of patient safety. A trainee having to learn the art of laparoscopic techniques during live surgery, although imperative to education, opens windows for error with complications from unskilled hands, prolonged surgical time, and subsequent prolonged time under general anesthesia. An article by Ziv et al. suggests that using medical simulation where applicable is an "ethical imperative" and that the implementation of simulation drills may help to ease the fundamental ethical debate over the delicate balance between patient safety and trainee education [4].

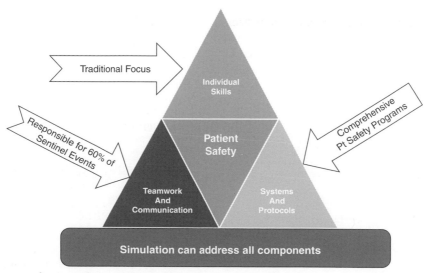

Figure 10.1 Components of patient safety.

Types of Simulators

Obstetric

Several obstetric specific simulators have been developed to develop skills including episiotomy, amniocentesis, spontaneous vaginal deliveries, operative vaginal deliveries, and even cesarean delivery. While some of these are task trainers, others are full-body mannequins that have the ability to simulate emergencies including postpartum hemorrhage, shoulder dystocia, umbilical cord prolapse, eclamptic seizures, and maternal cardiac arrest [2] (Figure 10.2).

Gynecology

For gynecologic procedures, there has been a greater focus on surgical trainers, and there are several options of both low- and high-fidelity simulators, even ones with virtual reality and haptics, available that allow for complete procedures to be performed as well. Some simulators are designed to depict the pelvis and to practice specific office procedures or basic skills like pelvic exams and intrauterine device (IUD) placement and removal. For more complicated surgical procedures, especially laparoscopic ones, there are several types of trainers to include everything from a simple "box trainer" to virtual reality and robotic surgical simulators (Figures 10.3 and 10.4). Several of the more advanced training tools provide instant individualized feedback that allows the operator to refine their technique on the spot. The goal for trainees is to be able to practice procedures so that they are more efficient in the operating room and improve their hand–eye coordination, dexterity with the instruments, efficiency in movement, and a better understanding of the flow of the surgical procedure [5].

Evidence For and Current Usage in Training

The evidence for the effectiveness of simulation to improve patient safety and outcomes continues to evolve. Although there are comprehensive articles that summarize the evidence for simulation in obstetrics, the best examples are for shoulder dystocia and umbilical cord prolapse [6].

Shoulder dystocia is an unfortunately common obstetric emergency that occurs in 0.2%–3% of all births [7]. Deering et al. tested the theory that simulation-based education could improve resident performance in the management of shoulder dystocia by randomizing residents to a control group with only standard didactic education to another group that received additional simulation training. The groups were then evaluated on a standardized shoulder dystocia scenario and graded on several factors including intervention timeline, performance of maneuvers, and time to delivery. Residents trained with simulation demonstrated superior performance in all areas measured [8]. Draycott et al. subsequently expanded on this concept and demonstrated a significant improvement in overall management of the dystocia as well as actual neonatal outcomes after implementing mandatory simulation training at the Southmead Hospital, Bristol in the United Kingdom [9]. After their training, use of McRobert's position drastically increased from 29.3% to 87.4% and they showed an overall decrease in head-to-body delivery time from 3 minutes to 2 minutes [9]. Neonatal outcomes were also shown to improve with a decreased incidence of neonatal injury at birth from 9.3% to 2.3% posttraining, including a decrease in the incidence of brachial plexus injury from 7.4% to 2.3% [7].

These findings have also been demonstrated in subsequent studies in the United States. A study by

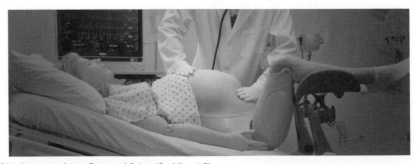

Figure 10.2 NOELLE birthing simulator, Gaumard Scientific, Miami, FL.

Grobman et al. showed a decrease in the incidence of brachial plexus at deliveries complicated by shoulder dystocia from 10.1% to 4.0% ($p < 0.001$) after implementing a standardized shoulder dystocia protocol and simulation-based training program [10]. After implementing a similar training program, Inglis et al. showed a decrease in the incidence of brachial plexus injuries with uncomplicated vaginal deliveries from 0.4% to 0.14% ($p < 0.01$) and after deliveries complicated by shoulder dystocia from 30% to 10.6% ($p < 0.01$) [11].

Simulation training has also been used to evaluate the adequacy of documentation after deliveries complicated by shoulder dystocia. Several reports have shown that significant deficiencies may be identified with simulation exercises, and that simulation training can help to improve documentation, which is important for both patient care and from a medical–legal standpoint [12–14]. Umbilical cord prolapse is another obstetric emergency where simulation training has demonstrated improvement in the care of pregnant women [15].

When an umbilical cord prolapse occurs, it is an indication for an expeditious delivery in order to ensure the best neonatal outcome possible. Simulation-based recognition of this obstetrical complication was undertaken by Siassakos et al., with an objective to determine if this training could affect the quality of care and decrease the time period between diagnosis and delivery in actual cases. The authors implemented a mandatory simulation-based training program for providers in the management of umbilical cord prolapse. They compared the diagnosis-to-delivery

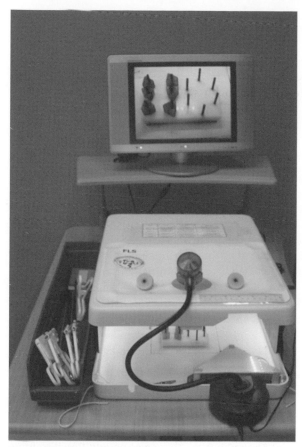

Figure 10.3 Laparoscopic simulators.

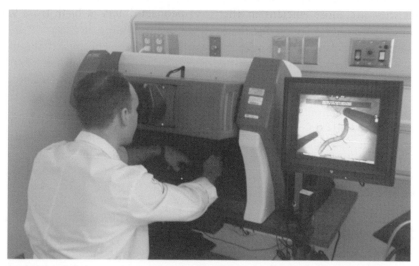

Figure 10.4 Robotic simulation trainer.

interval for all umbilical cord prolapse cases for the six years prior to and the six years after implementation of the training program. They found that the team was much more likely to take actions to alleviate cord compression (34%–82%, $p = 0.003$) after the training program and there was a significant decrease in the diagnosis to delivery interval from 25 minutes to 14.5 minutes ($p < 0.001$) [15].

For laparoscopic surgery, there have been multiple studies evaluating the effectiveness and validity of the simulators themselves, and some investigators have attempted to translate this to improved performance in the actual operating room.

In a randomized, blinded trial involving gynecology residents, Larsen et al. evaluated the impact of virtual reality simulator training for laparoscopic salpingectomy and how this translated to actual performance in the operating room [16]. The performance level of novices who underwent the training was increased to that of intermediately experienced laparoscopic surgeons and the median total operative time in the simulator trained group was 12 minutes (interquartile range 10–14 minutes) versus 24 (20–29) minutes in the control group ($p < 0.001$).

Another interesting simulation study looked at the use of a virtual reality (VR) laparoscopic simulator to "warm up" before performing an actual laparoscopic procedure in much the same way that athletes warm up before a game [17]. When surgeons were able to practice the procedure, in this case a laparoscopic cholecystectomy, just before going into the OR, they demonstrated significantly better performance as measured by a standardized assessment tool used by blinded observers. There is potential to apply this simulation training in our gynecology specialty, as there are VR simulators available for laparoscopic gynecologic procedures such as salpingectomy, tubal ligation, and laparoscopic-assisted vaginal hysterectomy.

A Cochrane review of VR laparoscopic training suggested that, in providers with limited laparoscopic experience, VR training results in an accelerated reduction in operating time, errors, and unnecessary movements than current standard laparoscopic training. They also identified that additional translational research was needed in this area [18].

Simulation and Teamwork Training

Traditionally, attempts to improve patient outcomes in obstetrics and gynecology have been directed at the individual provider level with a focus on honing technical skills and increasing medical knowledge. However, it is now recognized that the majority of complications and morbidity actually result from team and system failures rather than individual issues. The Joint Commission issued a Sentinel Alert in 2004 recognizing that most cases of perinatal death and injury are caused by problems with an organization's culture and communication failures [19]. A year later, another report highlighted that, despite awareness of the need to focus towards a movement to improve patient safety, there had not been a decrease in the death rate due to medical errors. They did note, however, that there were reductions in certain kinds of error-related deaths, including a 50% reduction in poor outcomes of preterm infants, when labor and delivery staff had participated in team training [20].

A 2010 systemic review of simulation for multidisciplinary team training in obstetrics performed a targeted focus on eight specific reported outcomes from 97 identified articles. Simulation multidisciplinary team training was found to be potentially effective in preventing errors and improving patient safety in acute obstetric emergencies, however additional studies were needed [21]. Riley et al. also addressed the use of teamwork training with and without simulation training in a study using three different hospitals. At one hospital, there was no additional training provided, another hospital implemented standard TeamSTEPPS® training only, and at the third hospital, they conducted TeamSTEPPS® training that incorporated simulation training. Over a three-year time period, they measured the weighted adverse outcomes score (WAOS) and found no improvement in the first two hospitals, but a 37% decrease in perinatal morbidity for the hospital that utilized teamwork and simulation training together [22]. A more in-depth discussion about teamwork training and patient safety can be found in Chapter 11.

Implementation: Planning and Costs

When reviewing programs that have demonstrated improvements in actual patient outcomes, Siassakos et al. noted that there were several commonly observed themes [23]. The essential components of effective simulation training programs reported included the following:

- Teamwork training was combined with clinical training in a multidisciplinary format. This training involved the entire team, including physicians, nurses, and even other specialties that interact during patient care.

- Relevant, "in house" training: Because of the difficulties with getting complete teams together at simulation centers located outside of the hospital, many successful institutions trained on their actual unit, or at least in their hospital. This resulted in multidisciplinary training being achieved more often and allowed for the identification of institution systems issues and real-time review of institutional protocols. Most importantly, these units were able to train the greater majority of their staff, and not just a select few.

- Developed local solutions: Successful programs took national guidelines and then evaluated their own systems and practices to create solutions that followed best practices and yet still worked within the capabilities of their institution.

- Utilized realistic training tools: With regards to simulators and training tools, high fidelity and engagement of the learners was found to be more important than having the most "high-tech" simulators available.

- Institution-level incentives: Besides strong support from leadership, hospitals with effective programs often were offered financial incentives including significant discounts on their malpractice premiums.

The expense of simulation training that encompasses simulators, physical space, technician time, and educator time is another common obstacle to implementation. Mannequins and training tools are the first obvious investment that most think of when simulation is mentioned. For obstetric simulation, simple pelvic models can be purchased for a few hundred dollars, and low-cost birthing simulators that a person can wear and train providers for vaginal deliveries and postpartum hemorrhage are less than $1,000 (Figure 10.5). Some of the most commonly used mid- to high-fidelity birthing simulators, which have been used in the studies discussed previously in this paper, range from $4,750 up to as much as $30,000. When considering which simulator to purchase, it is advisable to seek advice from other institutions that have implemented training as the most expensive mannequins are not always necessary.

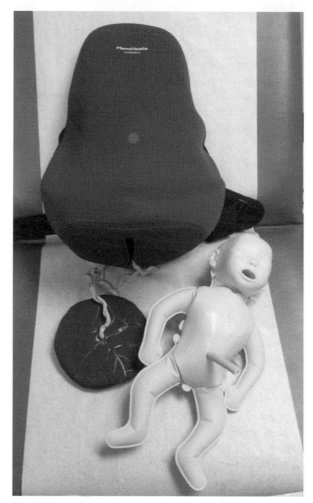

Figure 10.5 Mama Natalie, Laerdal.

For gynecologic simulators, there is a wide price range depending on what the training goals are. Simple laparoscopic box trainers, such as the ones used for the Fundamentals of Laparoscopic Surgery (FLS) courses, can be purchased for less than $2,000, while high-fidelity VR laparoscopic simulators can easily cost more than $200,000.

When considering the costs for simulation equipment, it is also important to consider the costs required for both support of the training in terms of a simulation technician, and the staff/instructor's time. For many of the low- to mid-fidelity obstetric simulators, the instructor is often able to act as the simulator operator as well as the instructor, while many of the laparoscopic simulators for gynecology can be used independently. Another consideration is the potential cost savings associated with implementation of simulation training and improved patient safety.

A review of monetary compensation for malpractice lawsuits demonstrated that over $3.6 billion dollars was awarded to patients across the United States in 2012, 24% of which were related to surgical complications and 11% were related to obstetrical complications [24]. According to a review of medical liability released by the ACOG, the average for all paid malpractice claims against obstetricians and gynecologists was $510,473 [25]. In light of these potential liability claims, the cost of training simulators seems relatively low. Iverson and Heffner reviewed the impact of a comprehensive patient safety program, which included obstetric simulation drills, and found that there was a 20% decrease per year on the amount of money set aside for reserved claims [26]. Another group that implemented a similar safety program with obstetric simulation drills showed a 99% drop from $27,591,610 to $ 250,000 on total claims paid from 2003 to 2009 [27].

Moreover, if there is truly a significant decrease in the risk of a brachial plexus injury with the implementation of shoulder dystocia simulation training as the data imply, avoiding just a single event could potentially save over a half a million dollars.

Credentialing and Licensure

Simulation use for training and licensure continues to expand in the world of medicine. Prior to matriculation into a residency program, both allopathic and osteopathic medical students are required to complete and pass a simulation-based examination known as the USMLE Step 2 Clinical Knowledge Examination and the COMLEX Level 2 Clinical Evaluation Examination. These examinations evaluate knowledge base, professionalism, interpersonal skills, and the ability of the student physician to effectively communicate with their patient. As of 2011, the ACGME began mandating several residency programs to require simulation training.

Anesthesiology residents are required to participate in at least one simulation experience annually while emergency medicine residents must report both patient care and simulation encounters. Internal medicine programs must provide access to a training facility for their residents and surgery residents must have a skills and simulation laboratory for the acquisition and maintenance of skills with a competency-based

evaluation protocol [22]. The American Board of Surgery currently requires the completion of three simulation-based courses in order to be eligible to sit for board certification: Advanced Cardiac Life Support (ACLS), Advanced Trauma Life Support (ATLS), and Fundamentals of Laparoscopic Surgery (FLS) [28].

As another example, the field of radiology has noted challenges in attaining diagnostic credentialing numbers because current requirements dictate that a resident must complete 100 diagnostic cervicocerebral angiograms prior to the postgraduate training for coronary stenting procedures. This has become increasingly difficult in the setting of the development of more sophisticated imaging, such as computed tomography angiography (CTA) and magnetic resonance angiogram (MRA), replacing the use of cervicocerebral angiograms for diagnosis. Future use of computer-based simulation is anticipated to balance education with patient safety, in addition to skill acquisition for many interventional radiology procedures [29].

Anesthesia has led the way in the incorporation of simulation-based education into training and evaluation for high-stakes exams. As of 2000, the American Board of Anesthesiology (ABA) licensing certificates were no longer a life-long certification and the mandate was set for simulation-based learning as a requirement for Maintenance of Certification for Anesthesiology (MOCA). In January of 2010, the ABA made simulation-based training a requirement for maintenance of certification and now all residents are required to participate in at least one simulated intraoperative experience annually [30]. The current goal is that by 2014, all newly graduated anesthesiologists seeking ABA certification will have to adhere to the new guidelines of mandatory simulation-based training as a prerequisite to licensure [24]. As of 2016, the ABA oral board examination will include simulation-based Objective Structured Clinical Examinations (OSCEs), which are similar to what the Israeli National Board of Anesthesiology Examination Committee incorporated into their licensing examinations in 2003 where five structured and standardized tasks using simulation must be performed to standard in order to pass the exam [31].

National Organizations

ACOG has committed to simulation training and supports its utility across our discipline for students,

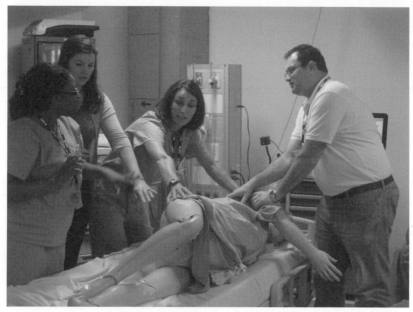

Figure 10.6 Teamwork training in obstetric emergencies. SMFM postgraduate course.

junior fellows, and fellows. Because of this, the ACOG Education Division created a Clinical Simulation Consortium that is working to expand simulation training for the specialty.

The SMFM recognizes the potential and promise of simulation as a teaching, learning, and evaluation tool and even debuted a postgraduate course featuring simulation by introducing models and procedures for education and management of obstetrical emergencies in 2010 (Figure 10.6). Subsequently, simulation was added as a component of a postgraduate course highlighting simulation in the context of patient safety.

The American College of Surgeons and the Society of American Gastrointestinal and Endoscopic Surgeons announced in 2012 the recommendation that all surgeons who perform laparoscopic surgery should be Fundamentals of Laparoscopic Surgery (FLS) certified. FLS was first launched in 2004 and is the first surgical assessment tool to be mandated by the American Board of Surgery in order to set the standard for safe laparoscopic surgery.

Case Resolution

In the case presented at the beginning of the chapter, several key points can easily be addressed. The regular use of drills, simulation, and team-directed training may potentially avoid such individual, team, and institutional system failures. For example, acquiring knowledge of a patient's medical history and prenatal course is essential. A drill on postpartum hemorrhage would allow this young physician in July to be aware of triggers that may predispose a patient to postpartum hemorrhage and help to better prepare for the aftermath if such a complication is encountered, including calling for assistance and back-up early, having uterotonics in the room and potentially two large-bore IVs if aggressive hydration and/or blood products are required. Communication would allow the providers to review the importance of closed-loop communication to address contraindications to specific uterotonics, doses, and routes of administration. This could have prevented the potentially life-threatening error of administering methergine to a hypertensive patient. Having the team present to review protocols and phone numbers for blood release may have sped the process where delay by mere moments may prove critical.

Summary

Simulation training is a critical component to any comprehensive patient safety program for obstetrics and gynecology. It has application in the acquisition of both technical skills and is irreplaceable in terms of training for teamwork and communication. The field has grown exponentially in the past several years, and this will continue for the foreseeable future. Although there is no substitute for actual clinical experience, there is every reason to be as prepared as possible when caring for actual patients, and simulation is the optimal method to provide this.

References

1 Quality Patient Care on Labor and Delivery: A Call to Action. Available at: www.acog.org/About_ACOG/ACOG_Departments/Patient_Safety_and_Quality_Improvement/~/media/F23BCE9264BF4F1681C1EB553DCA32F4.ashx (accessed December 20, 2013).

2 Improving America's Hospitals – The Joint Commission's Annual Report 2007. Available at: www.jointcommission.org/assets/1/6/2007_Annual_Report.pdf (accessed December 31, 2013).

3 American College of Obstetricians and Gynecologists, Preparing for Clinical Emergencies in Obstetrics and Gynecology, Committee Opinion No. 487 (April 2011).

4 Ziv A, Wolpe PR, Small SD, Glick S. Simulation-based medical education: an ethical imperative. *Simul Healthc.* 2006;1(4):252–256.

5 Deering S, Auguste TC. Obstetrics and gynecology In: Levine AI, DeMaria Jr S, Schwartz AD, Sim AJ, eds. *The Comprehensive Textbook of Healthcare Simulation, Obstetrics and Gynecology.* New York, NY: Springer Science/Business Media; 2013: 437–452.

6 Deering SH, Rowland J. Obstetric emergency simulation. *Semin Perinatol.* 2013;37:179–188.

7 American College of Obstetricians and Gynecologists Practice Bulletin Number 40: Shoulder Dystocia, November 2002.

8 Deering S, Poggi S, Macedonia C, Gherman R, Satin AJ. Improving resident competency in the management of shoulder dystocia with simulation training. *Obstet Gynecol.* 2004;103(6):1224–1228.

9 Draycott TJ, Crofts JF, Ash JP, et al. Improving neonatal outcome through practical shoulder dystocia training. *Obstet Gynecol.* 2008;112(1):14–20.

10 Grobman WA, Miller D, Burke C, Hornbogen A, Tam K, Costello R. Outcomes associated with introduction of a shoulder dystocia protocol. *Am J Obstet Gynecol.* 2011;205(6):513–517.

11 Inglis SR, Feier N, Chetiyaar JB, et al. Effects of shoulder dystocia training on the incidence of brachial plexus injury. *Am J Obstet Gynecol.* 2011;204(322):e1–e6.

12 Deering S, Poggi S, Hodor J, Macedonia C, Satin AJ. Evaluation of resident's delivery notes after a simulated shoulder dystocia. *Obstet Gynecol.* 2004;104:667–670.

13 Crofts JF, Bartlett C, Ellis D, et al. Documentation of simulated shoulder dystocia: accurate and complete? *BJOG.* 2008;115:1303–1318.

14 Goffman D, Heo H, Chazotte C, Merkatz IR, Bernstein PS. Using simulation training to improve shoulder dystocia documentation. *Obstet Gynecol.* 2008;112:1284–1287.

15 Siassakos D, Hasafa Z, Sibanda T, et al. Retrospective cohort study of diagnosis–delivery interval with umbilical cord prolapse: the effect of team training. *BJOG.* 2009;116:1089–1096.

16 Larsen CR, Soerensen JL, Grantcharov TP, et al. Effect of virtual reality training on laparoscopic surgery: randomised controlled trial. *BMJ.* 2009;338:b1802.

17 Calatayud D, Arora S, Aggarwal R, et al. Warm-up in a virtual reality environment improves performance in the operating room. *Ann Surg.* 2010;251: 1181–1185.

18 Gurusamy KS, Aggarwal R, Palanivelu L, Davidson BR. Virtual reality training for surgical trainees in laparoscopic surgery. *Cochrane Database Syst Rev.* 2009;1:CD006575.

19 Joint Commission on Accreditation of Healthcare Organizations. Sentinel Event Alert. Joint Commission on Accreditation of Healthcare Organizations, Issue No. 30; 2004.

20 Leape LL, Berwick DM. Five years after *To Err is Human*: what have we learned? *JAMA.* 2005;293:2384–2390.

21 Merien AER, van de Ven J, Mol BW, Houterman S, Oie SG. Multidisciplinary team training in a simulation setting for acute obstetric emergencies. *Am J Obstet Gynecol.* 2010;115(5):1021–1031.

22 Riley W, Davis S, Miller K, Hansen H, Sainfort F, Sweet R. Didactic and simulation nontechnical skills team training to improve perinatal patient outcomes in a community hospital. *J Qual Patient Saf.* 2011;37(8):357–364.

23 Siassakos D, Crofts JF, Winter C, Weiner CP, Draycott TJ. The active components of effective training in obstetric emergencies. *BJOG.* 2009;116:1028–1032.

24 Diederich Healthcare: 2013 Medical Malpractice Payout Analysis. Available at: www.diederichhealthcare.com/medical-malpractice-insurance/2013-medical-malpractice-payout-analysis/

25 ACOG: Medical Liability Climate Hurts Patients and OB/GYNs, September 2012. Available at: www.acog.org/About_ACOG/News_Room/News_Releases/2012/Medical_Liability_Climate_Hurts_Patients_and_Ob-Gyns (accessed December 23, 2013).

26 Iverson Jr RE, Heffner LJ. Obstetric safety improvement and its reflection in reserved claims. *AJOG*. 2011;205(5):398–401.

27 Grunebaum A, Chervenak F, Skupski D. Effect of a comprehensive obstetric patient safety program on compensation payments and sentinel events. *AJOG*. 2011;204(2):97–105.

28 The American Board of Surgery Training Requirements for General Surgery Certification. Available at: www.absurgery.org/default.jsp?certgsqe_training

29 Street T, Thompson KR. Credentialing for radiology. *Biomed Imaging Interv J*. 2008;4(1):e14.

30 Levine AI, Schwartz AD, Bryson EO, DeMaria Jr S. Role of simulation in US licensure and certification. *Mount Sinai J Med*. 2012;79:140–153.

31 Steadman RH, Huang YM. Simulation for quality assurance in training, credentialing and maintenance of certification. *Best Pract Res Clin Anaesthesiol*. 2012 Mar;26(1):3–15.

Rapid Response in Obstetrics

Allison R. Durica and Elizabeth S. McCuin

Case Scenario # 1 Prior to Institution of an Obstetric Rapid Response

While on call as attending physician, I walked past my chief resident as he was hanging up his blackberry and I saw the color draining from his face. I asked what was wrong. He stated that the phone call was from the Emergency Department (ED). A pregnant woman was in cardiac arrest. We both rapidly proceeded to the ED while I was calling our Labor and Delivery charge nurse so as to activate more help.

Upon entering the patient's room we learned that the ED staff had performed an ultrasound that confirmed the fetus was dead. Cardiopulmonary Resuscitation was being performed on the patient. We learned that she had been brought in by ambulance from home after a cardiac arrest. Her pregnancy was at term. The ED team was attempting to secure an airway. We immediately proceeded with a perimortem cesarean delivery in an attempt to facilitate the resuscitative efforts. Despite these efforts, this was not successful.

What are the Problems with this Anecdotal Case?

- The patient was already in the ED before the obstetricians were notified.
- The initial phone call was directed to the obstetric chief resident who had no experience with a maternal cardiac arrest.
- Obstetrical Nursing was notified by the obstetrical attending.
- The obstetrical nurse had to mobilize additional nurses, and also had to notify the newborn nursery personnel.
- There was no mechanism to easily mobilize a care team for this obstetric patient.

- Because we did not have an OB Rapid Response in place, patient care did not proceed as efficiently as might have.

Actual Case Scenario #2

You were on call covering your OB service, and have just delivered a 32-year-old woman, G2P2002 at 39 weeks estimated gestational age (EGA). Her prenatal course was notable for a placenta previa that resolved by 32 weeks EGA. The patient presented in labor, and required augmentation with oxytocin. She had an unremarkable labor and spontaneous vaginal delivery of an apparently healthy infant. Immediately postpartum she had significant vaginal bleeding.

You diagnosed uterine atony, and initiated uterine massage. Oxytocin infusion in the intravenous fluid was increased. Intermittent atony persisted despite giving doses of various uterotonic medications. You elected to move the patient to the OB operating room (OR) to gain better visualization to rule out a laceration. Anesthesia was also called to the OR to assist.

With the patient well-positioned in stirrups, and with optimal lighting and retraction, you confirmed the absence of vaginal or cervical lacerations as cause for the vaginal bleeding. The intermittent brisk bleeding continued despite all interventions employed.

The nurses in attendance, including the experienced nurse manager, inquired multiple times regarding the need to call back-up (perhaps the in-hospital Maternal Fetal Medicine physician who you helped train as a resident). You are an experienced OB provider, and believed that you had the situation under control. You were also embarrassed to admit that you might need some additional help or expertise. You reported to staff that back-up was not needed.

The anesthesiologist provided light sedation for patient comfort, and inquired regarding need to order blood products. You declined to do so, and instead, you ordered a STAT blood count and fibrinogen level to help guide your decision.

You were unaware of the amount of time that has passed since the delivery, but you believed it had been a short period of time. The anesthesiologist reported that the patient's vital signs were deteriorating. With this report, someone in the room called for back-up support from the in-hospital Maternal Fetal Medicine physician who was completing a delivery down the hall. Despite the extensive interventions, the vaginal bleeding continued. A laparotomy was initiated. Ultimately, a hysterectomy was performed. Blood product replacement had also been started concurrent with the decision to begin the laparotomy.

The patient was taken to the ICU following surgery, and required pressors and ventilator support. Labs confirmed coagulopathy during the surgery. Aggressive support was provided, but the patient was determined to be "brain dead" by EEG. Life support was discontinued on postpartum day #2. Severe brain injury and encephalopathy was believed to be due to extreme blood loss experienced during the postpartum hemorrhage.

You are an experienced and skilled provider, and you recognized that you misjudged the severity of the acute event. A central issue in this actual case was discomfort on the part of staff overriding the desire of an experienced attending physician in calling for assistance. Staff members and anesthesia colleagues may have been hesitant to do so, not wanting to insult a well-respected provider. Staff members also may have had some concern for retribution if they called for physician back-up without the primary provider's agreement. The attending physician did not recognize the extent of blood loss. He became preoccupied with "stopping the bleeding" and lost situational awareness. This led to underestimation of the amount of blood lost, as well as the duration of attempted interventions. Finally, in this case there was a lack of an organized approach to an emergency that would have helped enlist additional resources (blood, physicians, nurses, etc.).

A Rapid Response team was developed and implemented in part because of this case.

What is a Rapid Response System?

A Rapid Response system facilitates the identification of patients who show signs of deterioration and may require urgent intervention. This system mobilizes additional resources to help the patient at the time of initial signs of deterioration. The members of a Rapid Response team may vary based on the patient population targeted, as well as the resources in the hospital. Rapid Response teams may be physician- or nurse-led. Various terms are used to describe these teams, including: critical care teams, medical emergency teams, medical response teams, and rapid response teams [1,2].

Regardless of the term used, the components are similar:

- Criteria: The criteria needed to activate the rapid response system are often objective such as a change in vital signs or mental status, or complaint of chest pain or shortness of breath. However, subjective criteria also may serve as a trigger. A nurse who has cared for the patient may call a rapid response simply because, "he/she is worried about the patient's acute change in status." Regardless of reason for mobilizing the rapid response team, retribution in the event of a "false alarm" is unacceptable. Any staff members' perception of need for a rapid response should be respected if the system is going to work.

- Team Composition: An obstetric-specific rapid response team should be formed. Members should be chosen based on their ability to diagnose the clinical complication, initiate needed therapy, and have the authority to move the patient to the ICU if indicated. The expectations and duties of team members during response should be clearly explained and delineated prior to implementation of the system. There should be coverage available in-house 24/7.

- Activation: Following identification of patients in need of focused assistance, easy and rapid notification of response team members is crucial to maximizing the best patient outcomes. The goal is to notify all first responders simultaneously by text or page to the location and event. This should be a simple and straightforward message such as "OB Rapid Response, Room 1354." An identified team should be available for response 24 hours a day.

- System Evaluation: In continual efforts to improve the system and care provided, each response should be evaluated for opportunities for improvement. This may be done by collection of standard data such as time to response, need for blood products, or outcomes. This review may be done at a formal regularly scheduled meeting of team members or as a debriefing following an especially difficult event. The team should analyze their performance and identify areas where changes can be made to further improve the system.

Why is an OB Rapid Response Needed?

If we had a Rapid Response system for obstetrics in place at the time of the first scenario, one phone call by the Emergency Department personnel could have been made to the hospital operator prior to the patient arriving in the ED. The operator could mobilize the resources and staff needed. The team would be waiting in the ED as the patient arrived. (See Figure 11.1).

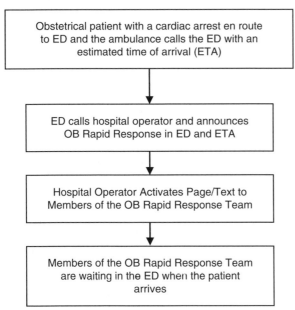

Figure 11.1 ER initiation of OB Rapid Response.

Experience with Rapid Response Systems

Use and description of Rapid Response systems/teams in the medical literature differ greatly. Most of the data and systems described focus on adult and pediatric populations and attempts to improve outcomes with regards to ICU admissions and respiratory/cardiac arrest [3,4]. The ability to measure efficacy or improvement in outcomes due to use of these response systems has proven difficult. This may

be due to the already severe acuity of the patients' illness, outcome measures identified, or heterogeneity in systems employed and studied. Regardless, institutions that have implemented these response teams suggest an overall improvement in care delivery and outcomes. The benefits of Rapid Response teams in critical obstetric care may be difficult to measure. The support and experience of team members for junior or lesser experienced staff/providers is important in optimizing patient safety. Also, with inpatient obstetric unit consolidations, fewer providers and staff are available to care for a greater number of patients. In these situations, it is especially important to have a system in place whereby an acute event requiring additional resources is identified, communicated, and acted upon.

Evidence of the use and efficacy of Rapid Response teams in obstetric literature is scant. With the recognition and endorsement of use of rapid response systems in OB care from the American College of Obstetricians and Gynecologists, the American Medical Association, and the Institute for Healthcare Improvement, hospital systems have turned their attention to ways in which this approach may improve outcomes for patients [5,6]. Previously, focused obstetric Rapid Response teams have been implemented following sentinel events in a hospital system such as maternal deaths. This is a reasonable and responsible response to such outcomes. Other hospital systems have proactively identified the Rapid Response system as a possible way to improve safety deficits noted during routine data collection. Review of the implementation of a Rapid Response system, Condition O, at a busy university hospital outlines the reasons for initiation of the system, protocol, outcomes, and challenges specific to an OB population [7].

Use of a similar system in a large city hospital noted improved outcomes, fewer maternal deaths, and improved patient safety measures after implementation of Rapid Response teams for postpartum hemorrhage. Formation of a multidisciplinary team in order to formalize a protocol and delineate duties in these events to specific team members allowed staff to respond in a more organized and effective way. Comparison of outcomes before and after the implementation of this system change showed better patient outcomes, including a significant reduction in maternal deaths. These effects were seen despite an increase in obstetric hemorrhage noted in the years following the addition of a Rapid Response team.

Such hemorrhages are believed to be related to the significant increase in pregnancies complicated by prior cesarean delivery [8].

Team training may be important to help implement an effective Rapid Response team. Simulation drills facilitate the group to learn to function as a team. It also helps the team to provide acute care in a protocol-driven, standard approach. Simulations focus on teaching team skills and coordination of care, but simulations ultimately may improve outcomes and safety as well. Use of simulation drills may also identify areas of adjustment needed in provider, staff, or system response in order to maximize patient outcomes [9,10].

Changes in Outcomes with Rapid Response Systems

Although resource optimization and mobilization may be obvious, the true impact of a Rapid Response system for obstetrics can be challenging to measure. Fortunately, severe adverse outcomes are rare. However, maternal and perinatal morbidities occur more commonly, as do near-misses. Developing appropriate process and outcome measures should be a part of the planning process for a Rapid Response program. Measures such as the adverse outcomes index can provide a useful starting point.

Specific OB Emergencies that may Benefit from Rapid Response Intervention

Specific role assignments should be determined by individual institutions, based upon their available staff and most effective response work flow. Assignment of roles is important to ensure that all critical tasks are addressed and flexibility in fulfilling these tasks should also be encouraged when indicated. A team leader should be identified within these team roles, and assignment of a physician or nurse leader should be determined by individual institutions based on their preferences.

Eclampsia

Eclampsia is a diagnosis of generalized seizures in the setting of preeclampsia with absence of any underlying neurologic cause. The incidence in developed countries is 1.6–10/10,000 deliveries. Eclampsia is expected in 2%–3% of patients with severe preeclampsia and up to 0.6% of patients with mild preeclampsia if prophylactic medical therapy is not given. Half

of all cases are preterm. Fifty-five percent of seizures are diagnosed antepartum, approximately 36% occur intrapartum, and up to 17% may occur within the first 48 hours after delivery [11].

Eclampsia is poorly predicted. In a study of patients readmitted post delivery with this diagnosis, 60% did not have prior findings of hypertension, and only 70% reported any headache. Correlation between development of eclampsia and severity of blood pressure elevation or symptoms such as headache and hyperreflexia is quite poor. Up to 40% of patients who experience eclampsia did not report any pertinent preceding symptoms such as headache, vision changes, or epigastric pain. Maternal/pregnancy complications may occur in the setting of eclampsia, and may include: placental abruption, acute renal failure, intracerebral hemorrhage, ischemic stroke, and death.

Recommended approach to management:

- With recognition of the event, call for help. Assistants are needed to start IV magnesium sulfate to reduce the likelihood of additional seizures, commence fetal monitoring, and begin maternal stabilization. Assigning the task of obtaining medications such as magnesium sulfate or antihypertensives to a nurse who responds as part of the team will allow the patient's primary nurse to maintain her role at the bedside in the initial stabilization and communication process with the gathering team members. The obstetrician may need to assist in determining fetal heart rate by bedside ultrasound if fetal monitoring is difficult or unclear following the seizure.
- Stabilize the patient with regards to airway, left lateral positioning, fall safety (bedrails, etc.), oxygen, and IV access. The patient's primary nurse will likely have initiated some of these interventions, but anesthesia may be assigned to ensure a stable airway and adequate IV access.
- Administer 4–6 g IV infusion of 20% magnesium sulfate over 15 minutes. Continue at 2 g/hour. If IV access is not available, give 5 g of 50% magnesium sulfate IM in each buttock. Continue with 5 g of magnesium sulfate in one buttock IM every 4 hours if no IV access is possible.
- Seizures are expected to be self-limited and usually last approximately 1 minute. They may, however, last up to 4 minutes. Repeated eclamptic seizures after appropriate magnesium sulfate

therapy are unlikely. If seizures continue despite appropriate magnesium sulfate serum levels, and the patient is stabilized, head imaging should be considered. Maternal head imaging is not considered part of the initial emergency response to eclampsia.

- Fetal heart rate evaluation is appropriate if the patient is still pregnant. Fetal bradycardia during the seizure is expected and common. This may last up to 3–5 minutes. Decreased variability and transient decelerations are not unexpected following the event.

- IV medication for severe blood pressure elevations should be given; 10 mg of labetalol IV or 5 mg of hydralazine IV may be given for systolic BP > 160 or diastolic BP > 110. Outcomes are not improved with treatment of mildly elevated BP. Rapid decreases in BP to low levels can actually worsen cerebral perfusion and outcomes.

- IV fluids, maternal oxygen, position change, seizure control, and discontinuation of oxytocin or other labor-inducing medication should be accomplished. Decreased uterine tone will facilitate intrauterine resuscitation of the fetus.

- Once the patient is stable, a decision regarding mode of delivery should be determined by the obstetrician. Eclampsia is not an indication for emergency cesarean delivery, and is also not a contraindication for vaginal delivery.

- Cesarean delivery should be performed if a patient has been stabilized, and a Category II or III, or otherwise non-reassuring fetal heart rate tracing persists greater than 15 minutes despite intrauterine resuscitative efforts.

- Serial labs including: liver function tests, LDH, platelets, and creatinine should be followed and urine output closely monitored during the labor and initial postpartum course. Discontinuation of serial lab testing is reasonable once a trend in values toward normal is noted. A standard protocol is to continue magnesium sulfate prophylaxis throughout labor and delivery and at least 24 hours postpartum.

Postpartum Hemorrhage

In general, postpartum hemorrhage is often defined as greater than 1,000 ml of blood loss, and continues to represent a significant cause of maternal morbidity and mortality. Specifically, level II hemorrhage is defined as acute blood loss of 1,200–1,500 ml, and may result in tachycardia, tachypnea, and orthostatic hypotension. Level III hemorrhage, 1,800–2,100 ml, will result in worsening maternal symptoms, and may represent as much as 35% of total blood volume lost. The approach to management for this complication depends upon the cause for blood loss. Many obstetric facilities have developed protocols to address management of excessive postpartum blood loss. Management of significant (level II and III) postpartum hemorrhage often requires participation from various care team members. Quick response and mobilization of resources is crucial for best patient outcomes.

Suggested approach to management of postpartum hemorrhage after delivery:

- Begin uterine fundal massage to encourage uterine contraction. The most common cause of postpartum hemorrhage is uterine atony.

- Ensure appropriate IV access, and run IV fluids at room temperature. Give oxygen.

- Administer oxytocin (40 units in 1 liter of normal saline), or increase rate if this solution is already running. Avoid an IV oxytocin bolus because this may precipitate acute hypotension and cardiac arrest.

- If blood loss is persistent despite these measures, consider moving the patient to the OB operating room for better lighting, assessment for lacerations, and possible need for laparotomy.

- If your hospital has an OB Rapid Response team, consider calling them as the patient is being brought back to the operating room. Otherwise, call for additional assistance (nursing, OB physician, Anesthesiology).

- Type and cross-match 4–6 units of packed RBCs, and transfuse 2 units if the patient is not stable, or bleeding is not stopped after 2–3 liters of IVF. Do not wait for laboratory blood counts to confirm this need. A quick test to assess clotting may also be done in the room: observe blood in a red-topped tube – if a clot forms and persists within 8–10 minutes, the fibrinogen level is normal.

- Ask Anesthesiology to provide needed medication for comfort during your evaluation and management. They may also help monitor vital signs and urine output. Place a Foley catheter with urimeter to monitor output precisely.

- Other medications that may be used to treat persistent uterine atony include: Methergine (methylergonovine) 0.2 mg IM (or directly into myometrium at laparotomy) in the absence of maternal hypertension, Hemabate (15 methyl-PGF2alpha) 250 µg IM (or directly into myometrium at laparotomy) in the absence of maternal asthma, or misoprostol (200–1000 µg) oral, sublingual, or rectally.
- If vaginal bleeding persists despite return of uterine tone, careful examination should be done for vaginal or cervical lacerations, and repair done. This evaluation may be done by the obstetrician in conjunction with uterotonic medications being administered by another team member. Lacerations should always be considered after operative vaginal delivery or cases of shoulder dystocia.
- Intrauterine tamponade with Bakri, Foley, or packing may be considered.
- Uterine artery embolization may be considered if available.
- Laparotomy may be needed for B Lynch stitch, uterine artery ligation, or hypogastric artery ligation.
- Hysterectomy should be performed if bleeding is not controlled by available measures in a reasonable amount of time.
- Cell saver may be used in some cases after consultation with anesthesia.
- Massive transfusion protocols are used in many hospitals, and vary somewhat. Remember the need for fresh frozen plasma (FFP) in addition to packed RBCs to prevent coagulopathies. Suggested ratios for administration are 6 RBC for each 4 FFP or 4 RBC for each 2 FFP. Cryoprecipitate should be given if the fibrinogen level is low or clotting is deficient. Make sure that the blood bank is informed that there is a significant obstetrical hemorrhage. Blood products require thawing and preparation (up to 45 minutes in some cases); ask for it sooner rather than later.
- Draw frequent serial labs for blood count and fibrinogen to establish need for further replacement as the patient is stabilized.

Shoulder Dystocia

Fetal shoulder dystocia is diagnosed when usual gentle downward traction of the fetal head is not sufficient to allow delivery of the anterior shoulder during delivery. In these cases, additional maneuvers are often needed to accomplish a safe delivery of the fetus. Unfortunately, although factors have been identified to suggest greater risk for this complication, such as fetal macrosomia in a diabetic mother, most cases occur without recognized risk factors present. The overall goal of intervention for shoulder dystocia is delivery of the fetus to prevent asphyxia while avoiding physical injury.

Suggested management of shoulder dystocia (specific order of maneuvers is provider-dependent):

- Additional assistance should be requested, and this may be done by calling an OB Rapid Response. The maneuvers necessary to safely resolve a shoulder dystocia often require multiple assistants. Also, accurate documentation during this event is necessary, and may be done by the charge nurse.
- Two people, in addition to the delivering obstetrician, are needed to flex the patient's legs at the hips, positioning the thighs against the abdomen. This McRoberts maneuver will maximize the pelvic diameter, and remove the sacral promontory as a possible obstruction to fetal delivery.
- An assistant may apply suprapubic pressure downward in conjunction with McRoberts maneuver. This assistant may require a stool to assist, and lowering the patient's bed is also often helpful. This maneuver may adduct the fetal shoulder, allowing delivery.
- The delivering obstetrician may employ other maneuvers such as delivery of the posterior fetal arm, Rubin (rotation of posterior fetal shoulder anteriorly), or Wood screw (posterior rotation of the anterior fetal shoulder under the maternal symphysis), if needed.
- The Gaskin maneuver may be used, placing the patient on hands and knees. Also, intentional fetal clavicular fracture has been used in some cases.
- The Zavenelli maneuver is used in extreme cases where other maneuvers have failed to effect fetal delivery. In this situation, the fetal head is replaced into the maternal pelvis. Nursing staff may be needed to administer a uterine relaxant such as terbutaline while the obstetrician is performing the fetal head replacement. Anesthesia is needed to provide pain control,

and ready the patient for an emergency cesarean delivery. Other staff members should be assigned to prepare the OR, transport the patient, alert pediatrics (if not yet done), record events, and inform the patient's family.

Maternal Cardiac Arrest

Cardiac arrest during pregnancy requires the expertise of both a code team and an obstetric team. The code team is necessary to manage the maternal resuscitation, but the obstetric team is needed for obstetrical interventions. Resuscitation of the pregnant woman should focus on stabilizing the patient, and delivery may be necessary to aid in this effort. Communication and coordination among Rapid Response team members is integral to maximizing maternal and fetal outcomes in this situation. Although most approaches to resuscitation in a pregnant patient are similar to the non-pregnant patient; the following aspects of this care should be considered:

- When performing chest compressions in the pregnant patient in the third trimester, hand placement should be more cephalad than in non-pregnant women to accommodate the upward displacement of the diaphragm by the gravid uterus. Chest compressions performed in the first half of pregnancy are done similarly to non-pregnancy.

- Caval compression in a pregnant patient in the supine position may result in a decrease in blood flow return to the heart, and further complicate the resuscitation efforts. Although supine positioning optimizes the vectors for effective chest compression in a non-pregnant patient, left lateral uterine displacement is necessary in a pregnant woman in order to minimize caval compression, optimize venous return, and generate cardiac output during CPR. Multiple methods are possible to achieve left lateral uterine displacement including: manual uterine displacement with the hand of a team member, tilt of the operating room table, placement of a resuscitation wedge, rolled up towels or blankets under the patient's hip, or tilting patient onto a rescuer (the rescuer sits on heels and places the patient on thighs as a wedge). A member of the Rapid Response team may be assigned the duty of ensuring this patient positioning is done during the resuscitation.

- IV access should be established above the diaphragm because any drugs administered via the femoral vein may not reach the maternal heart. If access is difficult to obtain, a member of the response team may be assigned the duty to place a central IV catheter, or contact personnel who are trained to do so within the institution.

- Continuous fetal heart monitoring is not necessary during the resuscitation of the patient because immediate intervention is focused on stabilizing the mother. If a monitor is already in place, or a team member is in the process of determining the presence of heart tones when defibrillation becomes necessary, all fetal monitors (both internal and external) must be removed prior to this intervention.

- Defibrillation and medication protocols are otherwise unchanged in the pregnant patient, and Advanced Cardiac Life Support (ACLS) drugs and doses are used. Do not delay defibrillation if indicated, and use usual recommended settings. Ventilate with 100% oxygen.

- Assess for hypovolemia and administer a fluid bolus if indicated. If blood loss is believed to be a contributive cause to the arrest, blood product repletion should be initiated as soon as possible during the event.

- In pregnancy, a difficult airway should be anticipated. An experienced provider is preferred for advanced airway placement, and should be assigned as part of any OB rapid response team. If the patient is receiving IV magnesium sulfate before the cardiac arrest, stop the magnesium and slowly administer IV calcium chloride 10 ml in 10% solution or calcium gluconate 30 ml in 10% solution over 5–10 minutes to reverse the effects of the magnesium.

- Irreversible brain damage can occur after 4–6 minutes of anoxia in the non-pregnant patient. Pregnant women become anoxic sooner than the non-pregnant because of their decreased functional residual capacity. A team member, often anesthesia, should be assigned to ensure a protected airway and provide oxygen for the patient.

- Despite uterine displacement, CPR may not restore spontaneous circulation or provide adequate cardiac output. Delivery of the fetus may relieve vena caval compression, and can result in a 60%–80% increase in cardiac output. If there has not been a maternal response to CPR measures after 4 minutes, and the uterus is greater than or equal to four fingerbreadths above the umbilicus (approximately 24 weeks estimated gestational age), consider expeditious perimortem cesarean delivery. In addition, intact fetal survival diminishes as the time between maternal death and delivery lengthens. Beginning delivery at 4 minutes into the resuscitation will more likely result in normal neonatal neurologic outcome.

- An emergency delivery kit should be located in labor and delivery and readily available. The duty to obtain this kit, and ensure that it is present at an OB rapid response, should be assigned to a team member. Often, this will be done by the OB charge nurse, as that individual will respond from the floor, and be an immediate team member present in most cases. Chest compressions should be continued without interruption during the perimortem cesarean delivery as should all other maternal resuscitative interventions in order to maximize fetal and maternal outcomes. Broad-spectrum antibiotics should be given to decrease the risk of maternal infection. It is also important to deliver the placenta and close the hysterotomy incision quickly to prevent further maternal blood loss.

- During a maternal cardiac arrest, identification and treatment of any possible precipitating causes is important. An algorithm suggested by the American Heart Association for this identification process is **BEAU – CHOPS** [12]:

Bleeding/DIC

Embolism – coronary/pulmonary/amniotic fluid

Anesthetic complications

Uterine atony

Cardiac disease – MI/ischemia/aortic dissection/ cardiomyopathy

Hypertension/preeclampsia/eclampsia

Other – differential diagnosis of standard ACLS guidelines

Placenta abuption/previa

Sepsis

Conclusion

An OB Rapid Response team allows an organized and quick response to emergencies, and focuses resources needed to benefit patient outcomes in areas of greatest need. The presence of two patients (mother and baby) in obstetrics, as well as unique physiologic changes inherent in pregnancy, may provide greater challenges in intervening in these cases. A trained team, with specific duties outlined, encourages a collaborative and efficient approach to these situations. Ensuring appropriate training for staff for these complications in obstetrics may require simulation drills or specific group instruction, and alterations in the process or duties assigned as indicated may be made as well. Each institution should design the team to meet their needs, and maximize the use of the staff resources they have available.

References

1 Devita MA, Bellomo R, Hillman K. Findings of the first consensus conference on medical emergency teams. *Critical Care Med.* 2006;34:2463–2478.

2 Jones DA, DeVita MA, Bellomo R. Rapid-response teams. *New Engl J Med.* 2011;365:139.

3 Kotsakis A, Lobos AT, Parshuram C, et al. Implementation of a multicenter rapid response system in pediatric academic hospitals is effective. *Pediatrics.* 2011;128(1):72–78.

4 Devita MA, Braithwaite RS, Mahidhara R. Use of medical emergency team responses to reduce hospital cardiopulmonary arrests. *Qual Saf Healthc.* 2004;13:251.

5 American College of Obstetricians and Gynecologists Committee on Patient Safety and Quality Improvement. American College of Obstetricians and Gyneocologists Committee opinion 353: medical emergency preparedness. *Obstet Gynecol.* 2006;108:1597–1599.

6 Berwick DM, Calkins DR, McCannon CJ, Hackbarth AD. The 100,000 lives campaign: setting a goal and a deadline for improving health care quality. *JAMA.* 2006;295:324.

7 Gosman GG, Baldisseri MR, Stein KL, et al. Introduction of an obstetric-specific medical emergency team for obstetric crises: implementation and experience. *Am J Obstet Gynecol.* 2008;198:367. e1–367.e7.

8 Skupski DW, Lowenwirt IP, Weinbaum FI, Brodsky D, Danek M, Eglinton GS. Improving hospital systems for care of women with major obstetric hemorrhage. *Obstet Gynecol.* 2006;107(5):977–983.

9 Clark EA, Fisher J, Arafeh J, Druzin M. Team training/simulation. *Clin Obstet Gynecol.* 2010; 53(1):265–277.

10 Deering S, Johnston LC, Colacchio K. Multidisciplinary teamwork and communication training. *Semin Perinatol*. 2011;35(2):89–96.

11 Sibai BM. Diagnosis, prevention, and management of eclampsia. *Obstet Gynecol*. 2005;105(2):402.

12 Vanden Hoek TL, Morrison LT, Shuster M, et al. Cardiac arrest in special situations: 2010 American Heart Association guidelines for cardiopulmonary resuscitation and emergency cardiovascular care. *Circulation*. 2010;122:S829–861.

Regulatory and Legal Implications

Mark S. DeFrancesco

Scenario #1: Moving procedures to the office: *You've recently started performing in-office procedures. You noticed that your first few patients were a bit uncomfortable when you did a global endometrial ablation, so you've contracted with a local anesthesiology group to come to your office and provide propofol sedation for your patients.*

You reason that you are not only providing an increased level of comfort for your patients, but you are also making the procedure more safe, as you will now have another physician present who can assist in the event of an emergency or an unusual reaction to the procedure or to medication administered.

Would it surprise you to learn that in many states in the USA you may have just broken the law and exposed yourself and your practice to prosecution and penalties?

Before the last 25 years or so, very little of what took place in the doctor's office was ever regulated by the government. The state did *license physicians* prior to that, as it does now, and the government regulated controlled drug dispensing ability, but regulating what physicians actually DO in the office, or HOW we do it, is a more recent phenomenon.

In 1967, the Clinical Laboratory Improvement Act (CLIA) was introduced. This act was largely the result of abuses in the cytology arena caused by overworked and/or less-than-proficient cytology technicians in some areas who missed significant diagnoses. After 21 years, it was amended to be more inclusive and provide better enforcement of the standards of the original Act. As a result, approximately 254,000 laboratories across the USA are now covered by CLIA, which in turn is overseen by the Centers for Medicare and Medicaid Services (CMS) or its designated accrediting agencies [1].

CLIA Waived tests: The CLIA amendment of 1988, which went into effect in 1992, clarified that certain tests that were simple and approved by the FDA for "home use" would be considered "waived" and not in need of a CLIA license for use in a medical office.

These include the following tests actually listed in the regulation [2]:

1. Dipstick or tablet reagent urinalysis (non-automated) for the following:

   - Bilirubin
   - Glucose
   - Hemoglobin
   - Ketone
   - Leukocytes
   - Nitrite
   - pH
   - Protein
   - Specific gravity
   - Urobilinogen

2. Fecal occult blood
3. Ovulation tests – visual color comparison tests for lutcinizing hormone
4. Urine pregnancy tests – visual color comparison tests
5. Erythrocyte sedimentation rate – non-automated
6. Hemoglobin–copper sulfate – non-automated
7. Blood glucose by monitoring devices cleared by the FDA specifically for home use
8. Spun micro-hematocrit
9. Hemoglobin by single analyte instruments with self-contained or component features to perform specimen/reagent interaction, providing direct measurement and readout (added on January 1, 1993).

Then in 1997, Congress further clarified that any test approved by the FDA for home use would automatically qualify for CLIA waiver. Some home tests have "professional versions" that must be approved for waiver, but generally these are granted expedited review. However, even if you are only performing CLIA-waived tests, you still need a CLIA "certificate of waiver" for your office.

Non-waived tests do in fact require a CLIA certificate, and these include "moderate complexity" tests and higher. The various types of certificates you can apply for are [3]:

Certificate of Waiver: This certificate is issued to a laboratory to perform only CLIA-waived tests.

Certificate for Provider-performed Microscopy Procedures (PPMP): This certificate is issued to a laboratory in which a physician, mid-level practitioner or dentist performs no tests other than the microscopy procedures. This certificate permits the laboratory to also perform waived tests.

Certificate of Registration: This certificate is issued to a laboratory that enables the entity to conduct moderate- or high-complexity laboratory testing or both until the entity is determined by survey to be in compliance with the CLIA regulations.

Certificate of Compliance: This certificate is issued to a laboratory after an inspection that finds the laboratory to be in compliance with all applicable CLIA requirements.

Certificate of Accreditation: This is a certificate that is issued to a laboratory on the basis of the laboratory's accreditation by an accreditation organization approved by the Health Care Financing Administration (HCFA).

In addition to CLIA, the Occupational Safety and Health Act (OSHA) has also become more involved in the medical office over the past quarter century. Enacted in 1971, OSHA was originally aimed at addressing safety in the workplace, particularly construction sites and chemical plants. Asbestos and related concerns were major drivers of OSHA's development.

However, with increasing awareness of AIDS, HIV, and blood-borne pathogens in general, there has been more focus on the medical office and other sites of healthcare provision since the 1991–2001 timeframe. A 2004 article cited a total of 480 violations of rules dealing with blood-borne pathogens in physician and dental offices resulting in penalties exceeding $285,000 [4].

Most of the regulations are things that we now take for granted: proper gloving and needle disposal and overall use of "universal precautions," for example, are "givens" in virtually all practices today, but there was a time when they were not, hence the need for the legislation and regulation.

OSHA and CLIA really pertain mostly to the physical plant and processes in the office, especially if any lab work is performed. OSHA, in particular, is seen as beneficial not only to patients but also to healthcare providers and staff. However, until recently, there was no real regulation of what could actually be performed in an office setting.

In addition to physical examinations and consultations, for instance, many primary care and specialty offices also provided treatment of "lumps and bumps," as they sometimes refer to very minor procedures, some not even requiring anything beyond local anesthesia. These could range from an incision and drainage of a furuncle or localized abscess to the removal of a skin tag or other questionable lesion, to the cleansing and suturing of a laceration. In most offices, these were very minor procedures and not a cause for alarm or concern.

However, as the mid-1980s saw the rise of the ambulatory surgery center (ASC) and more complex procedures were shifted from the hospital to the ASC, it was not exactly a quantum leap from the ASC to the office for some procedures that were more complex than what had traditionally been performed in the office venue. In addition, the managed-care industry, and the perceived need to lower the cost of care in general, added further pressure to move procedures to the office.

Liposuction was an early candidate for this move as many plastic surgeons (and some providers of other specialties) found it more convenient and more efficient to perform these procedures in the office setting. However, there were many tragically bad outcomes that focused the public's attention, and that of legislators at both the state and federal levels, on ambulatory safety.

In the ASC arena, this concern generally was resolved by facilities achieving accreditation from one of several nationally recognized and accepted accrediting agencies such as the American Association for Accreditation of Ambulatory Surgery Facilities (AAASF), the Accreditation Association for Ambulatory Health Care (AAAHC), and the Joint Commission. It has only been in the past few years that we've seen states require physician offices to be accredited to perform procedures requiring a certain level of anesthesia. According to data provided in a personal communication with the AAAHC in April of 2012, only 11 states currently require accreditation if certain thresholds (generally defined by the level of anesthesia in use) are met. These include Connecticut, Indiana, Nevada, New Jersey, New York, Ohio, Oregon, Pennsylvania, Rhode Island, South Carolina, and Washington State. There are several other states that, while they do not require accreditation, acccpt accreditation in lieu of state certification or licensing, again, if certain criteria are met. These include Arizona, California, Colorado, Florida, Indiana, Kansas, Kentucky, Louisiana, Massachusetts, North Carolina, Oregon, and Tennessee.

A key driver behind the move to enhance regulation of physician office activities has been a series of landmark studies over the past decade or so that have demonstrated significant (up to 10-fold!) and very worrisome differences in the incidences of severe adverse events and patient deaths when the performance of the same procedure by the same provider were compared in the offices versus the ASC [5].

The main takeaway point is that all physicians performing procedures in their offices really must be aware of all relevant state laws. For instance, you may be required to be licensed as a facility if you perform procedures requiring even moderate sedation. In at least 23 states you may be required to be accredited, licensed, or both in order to provide this level of care *legally*. Safety, however, is another issue. We are limiting our discussion in this chapter to only the regulatory and legal implications of in-office procedures. Other patient safety-related considerations are found elsewhere throughout this entire book.

Scenario #2: Embracing EMRs: *You've finally jumped onboard the train – you have embraced technology and are implementing an electronic medical record (EMR) and e-prescribing in your practice. You have spent countless hours discussing alternatives with various EMR vendors and are fully aware of all the great things these systems can do for you.*

To start with, your records and prescriptions will now be LEGIBLE! … and accessible even when you are at home or at the hospital. Patients' drug interactions and allergies will automatically pop up, enhancing patient safety and your own risk-management program in your practice. You'll be able to track abnormal lab results and be more certain that patients get the care they need, which is again good for the patient and good for your risk-management program!

In addition to the EMR and e-Rx capabilities, you have also created a site for your practice on a major social network and have a patient portal through which your patients can now interact with your practice. Patients will now be able to get their lab results, request refills and even schedule their own appointments. Finally, you will even have secure messaging available that will allow patients to ask you non-urgent questions when convenient for them and allow you to respond at a time convenient for you.

Through your social network site, you'll be able to post notices about changes in your practice providers, staff and/ or policies, as well as showcase some of the special services you may offer your patients. All this sounds very "cutting edge" and impressive …

However, there is a potential downside to technology too, and we must consider the risks attendant to the use of EMRs, e-Rx systems, and social networking sites.

There is no question that we are in an electronic world, and there are many useful tools that can make our offices more efficient and safer. Think about how labor-intensive a typical non-electronic office practice is. Everything is reduced to paper. Charts need to be filed, retrieved, and re-filed every time they are "touched" for anything, and they often are not where they are supposed to be when needed. Also, more than one person may need a particular chart at the same time. All in all, paper charts are very wasteful and inefficient.

When messages are generated over the weekend, it is also quite possible these messages may never be entered into a chart, particularly if you are covering for another physician or practice. If a patient is admitted to a hospital or seen in the emergency room anywhere while your office is closed, all of that information is not accessible, which could lead to tests being repeated at great expense to the system, or worse, some details of the medical history going unreported if the patient forgets to, declines to, or is unable to relate them.

An accessible, interoperable electronic health record (EHR) can solve virtually all of these problems. However, there are medico-legal risks attendant to the use of EHRs. This section will discuss what some of these risks are and suggest ways they may be avoided.

In addition to EHRs, there are many other electronic tools and social networking sites that can improve the efficiency and safety of a medical office practice. These include automated appointment reminders, secure messaging for lab results, interactive secure email for non-urgent questions, prescription refill requests, and even appointment scheduling. Think of how many things we all do in our daily life on the Internet: banking, investing, travel planning, and even courting our future mates; yet, we are way behind on allowing our patients to interact with our offices in the same way. Think of the time your staff could save if many of these routine tasks could be automated, and think of how much more satisfied your patients would be with your practice. Would you patronize a bank that discontinued all ATMs and forced clients to call or visit the bank to transact any business?

At present, we are slowly catching up as more practices are discovering the added value of electronic interactions with patients. This includes the judicious use of social networking sites like Facebook and Twitter. There are many policies being produced by organizations like the American Medical Association and the Federation of State Medical Boards to provide guidelines for physician–patient interaction on such sites, and the reader is referred to them [6,7].

Electronic prescriptions applications (e-prescribing) similarly offer substantial benefits. Improved legibility alone (as with EMRs) is a critical benefit of electronic prescribing, virtually eliminating issues with poor handwriting, shorthand, or names that may appear similar. Further, with built-in safety/decision support there is the reduced ability to write the wrong dosage, as the only options generally available are accepted dosages, and there is little or no chance of being off by a decimal point or more. Finally, many systems are linked to formulary checking software and drug interaction warning systems that can provide enhanced safety for patients.

Clearly, there are tremendous benefits to using electronic systems in the office for record keeping, prescribing and interacting with patients. However, there are also risks to doing so. First and foremost, security issues surrounding protected health information are far more complex. HIPAA violations are serious, and there is much greater opportunity for inadvertent violations with an electronic system than when all records were only in a paper chart that could be secured in locked file cabinets in a file room. Violations can result from simply faxing protected health information (PHI) to the wrong number or even releasing more information than was requested or needed to the proper location.

HIPAA is just one area where electronic systems may create susceptibility to litigation and malpractice liability. There are many ways the use of EMRs may actually raise the risk in a practice setting, particularly during the transition phase where there is a high learning curve involved. As Mangalmurti points out in an excellent article on the risks and benefits of going electronic, risks include the following [8]:

During initial implementation:

- Transition from paper to electronic may create documentation gaps.
- Failure to implement procedures that a prudent or reasonable provider would implement to avoid errors may leave physicians legally vulnerable.
- Inadequate training on systems may create error pathways.

- Errors by a new system may create incorrect or missing data entries.
- Failure of clinicians to use system consistently may lead to gaps in documentation and communication.
- System-wide EMR "bugs" and failures could affect clinical care adversely, leading to injuries and claims.

As systems mature in place:

- Email advice multiplies the number of clinical encounters that could give rise to claims and may heighten the risk of claims if advice is offered without thorough investigation and examination of the patient.
- More extensive documentation of clinical decisions and activity creates more discoverable evidence for plaintiffs, including metadata.
- Temptation to copy and paste patient histories instead of taking new histories risks missing new information and perpetuates previous mistakes.
- Failure to reply to patient emails in a timely fashion could constitute negligence and raise patient ire.
- Information overload could cause clinicians to miss important pieces of information.
- Departures from clinical-decision support care guidelines could bolster plaintiffs' case.

As EMRs and health information exchanges become widespread:

- Better access to clinical information through EMRs could create legal duties to act on the information.
- Widespread use of clinical-decision support may solidify standards of care that otherwise might be subject to debate.
- Rise of Health Information Exchanges may heighten clinicians' duties to search for patient information generated by other clinicians.
- Failure to adopt and use electronic technologies may constitute a deviation from the standard of care.

His article goes on to list generally agreed upon benefits that can and most likely will accrue:**After successful implementation:**

- EMR systems may lower discontinuities and errors in care, reducing adverse events and claims.
- EMR systems with integrated clinical-decision support may improve clinical decisions, reducing adverse events and claims.
- Better documentation of clinical decisions and activity – through user-entered data and metadata – may improve the ability to defend against malpractice claims when care was appropriate.

- Compliance with clinical-decision support care guidelines may constitute helpful evidence that the legal standard of care was met.
- Secure messaging may improve patient satisfaction and communication and reduce propensity to sue.
- Secure messaging could improve patient communication of clinically significant information, reducing adverse events and claims.

As EMRs and health information exchanges become widespread:

- Adherence to clinical-decision support recommendations may protect providers from liability.
- Rise of HIEs may facilitate sharing of information about cases, leading to better care and fewer claims.

It should be apparent, however, that given the newness of relative widespread use of electronic technology, much of the information in this section is opinion and theoretical. Hard evidence is lacking to substantiate some of the concerns or benefits expressed. At the very least, it would be prudent to be aware of these potential pitfalls and do your best to avoid falling into them.

Finally, the social networking phenomenon bears mentioning. Hardly a day goes by that you would not hear or see some reference to "liking us" or "following us" on one network or another. All practices can do the same thing, and many already do. Social networking can be a powerful way to market a practice, and maybe even have your patients help market you too. Keep in mind, though, that even without the use of social network sites, patients have always promoted (or not) our practice by "word of mouth." The nature of social networking can make these words travel much faster, and farther. So while such promotion hasn't changed, the format has, and patients now have a potentially huge megaphone with which to spread a specific message. Managing your practice's "online reputation" requires diligent oversight and care. Several companies now offer services to help monitor and manage your online presence and reputation.

An excellent article in the *Massachusetts Medical Law Report* from 2009 offered the following advice on how to avoid serious social media blunders [9]:

- *Be mindful of patient confidentiality.* As mentioned earlier, HIPAA concerns are very big, as violations can lead to significant compliance actions and/

or a lawsuit from an injured patient. Ironically, the patient may even be the actual source of the disclosed confidential information. Let's say a patient posts something on the physician's "wall," for instance, that unwittingly discloses her own medical information. Even though she was the source of the breach, she may still blame the doctor for allowing her to post it in the first place. As such, doctors are recommended to keep a firewall between their personal social media website pages and any patients', not allowing anyone to post on the practice's or physician's wall.

- *Remember that your patients are not your "friends."* The best approach to this issue is to set up a separate "practice" social network page and allow patients to "like" the practice.
- *Monitor your web presence regularly.* "Google yourself" is a good way to see what people are saying about you. Additionally, be wary of patients who might message you through a social network site, even if it is set up for your practice. You may have disclaimers warning patients against leaving important medical concerns, but some patients will invariably ignore such prohibitions and leave you serious messages. You cannot afford to miss an important message or even other important details from a patient's history of present illness or chief complaint, which could put you at serious medico-legal risk.
- *Take advice from online doctors' forums with a grain of salt.* There are many online chat rooms or bulletin boards exclusively for physicians where you may get a "curbside consult" on a particularly unusual case. Unless you actually know who is giving the advice, be wary about acting on the recommendations received in this way.
- *Be aware that you're never truly anonymous on the web.* Regardless of pseudonyms and screen names, anything you post can ultimately be traced back to you. It is generally good advice to never post anything anywhere that you would not want on the front page of the local newspaper or for that matter, on a 3' × 5' easel in a court of law!

The AMA has a succinct yet comprehensive policy on "professionalism" in the use of social media. It covers many of the same concepts outlined above and emphasizes the importance of appropriate boundaries when using any social media. It may be found at www.ama-assn.org/ama/pub/meeting/professionalism-social-media.shtml.

In this chapter we have explored the increasing regulatory role government and government-authorized proxy organizations play in the office practice. We have traced the history of some of the early examples of regulation within the office by OSHA and CLIA, and then discussed the evolution of a more formalized approach to patient safety in the office setting in response to the increasing complexity of procedures that we are now performing there on a regular basis. Regulatory agencies are playing a role in this legal formalization in many venues, and it is likely that all jurisdictions (if not the marketplace itself) will eventually demand proof of quality and safety in all healthcare settings.

Finally, the entire healthcare environment is changing. Our offices are becoming more complicated and also a lot busier. Technology, while disruptive in many ways, offers solutions that can help us care for more patients in a rational, efficient, and safe manner. However, as with any new tool, there is a learning curve and certain attendant risks. It is important that we recognize those risks and minimize them by education and appropriate accommodations in our workflow. Ultimately, the goal is to provide the best care we can for our patients.

References

1 CMS resources page. Centers for Medicare and Medicare Services website. www.cms.gov/Regulations-and-Guidance/Legislation/CLIA/index.html?redirect=/CLIA (accessed December 16, 2017).

2 FDA resources page. United States Food and Drug Administration website. www.fda.gov/MedicalDevices/DeviceRegulationandGuidance/IVDRegulatoryAssistance/ucm124202.htm (accessed March 17, 2013).

3 CMS resources page. Centers for Medicare and Medicare Services website. www.cms.gov/Regulations-and-Guidance/Legislation/CLIA/downloads//types_of_clia_certificates.pdf (accessed March 20, 2013).

4 Guglielmo W. A physician's guide to OSHA regulations. *Med Econ*. 2004;81:90.

5 Stumpf PG. Practical solutions to improve safety in the obstetrics/gynecology office setting and in the operating room. *Obstet Gynecol Clin N Am* 2008;35:19–35.

6 American Medical Association website. www.ama-assn.org/ama/pub/meeting/professionalism-social-media.shtml (accessed March 19, 2013).

7 Federation of State Medical Boards website. www.fsmb.org/pdf/nr-social.pdf (accessed March 20, 2013).

8 Mangalmurti SS, Murtagh L, Mello MM. Medical malpractice liability in the age of electronic health records. *N Engl J Med*. 2010;363(21):2060–2067.

9 Berkman E. Social Networking 101 for Physicians. *Massachusetts Medical Law Report*. October 19, 2009.

Patient Safety
A Patient's Perspective

Pamela K. Scarrow

Introduction

Patients who have a positive relationship with their physicians are often more compliant and consequently may have better outcomes than those who do not. In addition, studies have shown that when medical errors occur in patients with good relationships with their physician, they are less likely to seek legal intervention for an untoward outcome [1]. From a patient's perspective, there are several factors that are important, starting with communication.

Communication

Communication lies at the core of the physician–patient encounter. Research has shown that patient outcomes are improved with good communication [2]. In addition, poor communication is at the heart of the vast majority of complaints about clinicians' performance and a central factor in the large majority of medical errors. The Joint Commission has identified communication as one of the top three root causes of sentinel events from 2010 to 2012, and the second leading cause of maternal and perinatal events resulting in death and permanent loss of function from 2004 to 2012 [3]. Physicians should be aware that every time they walk into a clinical environment, the tone gets set for the patient and the team within seconds [4]. The patient's experience at the various encounters at the physician's office – on the phone, at intake at the front desk, with the nurse assistant, and the individual physician – will ultimately affect the patient's overall impression of the physician. The initial direct interactions with patients tend to strongly shape the experience and emotions that follow. For example, a woman presents to the office of her orthopedist in a wheelchair. She checks in with the receptionist, asks to use the facilities, and is given a key to the restroom with the assumption that her escort is a family member. In this particular case, the escort was a male taxi driver whom the patient clearly did not want taking her to use the restroom. Because physicians are ultimately responsible for the work of their staff, it is easy to see how a patient's opinion of a physician could be tainted by a negative encounter such as this.

By the time the physician enters the examination room, the patient has explained the reason for her visit to the nurse and then typically has to restate her presenting complaint to the physician. Too often, patients may be nervous or unprepared, not having notes or questions to refer to. Unfortunately, patients are commonly interrupted by the physician – as early as just 18 seconds into their conversation [5]. To optimize the physician–patient interaction, patients should be encouraged to ask questions; if there isn't enough time, another visit should be scheduled. Computer use also results in interruptions. With widespread use of electronic medical records, many physicians now enter data during the actual patient visit. It may be easier for the physician to look at the computer screen rather than the patient, thus diminishing the physician–patient dynamic. The physician may be able to access information more readily in an EHR, but the patient may miss the one-on-one interaction that is the hallmark of a personal visit.

Because of the power differential in knowledge and skills between patients and healthcare professionals, patients may only feel able to speak up and voice their concerns if they think the staff in charge of their care would be happy for them to do so [6]. The Agency for Healthcare Quality and Research (AHRQ) developed a campaign called "Questions are the Answer," which recommends that patients get more involved in their health care. In a DVD that physicians can show in their waiting rooms, Carolyn Clancy, MD, former AHRQ Director, states that "communication is a two-way street," suggesting that "sometimes Starbucks does a better job at this than we do in health care," in the way [baristas] take the order, repeat it back, and then give their colleague the order. In this way, she suggests, there is a kind of built-in error prevention.

Patient-centered Care

One of the six aims for improvement suggested by the Institute of Medicine (now known as the National Academy of Medicine) in its report *Crossing the Quality Chasm* is that healthcare should be patient-centered – providing care that is respectful of and responsive to individual patient preferences, needs, and values and ensuring that patient values guide all clinical decisions [7]. Put another way, three useful maxims of patient-centeredness are [4]: "The needs of the patient come first" [5]; "Nothing about me without me" [6]; "Every patient is the only patient" [8].

Being a patient is a profound social experience [4]. A major gap in the field of patient safety has been the absence of the patient's voice and perspective about her role in patient safety. Fortunately, this is beginning to change. Many physicians now consider patients and their families as part of the healthcare team, and incorporate patient-centeredness into their practices. Patient-centeredness is often explained in terms of patient satisfaction or the perceived social distance between the patient and the healthcare practitioner. In addition to the elements of patient-centeredness as defined by the Institute of Medicine, other components include information and education, emotional support, enhanced access to care, and involvement of family and friends [9]. Further, family-centered care amplifies person-centered care by recognizing and supporting the vital role of family caregivers.

One way to promote the concept of patient- and family-centered care is by establishing a patient and family advisory council, such as those at Massachusetts General Hospital. Massachusetts General incorporates the patient and family care experience into its planning and day-to-day operations through a variety of mechanisms, with the Patient and Family Advisory Councils (PFACs) serving as a primary vehicle for that collaboration [10]. In addition to the PFACs, patients and/or their family members serve on key service-based and hospital-wide committees. This approach provided for both frontline, grassroots involvement, as well as broad-based, hospital-wide impact.

The simple act of purposeful listening offers significant potential for patient-centered engagement and interaction. In 2008, the Consumers Advancing Patient Safety hosted the Chicago Patient Safety Workshop on consumer engagement in selected patient safety topics. Invitees included approximately 40 patients and family members, many of whom experienced harm because of healthcare systems failures, and equal numbers of other stakeholders and change agents. As part of this process, patients, family members, and healthcare professionals consented to be interviewed about their personal experiences with adverse medical events and any lessons learned. Comments from patients included:

> I want a doctor who is understanding. I want a doctor who is patient. I want a doctor who is going to sit there and listen to every word that I have to say.
>
> I'm a mother but I'm also a nurse, and so I'm thinking, I know what I'm talking about and they're not listening to me [9].

This study demonstrates the need for practitioners to reflect on their own capacity to listen, and why their beliefs, values, and practices might influence their understanding of patient-centered care [9]. The take-home message is that patient-centeredness means to listen, to be present, and to promote mutual understanding.

Cultural Sensitivity

The patient base for a given practice can contain significant ethnic diversity, which underlies the critical importance of understanding and sensitivity to cultural differences. Cultural awareness and sensitivity or competence is the knowledge and interpersonal skills that allow healthcare providers to understand, appreciate, and work with individuals from cultures other than their own. It involves an awareness and acceptance of cultural differences, self-awareness, knowledge of a patient's culture, and adaptation of skills [11]. Culture encompasses age, gender, faith, class, activity, profession, sexual orientation, disability, tastes, or any other practices or beliefs that individuals share. Lack of cultural awareness is one of many reasons why some groups receive inadequate medical care [12]. In the USA these include African-Americans, Hispanics or Latinos, other immigrant groups, migrant workers, and Lesbians/Bisexuals/Transgender populations. In maternity care, cultural sensitivity is particularly significant because many cultures have special traditions surrounding the birth of a child. The incorporation of cultural traditions can strengthen family ties and foster a better support system for the mother and her newborn.

Healthcare professionals may wish to consider using the 4 Cs of Culture as a mnemonic:

(1) What do you CALL your problem? This is another way of asking "what do you think is wrong?"

(2) What you think CAUSED your problem? This gets at the patient's beliefs regarding the source of the problem.

(3) How do you COPE with your condition? This is another way of asking "What have you done to try to make it better?"

(4) What are your CONCERNS regarding your condition? This is a way to ask the patient how the condition interferes with her life or her ability to function [13].

Situation: A couple has newly arrived in the United States and speaks no English. An interpreter is found, but appears to have difficulty interpreting the woman's symptoms. The couple apparently speaks a different regional dialect from the interpreter.

Solution: As soon as the physician notices that the interpreter is not able to communicate well with the couple, s/he needs to acknowledge the problem and seek an appropriate interpreter.

When patients have limited proficiency in speaking English, they may bring a friend or family member to serve as an interpreter. However, for a variety of reasons, including interpretation lapses and confidentiality, trained interpreters, rather than family members or friends, should be used for patients with limited proficiency in English. It is important that the patient feel confident that both she and her physician are correctly understood and that her confidentiality is maintained.

Health Literacy

A key aspect of patient-centered care is the concept of health literacy [4]. The Institute of Medicine uses the following definition of health literacy: the degree to which individuals have the capacity to obtain, process, and understand basic health information and services needed to make appropriate health decisions [14]. Simply put, health literacy is the ability to read, understand, and act on medical information. Health literacy can affect anyone regardless of educational level or socioeconomic background.

Accompanying his mother to her eye doctor appointment, the adult son initially didn't understand the surgical procedure, a trabeculectomy, recommended to treat his mother's glaucoma. The physician first explained the problem in complex medical terms. Only when she began to use analogies and simpler terms did the son grasp what the treatment would do. In this case, the son was an

obstetrician-gynecologist with years of medical training and practice, but who, despite his medical experience, did not know the optometric terms that explained his mother's surgery.

ACOG Today, April 2005

It is vital for patients to be proactive for themselves and to be their own advocate. However, physicians should encourage their patients to engage in the discussion by being a partner in the healthcare process. It is not enough for patients to ask questions; providers need to make sure they understand the answers. An algorithm for providing health-literate care in relation to the patient's experience can be found in Figure 13.1.

The American Medical Association has identified six steps to improve interpersonal communication with patients:

(1) Slow down. Communication can be improved by speaking slowly, and by spending just a small amount of additional time with each patient.

(2) Use plain, non-medical language.

(3) Show or draw pictures.

(4) Limit the amount of information provided, and repeat it. Information is best remembered when it is given in small pieces. Repetition further enhances recall.

(5) Use the "teach-back" technique.

(6) Create a shame-free environment: encourage questions [15].

The essential elements of the "teach-back" technique include the following:

- Do not ask a patient, "Do you understand?"
- Instead, ask patients to explain or demonstrate how they will undertake a recommended treatment or intervention.
- If the patient does not explain correctly, assume that *you* have not provided adequate teaching. Reteach the information using alternate approaches.

If the physician asks patients to "please tell me how you are going to explain this to your family" (using teach-back or return demonstration) [4], they are much more likely to demonstrate their lack of understanding.

At 30 years old, I went to the gynecologist and complained about part of this not working correctly. He said "we can repair that." Great! I didn't ask all the right questions. When I showed up two weeks later at the admissions office at the hospital, they put enough papers in front of me, I wasn't going to say "I don't read really

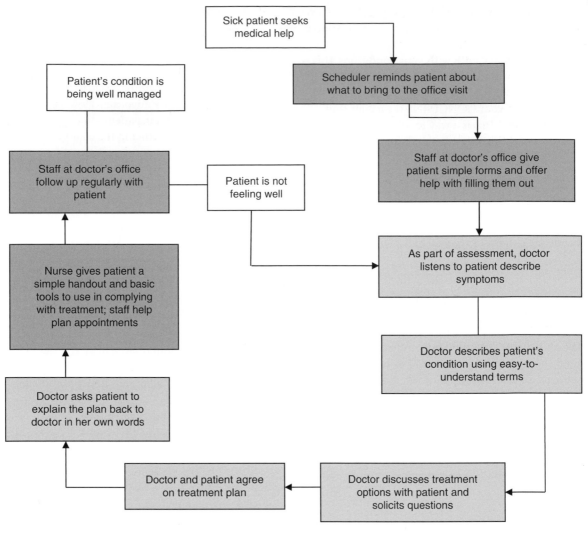

Direct action by doctor

Direct action by office or hospital staff

Effect on patient

Figure 13.1 Health-literate care: a patient's experience.

© Koh HK, Berwick DM, Clancy CM, et al. New federal policy initiatives to boost health literacy can help the nation move beyond the cycle of costly 'crisis care'. *Health Affairs* 2012;31:434–43.

well and I certainly don't read fast, and I'm concerned with some of these words" … and I wasn't going to reveal my sense of stupidity, so I signed everywhere they told me to sign, never read it, and then, a couple of weeks later in a follow-up office visit, the nurse said "how are feeling since your hysterectomy." I acted as normal as I could; inside [I'm thinking] how could I be so stupid as to allow somebody to take part of my body and I didn't know it.

Mrs. Cordell-Seiple
graduated high school; reads at 5th-grade level
Health literacy and patient safety:
help patients understand (AMA Foundation
2007) www.youtube.com/watch?v=cGtTZ_vxjyA

Informed Consent and Shared Decision-making

Patients scheduled for a surgical procedure or any of a number of treatments must provide their consent, having been advised of its risks, benefits, and alternatives, including not taking any action. Unfortunately, for various reasons, particularly medico-legal, many physicians focus more on the form documenting the consent rather than the informed consent process itself. If a patient has not been fully informed in advance of the procedure, she may not be able to honestly say, on the day of the surgery, that she understands its risks, benefits, and alternatives. Consequently, it is important that patients have a discussion with their provider, in advance of any procedure, about these elements. Decision aids may be useful, but the patient–physician conversation is also critical.

> **Actual Event:** When my mother was having cataract surgery, she was given a large packet of material to review in advance of the surgery. As her healthcare advocate, I read the material and shared with her all the pertinent information. When I returned the papers (one of them being an informed consent form) that needed to be signed to the manager in charge of scheduling the procedure, I mentioned to her that I was sure that Dr. Ophthalmologist realized that informed consent wasn't simply a form, but a process. Her response was to ask me whether I was a lawyer.

In recent years, the focus has expanded beyond informed consent to that of shared decision-making. Simple informed consent is appropriate in situations of significant risk, particularly when only one treatment option exists. Shared medical decision-making, however, applies when there are two or more reasonable medical options. Shared decision-making is a process in which the physician shares with the patient all relevant risk and benefit information on all treatment alternatives and the patient shares with the physician all relevant personal information that might make one treatment or side effect more or less tolerable than others [16]. Many patients appreciate being able to share in their treatment decision-making process. Oftentimes, the shared decision-making process leads to efficient healthcare and a more patient-centered model [9].

Tracking and Follow-up

Instead of being told that "no news is good news," more patients today are told how and when they will get their test results, laboratory work, or information from consultations. Unfortunately, systems failures may occur, which may have devastating results when test results are not relayed to patients in a timely manner. As a precaution, patients should be told that if they haven't received their test results within certain period of time, they should check back with the office. Many physicians' offices now have electronic portals through which patients can check on the results of their Pap tests and other routine tests. Regardless of the method for following up, patients should be encouraged to get the results of their tests – negative or positive.

Medication Safety

Medication errors are the leading cause of medical errors. Fortunately, many of these errors do not result in patient harm. Still, by virtue of sheer volume, significant numbers of patients suffer harm and even death due to medication errors every day. To reduce the likelihood of medication errors, for each medication prescribed, patients should be informed about its usage, dosage, expected benefits, and possible side effects, and every effort should be undertaken to ensure that this information is understood. Patients should be encouraged to ask about their medicines by asking the following questions:

- What is the medicine for?
- How am I supposed to take it and for how long?
- What side effects are likely? What do I do if they occur?
- Is this medicine safe to take with other medicines or dietary supplements I am taking?
- What food, drink, or activities should I avoid while taking this medicine [17]?

Patients are also responsible for informing their healthcare providers about the medications they currently take, including over-the-counter medicines and herbal supplements. They should be encouraged to keep a medication list that is updated on a regular basis. This list should include the name of the medication, the dosage, how it is taken (e.g., how many times per day, with meals, etc.), and its purpose. See more in Chapter 18 on Medication Safety.

Disclosure and Apology

Unfortunately, there will be times when a medical error occurs. Should an untoward event occur, the patient should be informed about what happened.

Patient Safety

Actual Event: It started with a sinus infection, although I was later told that this was simply an "incidental finding." Six months later, I was starting chemotherapy and radiation for Stage IIIA non-small cell lung cancer. I survived, but only because I was a proactive and engaged patient. I was never informed by a healthcare professional that there was a "worrisome" area on my lung. I learned this only because I asked for a copy of my chest x-ray report.

Upon receiving a copy of the report of my oncologist after having surgery, the otolaryngologist who initially ordered the chest x-ray and performed the outpatient sinus surgery called me to say simply, "I'm a good doctor." I was never given an apology.

As an informed patient, I knew to ask about the results of my chest x-ray. My father had died of lung cancer nearly 20 years earlier and I was a smoker. Had I not asked, I would never have known there were any issues until it was too late – when I was symptomatic.

Regardless of how a medical error occurs, whether by omission or by commission, how the patient is treated by her healthcare providers after the error will have a significant impact physically, emotionally, and psychologically as well.

Sorrel King's one-year old daughter died at Johns Hopkins Children's Center in 2001 as a result of a medical error. A fervent advocate for patient safety, she travels around the country telling her story to patients and providers alike. She says that families who have lost loved ones to medical mistakes want hospitals to do three things in the aftermath: Apologize. Tell the truth. And take steps to fix the problem [18]. For more, see Chapter 6 on Transparency and Disclosure.

A medical error may also have a serious impact on the provider. The unique problems facing second victims are addressed elsewhere in this publication.

Patient Rights and Responsibilities

According to Vincent and Coulter, the patient's perspective of quality includes access to care, responsiveness and empathy, good communication, clear information provision, appropriate treatment, relief of symptoms, improvement in health status, and, above all, safety and freedom from medical injury [19].

> **Box 13.1 The Patient's Role in Promoting Safety**
> The patient is involved in:
> - Helping to reach an accurate diagnosis.
> - Deciding on appropriate treatment or management strategy.

> - Choosing a suitably experienced and safe provider.
> - Ensuring that treatment is appropriately administered, monitored, and adhered to.
> - Identifying side effects or adverse events quickly and taking appropriate action.
>
> Vincent CA, Coulter A, Patient safety: what about the patient? Qual Saf Health Care 2002;11:76–80 [19].

Several organizations have developed formal positions about patient rights and responsibilities. Among them are the American Medical Association, The Joint Commission, and the National Patient Safety Foundation (NPSF). The NPSF's Universal Patient Compact (Table 13.1 includes principles of partnership between the healthcare partner and the patient). A central element among these position papers is the need for patients to provide full and honest information about their health status, including any medications they are taking, and ask questions as if they don't understand. The NPSF also promotes the *Ask Me 3* program, designed to enhance communication between healthcare providers and patients in order to improve health outcomes. The program encourages patients to understand the answers to three questions:

1. What is my main problem?
2. What do I need to do?
3. Why is it important for me to do this?

Patients should be encouraged to ask their providers these three simple but essential questions in every healthcare interaction. Likewise, providers should always encourage their patients to understand the answers to these three questions [20].

Conclusion

Patients come to their physicians during what may be vulnerable times in their lives. Various factors – including their presenting illness, pain, and the complexity of medical jargon – may affect their ability to understand and comply with recommended treatment and follow-up. Patients have certain responsibilities for providing information and complying with instructions; physicians should provide quality care and good service to their patients. Service has been defined as "the myriad characteristics that shape the experience of care for patients other than the technical quality of diagnostic and therapeutic procedures" [21]. Patients not only expect technical skills from their healthcare providers, but also dignity and respect. For example,

Table 13.1 National Patient Safety Foundation. The Universal Patient Compact™ Principles for Partnership © 2008 (reviewed and reaffirmed for Patient Safety Awareness Week 2011. Retrieved from www.npsf.org/?page=patientcompact, December 21, 2017.)

As your healthcare partner we pledge to:	As a patient I pledge to:
• Include you as a member of the team	• Be a responsible and active member of my healthcare team
• Treat you with respect, honesty, and compassion	• Treat you with respect, honesty, and consideration
• Always tell you the truth	• Always tell you the truth
• Include your family or advocate when you would like us to	• Respect the commitment you have made to healthcare and healing
• Hold ourselves to the highest quality and safety standards	• Give you the information that you need to treat me
• Be responsive and timely with our care and information to you	• Learn all that I can about my condition
• Help you to set goals for your healthcare and treatment plans	• Participate in decisions about my care
• Listen to you and answer your questions	• Understand my care plan to the best of my ability
• Provide information to you in a way you can understand	• Tell you what medications I am taking
• Respect your right to your own medical information	• Ask questions when I do not understand and until I do understand
• Respect your privacy and the privacy of your medical information	• Communicate any problems I have with the plan for my care
• Communicate openly about benefits and risks associated with any treatments	• Tell you if something about my health changes
• Provide you with information to help you make informed decisions about your care and treatment options	• Tell you if I have trouble reading
• Work with you, and other partners who treat you, in the coordination of your care	• Let you know if I have family, friends or an advocate to help me with my healthcare

correct medications and suture placements are issues of technical quality. Promptly answering questions to the patient's satisfaction in a clear, culturally relevant, easily understood manner is service quality [21].

The patient's perspective of patient safety and quality overall can be optimized by her real involvement in her own care. When she is viewed as an integral part of the healthcare team, compliance with treatment plans, her overall outcome, and general level of satisfaction will greatly improve.

References

1 Kraman SS, Hamm G. Risk management: extreme honesty may be the best policy. *Ann Intern Med.* 1999;131:963–967.

2 Roter DL, Hall JA. *Doctors Talking with Patients/Patients Talking with Doctors: Improving Communication in Medical Visits*, 2nd ed. Westport, CT: Praeger; 2006.

3 Sentinel event data: general information. Available at: www.jointcommission.org/assets/1/18/SE_General_Info_1995_4Q2012.pdf (retrieved December 21, 2017).

4 Leonard MW, Frankel A. The path to safe and reliable healthcare. *Patient Educ Couns.* 2010;80:288–292.

5 Groopman J. *How Doctors Think*. Boston, MA: Houghton Mifflin Company; 2007.

6 Davis RE, Sevdalis N, Jacklin R, Vincent CA. An examination of opportunities for the active patient in improving paient safety. *J Patient Saf.* 2012;8:36–43.

7 Institute of Medicine (US). *Crossing the Quality Chasm: A New Health System for the 21st Century*. Washington, DC: National Academies Press; 2001.

8 Berwick DM. What 'patient-centered' should mean: confessions of an extremist. *Health Aff.* 2009;28:w555–565.

9 Hovey RB, Dvorak ML, Burton T, et al. Patient safety: a consumer's perspective. *Qual Health Res.* 2011;21:662–672.

10 2017 PFAC Annual Report. Available at: www.massgeneral.org/patientadvisorycouncils/assets/pdf/MGH-PFAC-2016-17-FINAL.pdf (retrieved December 21, 2017).

11 Davis BJ, Voegtle KH. *Culturally Competent Health Care for Adolescents: A Guide for Primary Care Providers*. Chicago, IL: American Medical Association; 1994.

12 Institute of Medicine (US). *Unequal Treatment: Confronting Racial and Ethnic Disparities in Healthcare*. Washington, DC: National Academies Press; 2003.

13 Galanti G. *Cultural Sensitivity: A Pocket Guide for health care professionals*, 2nd edition. Oakbrook Terrace, IL: Joint Commission Resources; 2007.

14 Institute of Medicine (US). *Health Literacy: A Prescription to End Confusion*. Washington, DC: National Academies Press; 2004.

15 Weiss BD. *Health Literacy: A Manual for Clinicians*, 2nd ed. Chicago, IL: American Medical Association Foundation and American Medical Assocation; 2007.

16 Partnering with patients to improve safety. Committee Opinion No. 490. American College of Obstetricians and Gynecologists. *Obstet Gynecol*. 2011;117:1247–1249. (Committee Opinion No. 490 was reaffirmed in 2015).

17 Agency for Healthcare Research and Quality. 20 tips to help prevent medical errors. Patient Fact Sheet. AHRQ Publication No. 11-0089, September 2011. Agency for Healthcare Research and Quality, Rockville, MD. www.ahrq.gov/consumer/20tips.htm (retrieved December 21, 2017).

18 Niedowski E. From tragedy, a quest for safer care. *The Baltimore Sun*. December 15, 2003. www.baltimoresun.com/health/bal-te.sorrel15dec15,0,1054290.story (retrieved December 21, 2017).

19 Vincent CA, Coulter A. Patient safety: what about the patient? *Qual Saf Healthc*. 2002;11:76–80.

20 National Patient Safety Foundation. Ask Me 3™. www.npsf.org/?page=askme3 (retrieved December 21, 2017).

21 Kenagy JW, Berwick DM, Shore MF. Service quality in health care. *JAMA*. 2011;281:661–665.

Additional Resources

Agency for Healthcare Research and Quality. Questions are the answer. Rockville, Maryland. October 2011. www.ahrq.gov/questions/ (retrieved April 10, 2012).

American College of Obstetricians and Gynecologists. Patient Education Fact Sheet. Making the most of your health care visit. July 2011. www.acog.org/~/media/For%20Patients/pfs001.pdf?dmc=1&ts=20120408T1317492800 (retrieved April 8, 2012).

Consumers advancing patient safety. www.patientsafety.org/

Chapter

14

Safety Programs in a Community Hospital
Evidence-based Medicine Meets the Realities of Private Practice

Holly S. Puritz

Case Presentation

A 32-year-old woman, G2 P1, at 38 weeks gestation, requests elective induction in the next week as her husband is being deployed to Afghanistan. She had a previous uneventful 38-week delivery two years ago and has had an uncomplicated pregnancy. Her doctor is on call when she will be 38 5/7 weeks, but not yet full term. Given these circumstances, one could consider three different management scenarios:

1. Her attending obstetrician schedules her induction for his call day.
2. Her attending obstetrician attempts to schedule her induction, but the labor and delivery nurse refuses seeing that the patient is not yet 39 weeks gestation. The physician is told that the delivery cannot be scheduled for three more days and to discuss additional concerns with the unit medical director.
3. The attending obstetrician explains to his patient that he cannot schedule her induction until 39 completed weeks for safety reasons, and further explains that this is a hospital policy, which he supports. In addition, he provides a patient educational handout about obstetric safety, explaining the risks of late preterm birth.

Scenario 1 was the most common occurrence at our community hospital before an OB Safety Program was instituted 4 years ago. Scenario 2 was the initial response after the program was started. The hospital staff was quicker to adopt the requirement to avoid elective deliveries before 39 weeks gestation than many private physicians. With the safety program in place for four years, scenario 3 is now universally accepted as the new standard of care. Patients receive a unified safety message from both their attending obstetricians and the hospital staff with clear guidelines and explanations.

How did we get there and how can a community hospital get buy in for important safety programs from physicians in multiple private practices? Understanding physician behavior and what motivates that behavior is the key to instituting a successful safety program in a non-academic setting.

The Challenge of Behavior Change

Evidence-based guidelines are the mantra of medicine. The American College of Obstetricians and Gynecologists (ACOG) practice bulletins clearly spell out how we should care for our patients with specific clinical conditions and grades the strength of the evidence for those recommendations. Empirically, the implementation of such guidelines will improve the quality of care, and ultimately improve health outcomes for our patients. However, such implementation, with resultant clinician behavior change, remains a significant challenge. Most physicians try to keep up with the evidence, wanting to take the best care of their patients. Still, many physicians also believe that personal experience can supersede the need to follow guidelines, and that their patients are "different."

As such, there is commonly a significant gap between evidence-based guidelines and what occurs in daily practice. This chasm has been referred to as the "know–do gap" by both the World Health Organization and the Institute for Healthcare Improvement, and is increasingly recognized as an important research and improvement priority. Further, the adoption of research findings into practice among private practitioners can be particularly slow and haphazard.

It is often difficult to assess the quality of individual research studies and integrate appropriate changes into private practice. Even when physicians know what is right, the tools may be lacking to implement them into practice. For example, do we have the correct ratio of nurses to laboring patients in the hospital; do we have the right office policies and procedures or staff in place in the office setting to follow all the guidelines? Unfortunately, the answer for many in private practice and community hospitals is "no."

Another issue is getting physicians to accept change. When a complication is infrequent the chance of an individual physician encountering it is small. If the physician doesn't encounter a complication in his or her patients, they may minimize the concern with statements such as: "It's not my patient population" and "I don't have those complications." To change behavior we need to provide the physician with both accurate information and the skills and resources to allow implementation. We can only change behavior with clear messages that make sense to the target audience. Changes in physician behavior can also occur through their interaction with thought leaders and early adapters [1].

In certain instances, there are financial disincentives to adopt some of the necessary changes. Depending on the size of a practice, distance from the hospital and other logistics, it may be less safe to be on call and in the office simultaneously. On the other hand, the financial realities of a small practice may make it impossible to do otherwise. Consumer opinion plays a significant role in obstetrics. Birth plans, online blogs, and family involvement are common in our specialty. Local cultures can also be an obstacle to change. Anyone who has tried to implement changes to improve safety will have heard – "we've always done it this way and I have never had a problem" and "it's been good enough."

There is general agreement that there are significant lag times from when evidence-based guidelines become available and when they are observed in widespread practice. Even when there is general consensus about new guidelines, only 67% of physicians actually followed them. There is wide variation in the rates of acceptance of new guidelines among groups and between individuals within groups. Group practices seem more open to change than do smaller practices, and the addition of new physicians into a group can often bring new ideas and styles of practice. There is usually a culture of shared management in a group practice. Additionally, during the course of prenatal care, individual patients are co-managed by several providers in the group, and inpatient obstetric care often involves handoffs among different providers. This allows for review of the obstetric care given by any individual provider and inhibits any outlier behavior.

Regardless of the setting, deploying or posting guidelines by themselves without specific implementation strategies will typically end with failure. We know that practice guidelines alone simply do not work – the challenge is acceptance and implementation. Buy-in by the medial staff will be more likely if guidelines are developed collaboratively and with physician input. Multiple cohesive strategies are often needed, depending upon the scale of desired change. Among these, the use of academic detailers and enlisting local champions and opinion leaders can be particularly valuable [2–6].

Effective Strategies to Change Behavior

Engage Stakeholders – and Some Naysayers

The first step in setting up a safety program is the identification of local barriers to change and to engage stakeholders. Is there one powerful physician who is a naysayer? Is the head nurse not open to change? Is the hospital administration supportive of changes in practice and procedures? Is there adequate patient/family representation? Identifying these barriers and key stakeholders are early keys to program success.

Working with those most opposed to change may be difficult but it is critical for success. Engaging the naysayer in change may be a helpful strategy. Ask for their assistance in implementing a small part of the program that they may find acceptable. This strategy may lead to increased acceptance of the overall project. Flexibility in implementation across different facilities will also help. One hospital may start with one initiative, e.g., eliminating 39-week elective inductions, while another hospital may find physicians more interested in prevention of deep vein thrombosis. Finding common ground early will build a sense of community and collegiality that will enable more difficult issues to be tackled as the program matures. A hospital administrator must understand that programs that are successful on a medical floor may not necessarily work when used on a labor and delivery unit [7].

Use Different Strategies

Active Strategies

There are two types of strategies that have been used to change physician behavior – active and passive. Active strategies are the most effective and the more costly to implement. Two examples of an active strategy are the involvement of opinion leaders and academic detailers. *Academic detailers* are experts, often from the local medical schools, who would provide training and expertise on a new subject or change in practice pattern. Both of these strategies are active ways to target physicians by exposing them to experts [4]. Their knowledge of local solutions and problems will ensure the message is heard in a more favorable light.

Clinicians identified by their colleagues as being respected and effective communicators are needed to deliver the message and can serve as *opinion leaders*. An opinion leader can be seen as a change agent. She/he has significant social influence over others in the group. An opinion leader will have strong leadership skills and makes others want to follow. That person can facilitate local acceptance of a given intervention. They are the ones to help lead a new program and encourage early acceptance.

The use of academic detailing is a useful tool when used in conjunction with an opinion leader. Leaders from an academic setting are also well received and have a significant influence on the standard of care in the community and do well in the role of academic detailers. A physician from a research or academic setting is used to outline the new program based on the best available evidence. The detailer would meet with providers to give information with the intent of changing the physicians' behavior and performance. It can be done in a large group setting, but is also helpful when delivered *via* face-to-face time with small groups. When individual concerns are heard and addressed in a more private setting, acceptance of a new program increases dramatically [8]. Physicians feel especially valued when those meetings take place in their own office.

Passive Strategies

Passive strategies typically involve limited or no direct personal interactions, and are also useful behavior-changing tools in some settings. They have been shown to work very well on medical services but not as well in obstetrics. Common examples are chart reminders, audit and feedback initiatives, and educational programs. Mailings and continuing education reminders are also passive ways to improve knowledge by dissemination of important information and guidelines. They are often overlooked by busy physicians in private practice or dismissed as nuisances from medical records and not seen as valuable to the physicians.

Initiate Quality Improvement Methods

Other strategies that can be used include quality improvement methods, which bring together numerous tools and strategies to improve clinical processes, operations, or systems (see Chapter 9 on QI tools). There are a number of potentially high-impact methodologies available, including the Model for Improvement from the Institute for Healthcare Quality, Lean, Six Sigma, and many more. Further, many health systems now employ performance, safety, and quality improvement professionals. Importantly, these methods can be utilized across a broad array of settings, from very focused clinical processes, to larger systems-level improvements. A critical element of any improvement effort, yet one that often gets too little attention, is measurement. The design of metrics can be very simple, but it can also easily miss its mark. High-quality metrics are typically jointly derived from the input of key stakeholders, they are meaningful and important, they are obtainable, and they are specific. Simply measuring inputs and outcomes will often not suffice. Robust metrics for important clinical processes are commonly a cornerstone in any QI effort. See related chapters in this text, or plan to meet with your local improvement professionals.

Labor and Delivery Units are Very Different from Medical Units

Strategies that work well in other hospital departments may fail when they are utilized on a labor and delivery unit or similar venue. The high-acuity of intrapartum care, requiring intensive monitoring over a span of time that often includes multiple handoffs, is somewhat unique compared to many inpatient settings. There is also commonly an acute sensitivity to medico-legal concerns given the relatively high litigation risk with obstetric care.

The need to act quickly without time for reflection is the hallmark of many significant obstetric decisions, more akin to a trauma unit than a medical unit. Lastly, the patient's family is often intimately involved in decision-making, and, they are commonly present in the patient rooms and operating theaters. Nowhere else in the hospital does the family accompany a patient into the operating room. Additionally, patients report to the hospital when they are not sick in the traditional sense, so expectations are dramatically altered.

Many studies document what works to improve quality of care in obstetrics [9–11]. Audit and feedback worked well to reduce nosocomial infection rates. Opinion leaders reduced cesarean delivery rates. The most effective way to change behavior on a labor and delivery unit was a combination of an opinion leader, academic detailing, educational sessions, and use of audit and feedback. This can save significant time when designing a new program in an obstetric unit of a community hospital. Knowing the local culture and having an opinion leader set the stage for a desired change are good first steps. One effective means of understanding local culture is to use a safety culture or attitude survey, such as the one available from the Agency for Healthcare Research and Quality. Not only can this provide an idea of the degree of challenge ahead, but it can also highlight some important deficits that may need to be addressed foremost. Understanding and addressing local barriers to change is paramount for a safety program to be successful. Some examples of barriers include resistance of a key physician leader, hospital policies that make change difficult to implement, poor team culture, or lack of understanding as to why the change is important or needed.

Finally, when choosing to embark on an improvement program, it may be useful to begin with a small-scale project with readily accessible metrics and with a high likelihood of success. Doing so will likely generate increasing enthusiasm for such work, and the momentum to move onto more challenging improvement projects.

The "OB Right" Program

Sentara Health System, a multihospital system in Virginia, initiated an obstetrical safety program in 2006. Only one of the hospitals was an academic center. The other five were community hospitals with separate staffs. From the outset, we sought and received buy-in from nurse managers and physician leaders in each of the hospitals. Critical for success, there was financial and staff support from the health

system. A program manager was hired at the beginning of the process to help implement and disseminate the new program to each of the hospitals. Physicians relied on a strong support staff to implement the variety of projects discussed at interactive meetings and brainstorming sessions. The hospital concurrently had purchased an Electronic Medical Record system (EMR), which, through the use of templates, helped standardize protocols and documentation.

A website was started to promote education and near-miss reporting. Interested physicians from all practices were welcomed on any and all committees. Financial reimbursement was provided to individuals to compensate them for their time spent in meetings, demonstrating that their contributions were valued. There was a kick-off dinner to introduce the concept of "safety first and sharing a culture of safety" with excellent attendance by nursing and medical staff. The program was not without its problems. Many of the physicians did not initially feel that a change was needed, or that there was any perceived benefit to the change.

Elective Induction Bundle – the Program and the Evidence

The group decided to address elective induction labor and oxytocin protocols as their first safety initiative. Induction of labor is one of the most common practices in obstetrics, and there are many reasons for elective induction of labor. These include patient desire, physician convenience, improved chances for attendance by their own physician, avoidance of prolonged pregnancy and possibly stillbirth, and daytime delivery with more perinatal personnel. However, such practices do not come without risk. Specific risks include perinatal morbidities associated with late preterm and early term deliveries. Also, the consequent use of oxytocin and other induction methods heralds additional risks, including maternal or fetal compromise, particularly without adherence to strict protocols.

There is compelling evidence that a standardized oxytocin protocol would improve outcomes [12,13]. There also was mounting evidence supporting improved outcomes through reducing late preterm and early term deliveries.

Practically speaking, the actual scheduling of inductions at many community hospitals created extra nursing activities that took the nurses away from

Table 14.1 Calculating Bishop score.

The higher the score, the more favorable the cervix with the clinical trial showing a score of 9 or more associated with 100% successful inductions

Criteria	0	1	2	3
Dilation	0	1–2	3–4	5–6
Effacement (%)	0–30	40–50	60–70	80
Station	–3	–2	–1	+1, +2
Consistency	Firm	Medium	Soft	
Position	Posterior	Middle	Anterior	

direct patient care. These activities included scheduling and rescheduling when the unit was busy, often requiring the nurses to call both the patients and the physician offices multiple times. Prior to the OB Right program, elective induction of labor not uncommonly occurred before 39 weeks gestational age. The attending physician was the final arbiter for all clinical decisions. The culture discouraged questioning of these decisions by the nursing staff. Many units were understaffed, and elective inductions of labor exacerbated this situation, raising concerns among nurses regarding safety. Many elective inductions of labor were being done at great expense and inefficient use of limited staff. Patients were often in the hospital for two to three days for inductions due to an unfavorable cervix (see Table 14.1).

Newborn Intensive Care Unit (NICU) admissions increased among patients who were induced and required cervical ripening agents [14]. Cesarean section rates were increased among multiparous patients who were induced and were highest when cervical ripening agents were used. The costs to the Sentara hospitals were 17.4% higher among patients who were induced. Patients should be informed of these risks when they are offered or request an elective induction of labor especially with an unfavorable cervix. Avoiding elective labor inductions that may have significant risks and unproven benefit may aid efforts to reduce the primary section rate and make for a safer labor and delivery unit.

Recommending an induction labor to a nulliparous patient increases her likelihood of a cesarean section by an average of 10%. Maternal morbidity may not occur at the index delivery, but is more likely with subsequent deliveries. Gestational age and Bishop score should both be considered before scheduling an elective induction of labor. A Bishop score greater than 9 has been recommended as the cutoff to be used for allowing elective induction. Elective induction of labor with a Bishop score of < 5 should be especially discouraged for women over 30 years of age and/or a body mass index (BMI) greater than 30 because of an increased risk for cesarean section.

How was the Evidence about the Risk Benefit Ratio for Elective Induction used in an OB Safety Program?

Opinion leaders within the community hospitals and academic detailers (Maternal Fetal Medicine (MFM) attendings) presented the evidence regarding issues with elective induction of labor at department meetings and at individual practices. Community-based lectures, eligible for Continuing Medical Education credit, were also archived and available on the OB Right website. Once the evidence was reviewed, an elective induction bundle was created by the OB Right program. It was endorsed by all the community hospitals and is now standard of care in all Sentara hospitals. The elective induction bundle consists of four separate entities, all of which must be in place before an elective induction of labor can occur. The bundle includes:

1. Assessment and documentation of gestational age greater than 39 weeks
2. Monitoring and assessment of the fetal heart rate prior to initiation of oxytocin
3. Pelvic assessment and cervical exam documented by the physician within 72 hours of admission or at time of admission
4. Standardized protocols for administration of oxytocin and diagnosis and management of hyperstimulation.

When a physician's office now calls to schedule an elective induction of labor, the patient must be at least 39 weeks 0 days gestation on the day of admission. Elective inductions cannot be scheduled more than 2 weeks in advance. If the patient will not be at least 39 weeks gestation at the time of the scheduled admission, the induction is not scheduled. Instead, the physician's office is told that the medical director of the unit will call and personally speak to the admitting physician. It was remarkable to observe how effectively that simple step changed physician behavior. Very few physicians wanted to defend themselves to their colleague when it was clear that the bundle was not being followed. Instead, they would often reschedule the induction to a more appropriate date.

The physician was also required to document fetal position, estimated fetal weight, and pelvic assessment and cervical exam as part of their admission note – a simple request that forced physicians to reconsider the need for an elective induction. With a multidisciplinary committee overseeing the program, an improved working relationship between the nurses and physicians developed. The implementation of common policies and procedures also helped the nurses. The nurses felt more comfortable to speak up and question a physician if it appeared that an induction was not indicated or a policy was not being followed. Nurses were encouraged to advocate on behalf of the patient as well as educate the patient as to the risk of late preterm delivery.

The rate of elective induction of labor fell sharply in the four years since this program has been implemented. A recent Leapfrog Hospital Survey reviewed hospital rates of deliveries prior to 39 weeks gestational age. The national average was 18%, the Virginia State Average was 19%, and the six Sentara Hospitals with the OB right program had rates of 0%–3%.

Similar protocols have been put in place for elective cesarean section. They cannot be scheduled prior to 39 weeks and 0 days. They can be scheduled 60 days in advance, but the nurses review the prenatal record carefully for appropriate gestational age prior to the patient being admitted. Nurses are empowered to send patients home (with their physician's approval) when a patient arrives for her cesarean section that has been mistakenly scheduled too early. They and the physicians have become strong advocates of avoiding late preterm birth. Physicians and nurses are now able to discuss the concerns with the patient with a clear and consistent message so that the patients are willing to delay a scheduled cesarean delivery.

There will always be unanticipated issues once a new system is implemented. For example, one such concern was related to cervical ripening with prostaglandin. Could a patient be admitted at 38 weeks and

6 days for cervical ripening with the induction starting the next day? It is certainly a small point, but physician behavior has changed in such a way that it was brought up for discussion at the ongoing meetings of the OB Right Program Committee. Physicians wanted clinical practice to be standardized. The decision was made that a patient could not be admitted until she completed 39 weeks gestation. Future areas for discussion include mandating that the Bishop score be part of the elective induction bundle and screening all medically indicated inductions using similar criteria currently used to screen elective inductions. There is also ongoing collaboration with the MFM department about their current recommendation to deliver even a well-controlled gestational diabetic at 39 weeks gestation regardless of her Bishop score.

How was the Information Disseminated?

Opinion leaders (usually the local medical director of the obstetrical unit) as well as academic detailers personally reviewed the patient data with individual groups at department meetings and group practices. The evidence was reviewed without making it personal. We shared with them the concept that everyone is responsible to discourage elective induction of labor. We all should provide women who desire such intervention an accurate assessment of the anticipated labor course, the risk of complications related to labor induction as well as the anticipated benefits of watchful observation. We were respectful of their observation that many of their patients had done well when electively delivered earlier than 39 weeks but noted that the potential risks were clear. Physicians felt it was helpful to be able to tell their patients that hospital policy prevented them from making exceptions regarding elective induction of labor.

We used additional educational material in the form of a newsletter and web page to disseminate information. We also tracked rates of induction, numbers of elective inductions prior to 39 weeks and induction requiring multiple days. Near-miss reporting forms were placed on all units for anyone to complete. The reported events were analyzed by a committee of physicians and nurses. Lessons learned were communicated to all the obstetrical staff. Educating the hospital coders improved the accuracy of reporting. This gave the physicians more confidence that reported events were correct and useful as a reasonable quality indicator.

Over time we changed the culture of the different units and the behavior of the physicians. Our elective induction rate < 39 weeks now approaches 0% in all Sentara hospitals. We consistently disseminated clear and consistent messages of any changes before they took place. Feedback was solicited when any new policy was implemented. Appropriate changes were made when warranted. The medical directors of each unit were very responsive to any physician when there was a concern or a question about changes that were being instituted. Nurses referred physicians' questions to the medical director so that a doctor to doctor conversation could be held to explain new programs. Larger group practices were asked to be more accommodating when it came to scheduling inductions so that small groups or solo practitioners could have elective patients come in earlier in the day. It was easier for a larger group to have patients come in later in the day to start an induction when the doctor on call had the next day off. Nurses were empowered to question the reasons for inductions. They had clear-cut guidelines to cite when they were questioned by a physician.

Monthly multidisciplinary meetings were scheduled in each unit with representatives from all concerned parties: obstetrics, pediatrics, anesthesia, nursing, and hospital administration to help resolve issues collaboratively. We encourage physician and nursing involvement on all committees. Individual concerns were addressed directly by the medical director who is an opinion leader and academic detailer.

We also provided multiple CME opportunities supported by the hospital system to help standardize communication. Even simple issues, such as the definition of hyperstimulation, varied widely prior to these educational programs. Programs have included interpretation of fetal heart rate tracing, shoulder dystocia training, fetal acid base physiology, maternal haemorrhage, and maternal infections. Physicians and nurses are required to take these courses for staff privileging. Simulations are also being planned. Malpractice rate reductions for participation in OB Right were established. Physicians saw a positive and direct benefit from their participation in the new safety program.

Summary

Physicians have learned to discuss new issues before embarking on a course of action that might be detrimental to patient safety. They have embraced standardized protocols that ultimately protect them and

their patients. Collegiality improved between physicians and nurses as the goal of our maternity units become clear – to care for mothers and babies in a safe environment where evidence-based guidelines and standardization inform the care we provide.

References

1 Doumit G, Graham I, Grimshaw J, Smith A, Wright F. Opinion leaders and changes over time: a survey. *Implementation Sci.* 2011; 6:117.

2 Flodgren G, Parmelli E, Doumit G, et al. Local opinion leaders: effects on professional practice and health care outcomes. *The Cochrane Database of System Rev.* 2011; issue 8:CD000125.

3 Holmgren S, Silfver K, Lind C, Nordström L. Oxytocin augmentation during labor: how to implement medical guidelines into clinical practice. *Sex Reprod Healthc.* 2011;2:149–152.

4 Honigfeld L, Chandhok L, Spiegelman K. Engaging pediatricians in developmental screening: the effectiveness of academic detailing. *J Autism Dev Disord.* 2012;42:1175–1182.

5 Wright S, Trott A, Lindsell C, Smith C, Gibler W. Creating a system to facilitate translation of evidence into standardized clinical practice: a preliminary report. *Ann Emerg Med.* 2008;51(1):80–86.

6 Nast A, Erdmann R, Hofelich V, et al. Do guidelines change the way we treat? Studying prescription behaviour among private practitioners before and after the publication of the German Psoriasis Guidelines. *Arch Dermatol Res.* 2009;301:553–559.

7 Davies K. Evidence-based medicine: is the evidence out there for primary care clinicians? *Health Inform Libraries.* 2011;28:285–293.

8 Simpson F, Doig G. The relative effectiveness of practice change interventions in overcoming common barriers to change: a survey of 14 hospitals with experience implementing evidence-based guidelines. *J Eval Clin Pract.* 2007;13:709–715.

9 Penney G, Foy R. Do clinical guidelines enhance safe practice in obstetrics and gynaecology? *Best Pract Res Clin Obstet Gynaecol.* 2007; 21(4): 657–673.

10 Main EK, Morton CH, Hopkins D, Giuliani G, Melsop K, Gould JB. *Cesarean Deliveries, Outcomes, and Opportunities for Change in California: Toward a Public Agenda for Maternity Care Safety and Quality.* Palo Alto, CA: CMQCC; 2011.

11 Althabe F, Bergel E, Belizan JM, et al. A cluster randomized controlled trial of a behavioral intervention to facilitate the development and implementation of clinical practice guidelines in Latin American maternity hospitals: the Guidelines

Trial: Study protocol. *BMC Womens Health.* 2005;5(1):4.

12 Jonsson M, Nordén-Lindeberg S, Östlund I, Hanson U. Metabolic acidosis at birth and suboptimal care – illustration of the gap between knowledge and clinical practice. *BJOG.* 2009;116:1453–1460.

13 Clark S, Belfort M, Dildy G, Meyers T. Reducing obstetric litigation through alterations in practice patterns. *Obstet Gynecol.* 2008; 112(6):1279–1283.

14 Ehrenthal D, Hoffman M, Jiang X, Ostrum G. Neonatal outcomes after implementation of guidelines limiting elective delivery before 39 weeks of gestation. *ACOG.* 2011; 118(5):1047–1055.

Improving Perinatal Safety in an Integrated Healthcare System

Hans P. Cassagnol and Harry Mateer

Safe and Reliable Obstetrical Care

Providing safe and reliable care is the goal of every healthcare provider, especially in obstetrics. The field of obstetrics is currently in a state of crisis. It is under attack by numerous forces: lack of access to care, finances, depletion of the work force, and provider burn out, just to name a few. In this chapter, we will make the argument that an Integrated Healthcare Delivery System is one of the novel ways to improve safety and reliability in obstetrics in the face of all these challenges [1–4].

Our experience stems from working at Geisinger Health System for greater than 10 years. The system provides care for about 5,000 pregnancies and more than 4,500 deliveries per year. It has a robust electronic medical record (EMR). In the Geisinger Women's Health Service Line (WHSL), there are 76 Clinicians (30 MDs, 12 Residents, 10 Midwives, 14 NPs, 10 PAs), 24 Clinic Sites, and five Hospitals (two non-Geisinger). The coverage area is about 20,000 square miles in northeastern Pennsylvania. The system is deeply involved in redesigning care in order to increase efficiency, improve outcomes, and decrease costs. The episodic care provided to pregnant patients is an example of one such model of care. Recent analyses of our outcomes were conducted for the target areas of C-section rates, Diabetes, Preterm Labor & Delivery, Maternal Wellness, Fetal & Newborn Wellness, Preeclampsia & Hypertension, Induction of Labor Rate, Smoking Cessation, and Postpartum depression. The most significant findings, which directly impact costs, include NICU admissions rate decrease of about 33%, NICU length of stay decreased by two days, and birth trauma rate decreased to 0.59/1,000 from 2/1,000 (vs. national rate 2.31/1,000). We also offer VBAC, Lactation services, Nutrition counseling, Mental Health Services, Dula services, and Midwifery Program. Over the past five years, we have been using our proprietary ProvenCare model designed by our team, which has helped improve quality metrics. We have maintained our net profit margin in obstetrical services in the face of decreases in reimbursement and a 15% increase in labor costs.

Market Forces Impacting Safety

The profit margin for a healthcare entity involved in women's health offering the entire scope of women's healthcare services has been diminishing, while at the same time, niche services such as outpatient surgery programs, surgical centers of excellence, and minimally invasive surgical programs are demonstrating growth in profit margins. These surgical centers have grown by 45% over the past 10 years, to a current number of about 300 in Pennsylvania. Medical malpractice premiums for a full-scope practicing Ob/Gyn is one of the highest of all medical subspecialties in most states, having increased by at least 95% over the last 10 years in Pennsylvania. Since 1997, the number of obstetricians has declined by 15%–25% in various regions of Pennsylvania. As a result, almost 40 hospitals have stopped offering obstetrical care in Pennsylvania. This is a decrease of about 30% in obstetrical capacity. During this same period, the specialty has seen continuous decreases in reimbursement for services. Meanwhile, demand for these services continues to rise. One-fourth of hospital discharges in the US are related to childbearing. New healthcare laws will increase the percentage of the population with insurance. The US birth rate is on the rise [US – CDC, increase in > 40 y/o and slowing of decline in all other age groups (16–17)]. Our catchment area can support at least an additional 25 Providers. The current wait time for a new patient to see a provider is approximately 8 weeks (range: 6–14 weeks). Yet, more hospitals are planning to discontinue obstetrical services. Confounding these facts, the new healthcare law will invariably cut reimbursement for these services in the near future.

For obstetrical services, we would expect less competition. Although this may initially appear enticing, the details are in fact troubling when reviewed further. The brunt of the negative impact (delivery of care cost, revenue, and liability) will be borne by obstetrical providers. Furthermore, niche markets are likely to proliferate due to the more favorable bottom line (less cost for delivery of care, much less liability, and positive profit margin). This means more outpatient surgery programs, surgical centers of excellence and minimally invasive surgical programs. Such growth driven programs will compete with obstetrical services for the profitable portion of women's health services. Recruitment and retention of obstetrical providers will be a major challenge. Without adequate numbers of providers, operational efficiency and quality of obstetrical services will be difficult to maintain.

How do you deliver safe and reliable care with less providers, cover a large geographic area, and at a lower cost?

The Geisinger Experience

In 2005, Geisinger Health System's (GHS) executive leadership accepted the challenge to demonstrate that a large integrated healthcare delivery system, supported by an electronic health record (EHR), could successfully re-engineer a complicated clinical process, reduce unwarranted variation, and reliably deliver evidence-based care for a subpopulation of patients. The program was named ProvenCare®. Starting with elective coronary artery bypass graft (CABG), we demonstrated that embedding evidence-based medicine into the workflow, applying the principles of reliability science (standardization, error proofing, and failure mode redesign) to the care redesign process, and engaging patients in their care, the right care was delivered 100% of the time, resulting in better patient outcomes [2]. This model has been replicated for elective total hip replacement and cataract surgery. In 2007 GHS applied the model to the new percutaneous coronary intervention (PCI) mesosystem, which has subsequently attained similar levels of reliability. Clearly the ProvenCare® model works for acute inpatient interventions, but we wondered if it was adaptable to more complicated, longer-term conditions of "wellness" such as perinatal care.

Unwarranted variation in care, the major driver of poor quality and safety [5–7], can lead to devastating outcomes for mother and child. In 2005 the Institute of Healthcare Improvement (IHI) launched the Idealized Design of Perinatal Care collaborative in an effort to improve care during labor and delivery through process redesign and implementation of an induction and an augmentation bundle of care. In 2007 WHSL leadership determined that they would incorporate this initiative into a Perinatal ProvenCare pathway to support the delivery of evidence-based care for patients throughout pregnancy and the postpartum period. Unlike previous ProvenCare initiatives, the perinatal initiative encompassed both inpatient and outpatient care, and involved a significantly larger number of practice sites and clinicians [8].

Paul Batalden, MD proposes that purposeful integration of generalizable scientific evidence into the "local" care system with a focus on measurable outcomes can affect an improvement in daily patient care. We suggest that the application of Batalden's model to the perinatal population catalyzed an evolution of the established ProvenCare model to one more broadly applicable [9].

All ProvenCare initiatives rely on evidence-based medicine. The perinatal initiative extensively utilized the American College of Obstetricians and Gynecology (ACOG) guidelines (also American Academy of Pediatrics (AAP), Institute for Healthcare Improvement (IHI), Institute for Clinical Systems Improvement (ICSI), Centers for Disease Control and Prevention (CDC)), making elements of care generalizable across all 24 OB practices (spanning 30 counties and 200 miles east to west). All elements were transferable across practice types regardless of variation of patient population across counties and how clinics tailor their care to meet specific patient needs. ProvenCare Perinatal incorporates all prenatal clinic visits, delivery and inpatient care, and postpartum care; an average of 13 clinic visits for each pregnant patient plus her inpatient stay. The breadth and depth of the evidence far exceeded prior ProvenCare initiatives, driving changes in our process for establishing staff engagement from across the system and in how we used the EHR to support the work [10–14].

ProvenCare Perinatal differed from prior GHS initiatives in geography and scope as well as its fundamental definition and local context. Unlike patients with acute problems like hip degeneration (which requires hip replacement) or blocked arteries (which may require CABG surgery), pregnancy is a state of wellness and is typically an exciting time for this cohort of patients. Patients are followed in 24 Geisinger sites, some of which are high-volume clinics dedicated solely to women's health and others that are low-volume primary care sites with visiting obstetricians. Babies are delivered at two GHS tertiary care centers and two non-GHS community hospitals.

Significant workflow differences existed in both the clinic and hospital environments.

The large volume of pregnant patients who come through our system (approximately 4,400 each year) combined with the sheer number of best practice measures (BPM) and multiple visits drove the process of incorporating data fields into the EHR and the development of a reporting mechanism to track performance outcomes. One hundred and three unique BPMs were pulled from the literature and hard-wired into the perinatal process. As many as 300 opportunities to deliver these BPM exist per patient, if the mother begins her care within the first trimester and continues through postpartum visits. All measures were included for one ultimate goal: to ensure mother and baby receive evidence-based care for optimal outcomes. With varying levels of activities geared to build engagement, each team member clearly recognized the importance of the task at hand.

The 103 BPM were grouped into clinically relevant bundles. Each patient will have a customized set of applicable BPM based on the gestational age at which they enter/exit the system and their clinical condition. Monitoring the reliability of executing the BPM reports in the aggregate, clinic, and individual provider levels needs to be created in quick-time.

Finally, new strategies in system redesign, new strategies for involving and motivating staff and patients, and a new willingness to reexamine every aspect of operations were required to achieve safe and reliable care. A key foundational element of this project was workflow redesign and optimization supported by a thoughtfully designed EHR. Bataldens model provided the foundation and context for the establishment of an eight-step methodology for multisite improvement initiatives. Application in this context marked a significant, more ambitious shift from prior Geisinger ProvenCare programs.

Table 15.1 ProvenCare perinatal best practice measures.

	Components of care	Evidence-based	Guideline/consensus-based	Evidence/guideline
1	Pregnancy confirmation			ACOG
2	Menstrual history	X	X	ACOG, ICSI 13
3	Pregnancy history		X	ACOG
4	Chronic disease		X	ACOG
5	Thyroid dysfunction		X	ACOG
6	Tobacco/drug/alcohol use	X	X	ACOG
7	Hepatitis		X	ACOG
8	Depression		X	ACOG
9	Postpartum depression		X	ACOG
10	Allergies		X	ACOG
11	Rh sensitization		X	ACOG
12	Breast		X	ACOG
13	Gyn surgeries		X	ACOG
14	Complications from anesthesia		X	ACOG
15	Abnormal pap		X	ACOG
16	Infertility		X	ACOG
17	Trauma or violence	X	X	ACOG
18	Thalassemia, history		X	ACOG
19	Neural tube defect, history		X	ACOG
20	Congenital heart, history		X	ACOG
21	Down syndrome, history		X	ACOG
22	Tay Sachs, history	X	X	ACOG
23	Canavan disease, history		X	ACOG

(continued)

Table 15.1 (*cont.*)

	Components of care	Evidence-based	Guideline/consensus-based	Evidence/guideline
24	Familial dysautonomia, history		X	ACOG
25	Sickle cell disease or trait, history		X	ACOG
26	Hemophilia/other blood disorder, history	X	X	ACOG
27	Muscular dystrophy, history		X	ACOG
28	Cystic fibrosis, history	X	X	ACOG
29	Huntington's chorea, history		X	ACOG
30	Mental retardation, history	X	X	ACOG
31	Maternal metabolic disorders (PKU)		X	ACOG
32	Recurrent pregnancy loss	X	X	ACOG
33	Other fetal anomalies		X	ACOG
34	Medication history	X	X	ACOG, ICSI 12
35	TB exposure	X	X	ACOG
36	Patient/partner with genital herpes	X	X	ACOG
37	Rash or viral illness since last menses		X	ACOG
38	Hepatitis B	X	X	ACOG
39	History of STD	X	X	ACOG
40	HIV (including partner hx)	X	X	
41	BP	X	X	ICSI 6
42	Calculate body mass index	X	X	ICSI 5
43	Fetal heart tones, 10 weeks+	X	X	ICSI 27- at 10-12 weeks and every visit after, ACOG
44	Physical exam: HEENT		X	ACOG
45	Physical exam: Teeth	X	X	ACOG
46	Physical exam: Thyroid		X	ACOG
47	Physical exam: Breasts		X	ACOG
48	Physical exam: Lungs		X	ACOG
49	Physical exam: Heart		X	ACOG
50	Physical exam: Abdomen		X	ACOG
51	Physical exam: Extremities		X	ACOG
52	Physical exam: Skin		X	ACOG
53	Physical exam: Lymph nodes		X	ACOG
54	Physical exam: Vulva		X	ACOG
55	Physical exam: Vagina		X	ACOG
56	Physical exam: Cervix		X	ACOG
57	Physical exam: Uterus size		X	ACOG
58	Physical exam: Adnexa		X	ACOG
59	Physical exam: Assessment of bony pelvis		X	ACOG
60	1st trimester screening		X	ACOG
61	CBC	X	X	Physician consensus, ACOG, ICSI 1 5
62	Urine culture	X	X	ICSI 18, ACOG
63	Type/Rh	X	X	ICSI 16, ACOG

Table 15.1 *(cont.)*

	Components of care	Evidence-based	Guideline/consensus-based	Evidence/guideline
64	Antibody	X	X	ICSI 16, ACOG
65	Rubella IgG	X	X	ICSI 8, ACOG
66	Chlamydia	X	X	ICSI 4, ACOG-risk assessment
67	Gonorrhea	X	X	ICSI 4
68	Hepatitis B sag	X	X	ICSI 25, ACOG
69	HIV	X	X	ICSI 19, ACOG
70	Pap		X	ACOG
71	Syphilis (RPR)	X	X	ICSI 17, ACOG
72	Cystic Fibrosis screening offered		X	ACOG
73	Thalassemia (if history warrants)		X	ACOG
74	Tay Sachs (if history warrants)		X	ACOG
75	Canavan (if history warrants)		X	ACOG
76	Smoking cessation	X	X	ICSI, ACOG
77	Nutrition counseling for obesity	X	X	ACOG, WHO, ICSI
78	Antenatal education	X	X	
79	Influenza	X	X	ICSI 26, ACOG, CDC
80	Domestic abuse questioning	X	X	ACOG, ICSI
81	Establish EDD		X	ACOG
82	Birthing class offered	X		ACOG
83	Fetal aneuploidy screening	X	X	ICSI 23
84	Urine 2-dip		X	ACOG
85	Quad screening offered (15-20 wks)		X	ACOG
86	Glucola (26-28 wks)	X	X	ACOG, ICSI
87	Rh– mothers, repeat type and screen and administer rhogam (28 wks)	X	X	ACOG, ICSI
88	Ultrasound offered (18-22 wks)	X	X	ACOG, consensus
89	Fundal height (after 20 wks)	X	X	ICSI, ACOG
90	Fetal movement	X	X	ICSI, ACOG
91	Bleeding assessment	X	X	ACOG
92	Presentation		X	ACOG
93	Preterm labor signs/symptoms		X	ACOG
94	Labor education		X	ACOG
95	Edema		X	ACOG
96	Pain scale		X	ACOG
97	Elective induction bundle		X	IHI
98	MMR administration for rubella negative patients (as determined by the 1st prenatal labs)	X	X	ACOG, consensus
99	Rhogam administered prior to discharge to nonsensitized Rh– pts with Rh+ babies	X	X	
100	Episiotomy repair		X	ACOG
101	Review birth control		X	ACOG
102	Uterine involution		X	ACOG
103	Postpartum depression assessment	X	X	ACOG, ICSI, literature

ProvenCare Perinatal

ProvenCare Perinatal began with an engagement meeting that included executive and administrative leadership from WHSL and the quality improvement team from the Division of Quality & Safety. Rules of staff engagement, roles, and expectations were discussed and the timeline was established. Recognizing the scope of the initiative (76 providers, 24 sites, four hospitals, and the duration of the pregnancy episode) required a new communication and management structure; a steering committee, mesosystem team, and local microsystem teams were formed. The steering committee included: three physician champions from across the WHSL (a physician from each Geisinger service region); a senior nurse; the WHSL administrative VP; EHR programming staff; and a quality improvement specialist. Critical factors for success included highly engaged leadership, diligent planning, and committed local champions. A larger team of mesosystem delegates was assembled comprising: six physicians and one midwife (representing all 24 clinic sites), one nurse from each clinic, operation managers, a front-line workflow expert, and representatives from the EHR team and quality improvement. Finally, each of the 24 local microsystems participated. This resulted in drastic changes in the workflow, especially in our EMR (result console, best practice alerts, trending reports, alerts for at-risk populations, patient education, and communication tools).

The purpose of the new structure was to create an effective communication pathway across all practice sites. This allowed all aspects of the redesign process to be shared and influenced equally, expanded the pool for innovative ideas, and ultimately facilitated rapid adoption of changes as the final redesign was deployed.

Perinatal ProvenCare methodology steps:

Step 1: Map out the current process

Step 2: Establish best practices

Step 3: Identify barriers to meeting best practice standards reliably

Step 4: Identify available resources to overcome barriers

Step 5: Optimize participation in given tasks by utilizing small and large work groups

Step 6: Provide just-in-time training and continuous issue resolution

Step 7: Measure reliability consistently and provide quick-time data feedback

Step 8: Emphasize project ownership and accountability with front line groups

Measuring Quality

As with all ProvenCare initiatives, all-or-none bundles are both the goal and the expectation. In other words, each bundle was considered a single unit, and included all critical processes. With up to 300 opportunities to provide best practice for each patient, evaluation is a very challenging task. We developed clinically relevant bundles that group the BPMs in a logical manner. These bundles provide a quick reference for process reliability. They are also important for evaluating specific clinical outcomes and how they correlate with specific BPM. A large component of this ProvenCare initiative centered on how to collect, analyze, and provide meaningful feedback to the teams. This work began with the development of the new workflow and ensuring that each BPM was designed in the appropriate format for easy data retrieval. It has continued on through the development of an interactive dashboard where the user is able to identify what information they want to review, i.e., data for the entire service line or a single clinic, one bundle or the all-or-none data. Global data are reviewed quarterly, while specific processes that may lead to preventable harm are reviewed weekly or even daily, such as elective delivery at less than 39 weeks.

Quality Outcomes

We established standardized processes and workflows that were instituted across 24 diverse practice sites, on time and with minimal problems. The application of consistent processes yielded significant efficiency gains. One example is the amount of nurse time that was saved during the first prenatal clinic visit. At our largest clinic, we saved an average of 13 minutes per first prenatal visit. Based upon the volume of new prenatal visits and the nurse time saved, we were able to hire an additional physician without needing to hire the usual compliment of new nurses. Consistent with our philosophy that efficiency and quality care are not mutually exclusive, the team identified patient outcomes metrics that they expected to influence. With the inclusion of the IHI elective induction bundle, our team has reduced primary c-section rates by 26% to a rate currently below

Table 15.2 BPM bundle table.

Examples of ProvenCare Perinatal bundles with associated BPMs and number of times each measure must be satisfied in the care pathway. Additionally, potential outcomes that may be affected by reliable execution of all BPMs within the bundle are indicated.

Bundles	BPMs (examples)	#Opportunities*	Possible impacted outcomes
Diabetes	28 week Glucola	1	Decreased maternal/fetal complications related to uncontrolled and late diagnosed gestational diabetes
	Urine dip – glucose each visit	13	
	Weight gain	13	Decreased incidence of LGA babies
	Fundal height 20 week and each visit after	10	Decreased incidence of insulin-dependent gestational diabetes
			Decreased NICU admission rate
			Decreased NICU LOS
Preeclampsia/ eclampsia/HELP	Urine dip – protein each visit	13	Delayed on set or prevention of eclampsia/ HELLP syndrome
	Edema each visit	13	
	Smoking cessation screening and intervention	13	Decrease number of newborns born with complications associated with late diagnosis of preeclampsia/eclampsia/ HELLP
	Weight gain	13	
	BP each visit	13	Decreased NICU admission rate
			Decreased NICU LOS
Preterm labor	Fundal height each visit post 20 wks	10	Decreased incidence of early delivery
	Smoking cessation screening and intervention	13	Decreased NICU admission rate
	Establish EDD	1	Decreased NICU LOS
	Fetal movement assessment	12	
Induction/ augmentation bundle (IHI)	Assessment of gestatinoal age and dating criteria	1	Decreased rate of primary cesarean section
	Monitoring fetal heart rate for reassurance	1	Decreased cost of care (length of stay)
	Pelvic Assessment	1	Decreased time laboring
	Monitoring and management of hyperstimulation	1	
	Bishops score	1	
Maternal and fetal wellness	Rhogam administered prior to discharge to nonsensitized RH– pts with Rg + babies	1	Overall maternal and fetal wellness
	Rubella sensitization screening and intervention	1	Decreased NICU admission rate
	Obesity intervention	1	Decreased complication rate associated with childbirth
	Smoking cessation screening and intervention	13	
	Postpartum visit bundle (episiotomy evaluation, uterine involution assessment, contraception discussion)	1	
	Influenza vaccination for mom	1	Decreased incidence of newborn admissions related to influenza, birth–3 months
	Postpartum Depression Tool Edinburgh Scale	1	Decreased severity of postpartum depression by appropriate identification and action
			Increased appropriate referrals to psychiatry

* Number of opportunities for a patient who has one clinic visit in the first trimester, delivers at 40 weeks gestation, and attends all scheduled appointments.

the national average. The reliability of executing each measure for every patient is also tracked. Postpartum depression screening, which was highly variable before ProvenCare, has been reliably provided to 98.5% of our patients since implementation. Our NICU admission rate has deceased by 33%. Our birth harm score

has decreased to well below the national average. Our NICU length of stay has decreased by two days. And our preterm delivery rate has decreased by 25%.

Outcome Tables and Figures

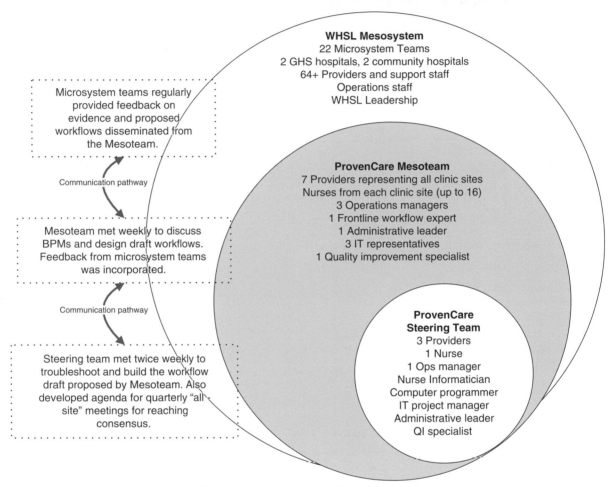

Figure 15.1 Improvement of primary c-section rates through application of ProvenCare methodology.

Table 15.3 Birth trauma rates (based on PSI 17 criteria).

GWV	# of births	# of birth trauma cases	Birth trauma rate (per 1000 babies)	Chi-square *p*-value (compared to baseline)
July07–June08	1010	2	1.98	Baseline
July08–June09	1196	2	1.67	0.865
July09–Sept10	1687	1	0.59	0.295

Table 15.4 Reliability in providing best practice measures.

Best practice measures and/or process steps	Pre-ProvenCare (N = 101)	Post-implementation (N = 1,010)	Pearson's Chi-square p-value
Diabetes bundle (All-or-none)	30.89%	79.02%	0.00
Preeclampsia bundle (All-or-none)	42.63%	67.83%	0.00
Postpartum visit bundle (All-or-none)	61.63%	97.62%	0.01
Smoking cessation intervention	45.27%	88.50%	0.00
Intervention for obesity offered	3.51%	77.47%	0.00
Rh blood factor initial screen and Rhogam administration	91.53%	100.00%	0.53
Rubella sensitization initial screen and MMR administration	88.07%	98.88%	0.43
Postpartum depression screening	n/a	100.0	n/a

Table 15.5 Clinically relevant measures and bundles were identified by physicians on the ProvenCare mesoteam. These reliability data correspond to Table 15.4, which provides the details behind each measure and bundle.

GHS patients	Total GHS babies	GHS NICU admissions	Percent NICU admissions	NICU babies born to mothers with insulin-dependent gestational diabetes	Percent insulin-dependent gestational diabetes
Pre-ProvenCare	4,526	427	9.43	18	4.2
Post-ProvenCare	3,738	271	7.25 (p < 0.01)	4	1.5 (p = 0.04)

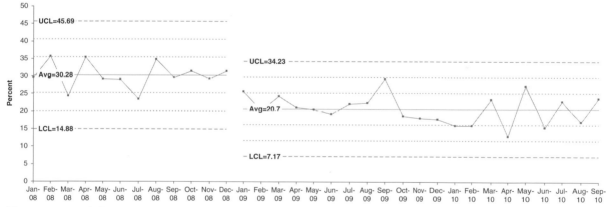

Figure 15.2 Trend of primary C-section rates pre- and post-Perinatal ProvenCare implementation.

Discussion

Over the past five years, we have realized significant gains in both patient safety, economic performance, and operational efficiency. We attribute the resulting positive clinical outcomes and cost savings to the realized workflow redesign. This improvement initiative was significantly more complex than prior ProvenCare endeavors in terms of breadth, scope, and duration. A strength of this project was that the decision-making framework effectively aligned a diverse group of providers with a common purpose and vision to affect a redesign that provided a standardized, evidence-based pathway to pregnant women across multiple sites. This is exactly the idea behind the concept of integrated care in a continuum. The entire concept of an Accountable Care Organization (ACO) fits well within this model.

Two clear requirements for effective execution of such a process are committed leadership and engaged care providers. Additionally, the inability to provide dedicated quality improvement specialists to guide and oversee initiatives of this size may prove limiting. The return on investment has been realized through reduced educational materials, freeing 20–30 minutes of provider time per clinic each day, and efficiency leading to preservation of margin per case despite decreased reimbursement and increased labor costs.

In conclusion, we have proven with hard work, the willingness to analyze all aspects of the care delivered, and the ability to re-engineer workflow using a robust

EMR, anyone can improve their quality metrics, reliability of care delivered, and decrease cost.

EMR Process Redesign Examples

eForms now enable nurses and providers to complete documents electronically

- Care Coordination Record
- Home Health Referral for Healthy Beginnings
- OBNA for MA insurance
- Cervical Ripening – Scheduled Induction

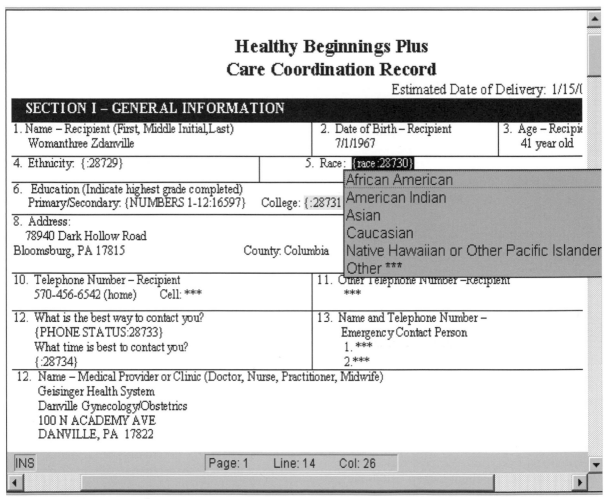

Figure 15.3 The infrastructure was designed to create an effective communication and management pathway across all practice sites.

Smoking Cessation Intervention Barriers identified
- difficult and timely documentation were preventing team members from executing

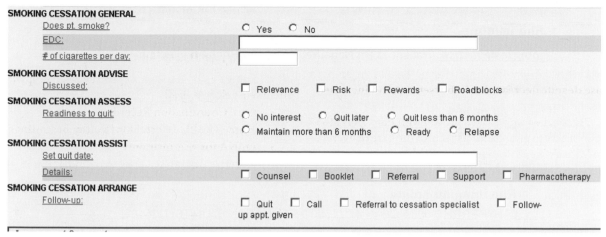

SMOKING CESSATION GENERAL
Does pt. smoke?   ○ Yes   ○ No
EDC:
# of cigarettes per day:

SMOKING CESSATION ADVISE
Discussed: □ Relevance   □ Risk   □ Rewards   □ Roadblocks

SMOKING CESSATION ASSESS
Readiness to quit: ○ No interest   ○ Quit later   ○ Quit less than 6 months
                      ○ Maintain more than 6 months   ○ Ready   ○ Relapse

SMOKING CESSATION ASSIST
Set quit date:
Details: □ Counsel   □ Booklet   □ Referral   □ Support   □ Pharmacotherapy

SMOKING CESSATION ARRANGE
Follow-up: □ Quit   □ Call   □ Referral to cessation specialist   □ Follow-
up appt. given

Figure 15.4 Process around smoking cessation documentation and counseling was in-bedded in the workflow.

- Standardization improves execution and facilitates optimal data collection for comparison
- Process is replicated in the Pediatric offices
- Psych department was educated about the instrument and the revised process

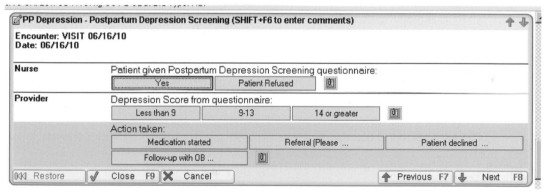

Figure 15.5 Depiction of the process and tool used for postpartum depression screening and intervention.

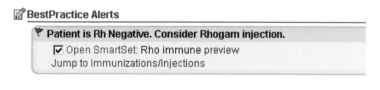

Figure 15.6 An example of an electronic tool built for 100% reliability while avoiding hard stop fatigue.

141

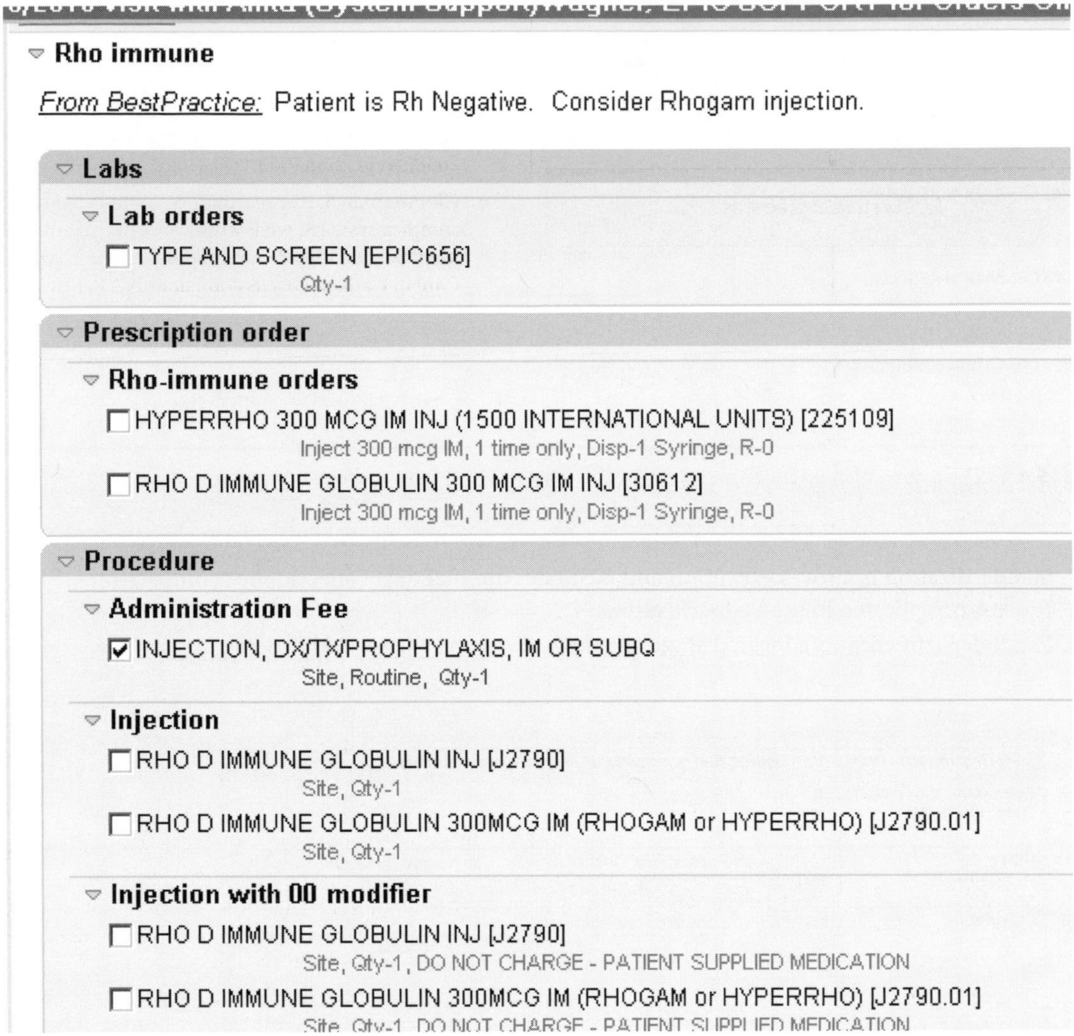

▽ Rho immune

From BestPractice: Patient is Rh Negative. Consider Rhogam injection.

▽ Labs

▽ Lab orders

☐ TYPE AND SCREEN [EPIC656]
Qty-1

▽ Prescription order

▽ Rho-immune orders

☐ HYPERRHO 300 MCG IM INJ (1500 INTERNATIONAL UNITS) [225109]
Inject 300 mcg IM, 1 time only, Disp-1 Syringe, R-0

☐ RHO D IMMUNE GLOBULIN 300 MCG IM INJ [30612]
Inject 300 mcg IM, 1 time only, Disp-1 Syringe, R-0

▽ Procedure

▽ Administration Fee

☑ INJECTION, DX/TX/PROPHYLAXIS, IM OR SUBQ
Site, Routine, Qty-1

▽ Injection

☐ RHO D IMMUNE GLOBULIN INJ [J2790]
Site, Qty-1

☐ RHO D IMMUNE GLOBULIN 300MCG IM (RHOGAM or HYPERRHO) [J2790.01]
Site, Qty-1

▽ Injection with 00 modifier

☐ RHO D IMMUNE GLOBULIN INJ [J2790]
Site, Qty-1, DO NOT CHARGE - PATIENT SUPPLIED MEDICATION

☐ RHO D IMMUNE GLOBULIN 300MCG IM (RHOGAM or HYPERRHO) [J2790.01]
Site, Qty-1, DO NOT CHARGE - PATIENT SUPPLIED MEDICATION

Figure 15.7 Triggered best practice alert for Rh negative patients.

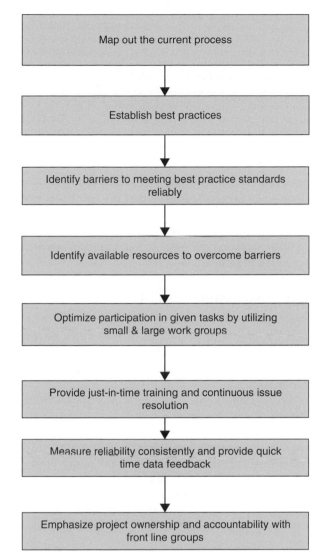

Figure 15.8 Perinatal ProvenCare methodology steps.

References

1 Berry SA, Laam LA, Cassagnol HP, et al. ProvenCare Perinatal: a model for delivering evidence/guideline-based care for perinatal populations. *Joint Comm J Qual Patient Saf.* 2011;37(5):229–239.

2 Berry SA, Doll MC, McKinley KE, Casale AS, Bothe Jr A. ProvenCare: quality improvement model for designing highly reliable care in cardiac surgery. *Qual Saf Healthc.* 2009;18:360–368.

3 McKinley KE, Berry SA, Laam LA, et al., Clinical Microsystems, Part 4: building innovative population-specific mesosystems. *Jt Comm J Qual Improve.* 2008;34(11):655–663.

4 Glouberman S, Zimmerman B. Complicated and complex systems: what would successful reform of Medicare look like? Commission on the Future of Health Care in Canada Discussion Paper No. 8, July 2002.

5 Fisher ES, Wennberg JE. Health care quality, geographic variations, and the challenge of supply-sensitive care. *Perspect Biol Med.* 2003; 46(1):69–79.

6 Fisher ES, Wennberg DE, Stukel TA, et al. The implications of regional variations in Medicare spending. Part 1: the content, quality, and accessibility of care. *Ann Intern Med.* 2003;138(4):273–287.

7 Fisher ES, Wennberg DE, Stukel TA, et al. The implications of regional variations in Medicare spending. Part 2: health outcomes and satisfaction with care. *Ann Intern Med.* 2003;138(4):288–298.

8 Nolan TW. *Execution of Strategic Improvement Initiatives to Produce System-Level Results.* IHI Innovation Series white paper. Cambridge, MA: Institute for Healthcare Improvement; 2007 (available at www.IHI.org).

9 Batalden PB, Davidoff F. What is "quality improvement" and how can it transform healthcare? *Qual Saf Healthc.* 2007;16(1):2–3.

10 Asch SM, Kerr EA, Keesey J, et al. Who is at greatest risk for receiving poor-quality health care? *N Engl J Med.* 2006;354:1147–1156.

11 Mangione-Smith R, DeCristofaro AH, Setodji CM, et al. The quality of ambulatory care delivered to children in the United States. *N Engl J Med.* 2007;357:1515–1523.

12 Bogner MS. Revisiting *To Err Is Human* a decade later. *Biomed Instrum Technol.* 2009;43(6):476–478.

13 Nolan T, Resar R, Haraden C, Griffin FA. *Improving the Reliability of Health Care, IHI Innovation Series White Paper.* Boston, MA: Institute for Healthcare improvement, 2004 (available at www.IHI.org).

14 Resar RK. Making noncastastrophic health care processes reliable: learning to walk before running in creating high-reliability organizations. *Health Ser Res.* 2006;41(4):1677–1689.

Chapter

16

Fatigue and Safety

Peter A. Schwartz, James W. Saxton, and Maggie M. Finkelstein

Case #1

You're 45 minutes away from the end of your shift on labor and delivery when two patients get admitted simultaneously for term labor. During this one night-float shift, you did three vaginal deliveries, two cesarean sections (one an emergent section for fetal distress and the other complicated by a postpartum hemorrhage), and managed one term fetal demise, which took up most of your time. The other resident on call with you had been back and forth to the emergency room, and you thought asking the chief resident for help would be an admission that you couldn't handle the workload.

Exhausted from being on nights for the last 2 weeks, you look for the 5 AM surge to carry you through the rest of the morning, knowing full well that your co-intern would be relieving you in less than an hour. You work under stress and exhaustion all the time, so what difference would an hour make? To make things easier, all you had left were two admissions, which you could do with your eyes closed.

The first patient was relatively uncomplicated; she was a nulliparous woman with no medical problems and an uncomplicated prenatal course. She was in early labor without any complaints. The second woman was multiparous and carrying vertex/vertex twins. She reported occasional headaches which she attributed to tension and denied any other problems. Her vital signs were normal and her fetal heart tracing was a category I. Thinking that she would tell you if there was something wrong, you proceed with the usual order sets and continue with expectant management.

Once sign out is done you go home and sleep the day away. Feeling better, you return later that night for your shift. You immediately note that there is a patient in the Surgical Intensive Care Unit (SICU). The patient with twins you had admitted earlier in the day had undergone an emergent primary

cesarean section secondary to eclampsia. Review of her prenatal records showed that she had had a history of elevated blood pressures for the past 3 weeks and her last 24-hour urine which was processed and in the system an hour prior to her admission showed 5,500 mg of protein.

Case Discussion

The first year of residency is often the most challenging. The enormous amount to learn, number, variety, and complexity of new patient experiences are augmented by sleep deprivation, fatigue, lack of confidence, and non-medical demands on your time and emotions (family, etc.). Although the responsibilities change, the fundamental burden of so much to learn in a finite amount of time makes fatigue and sleep deprivation unremitting throughout the four years of training. Before you know it, if you're not paying attention, the chance of making a mistake that may seriously harm or injure a patient increases exponentially. Everyone knows that physicians work demanding hours; but for some reason, exhaustion and sleep deprivation are accepted as the norm rather than tolerated as the exception.

Most Americans sleep for approximately 7 hours a night, which is one hour less than the amount recommended by the National Sleep Foundation. Surgical residents average less than 6 hours of sleep per night, even when overnight call shifts are scheduled every fourth night [1]. When adults sleep less than 5 hours per night, language and numerical skills, retention of information, short-term memory and concentration are all noted to decrease on standardized exams [2]. Additionally, sleep-deprived adults tend to exhibit impaired complex problem-solving skills [2]. Sleepiness is commonplace among house staff; 10% of residents perceive sleepiness as an almost daily occurrence for themselves [1].

To assuage this problem, the Accreditation Council for Graduate Medical Education established limits on resident work hours in July 2003 and further modified these limits in June 2011. Although these limits emphasized the importance of faculty supervision, handover processes, and management of alertness, there is no clear evidence that restricting work hours improves patient outcomes. In the residency setting, work-hour restriction has resulted in utilizing a night-float system, which has not been shown to decrease fatigue [2]. Adjustment to night-shift schedules or readjustment from sequential night-shift may take up to 3 to 4 days [3]. Moreover, a recent study of night-float-protected interns showed that trainees with protected time for sleep often failed to use the time to sleep, leading to sustained levels of fatigue [1].

There are four recognized components of fatigue:

1. Acute continuous sleep deprivation (less than 4–6 hours of sleep per night)
2. Chronic partial sleep deprivation
3. Cumulative sleep debt (accumulation of owed sleep from days of inadequate sleep)
4. Sleep inertia, exhaustion and workload and circadian rhythm disruption.

Acute sleep deprivation has been shown to lead to an increasing amount of sleep debt which is associated with decreased performance in psychological tests [3, 4]. Additionally, a meta-analysis examining laboratory-based sleep loss studies estimated that the mean cognitive performances of healthy young adults who are sleep deprived (both short-term and chronic) are 1.3 SDs or more below the mean [1]. Studies in sleep laboratories have shown that both at base line and after on-call duty, levels of daytime sleepiness in residents are similar to or higher than those in patients with narcolepsy or sleep apnea [5].

Studies regarding the effect of fatigue on resident surgical skills have been contradictory. However, recently, Landrigan et al. [6] conducted a single-center randomized crossover-controlled trial of 20 interns during critical care rotations. During the course of a year, interns worked a traditional schedule of every third night on call (i.e., > 24-hour shifts), and an intervention schedule that split the on-call shifts between two residents. This modification limited work shifts to 16 hours or less and reduced the total number of hours worked per week to 61 hours. While the residents worked according to the intervention schedule, they slept significantly

more than when they worked according to the traditional schedule (7.4 ± 0.9 h/ day vs. 6.6 ± 0.8 h/ day, $p < 0.001$). Moreover, residents working according to the traditional schedule showed a significant increase in failures of attentiveness when compared with the intervention schedule. During night work the incidence of these events was more than doubled ($p = 0.02$); during the day their incidence was increased 1.5 times ($p = 0.07$).

To assess the associated risk to patient safety, Landrigan et al. [6] further evaluated the same residents with respect to their propensity to commit medical errors under both schedules. While working the traditional schedule, residents committed 35.9% more serious medical errors ($p < 0.001$) while residents working according to the traditional schedule made 57% more non-intercepted serious ($p < 0.001$) and 5.6 times as many serious diagnostic errors ($p < 0.001$) compared with when they were working according to the intervention schedule [4].

However, perhaps the most relevant data come from resident perception of the effect of fatigue and sleep deprivation on errors. Residents identified fatigue as a major contributor to their worst errors. Residents in the United States working more than 80 hours per week reported that they were more likely to make a significant medical error than residents working less than 80 hours per week. The majority of studies, which include surveys and observation studies, have provided indirect evidence that the traditional system of on-call shifts longer than 24 hours is not ideal. Some have also provided unequivocal evidence that mood is worsened by fatigue, as indicated by increased scores on measures of depression, anxiety, confusion, and anger, and that psychomotor performance is impaired in sleep-deprived residents. One survey using the Maslach Burnout Inventory found one-third of residents had emotional exhaustion, more than half had high levels of depersonalization, and just less than half had a positive depression screen [3].

Residents working extended duty shifts are faced with increased risk of experiencing occupational injury. They have nearly twice the risk of a needle-stick injury when they are post call. There is a substantially increased risk of a "fall asleep" vehicle crash when a resident is driving home from a call shift compared with normal shifts [7]. Additionally, it was found that 24 hours of constant wakefulness impaired hand–eye coordination to the same degree as a blood-alcohol concentration of 0.10%, a level above the legal driving limit in every state of the US [4].

Residents, feeling fatigued at or near the end of an overnight shift, are at increased risk of making an error in patient care. Caregivers must recognize that asking for help when fatigued is not a sign of inadequacy but is an important patient safety strategy.

Case #2

Three years after completing your residency you joined a small practice with a large patient volume. After delivering three patients between the hours of 10 PM and 12 AM, a woman with a ruptured ectopic pregnancy requiring immediate surgery presented to the emergency room. You rushed her to the operating room and performed a unilateral salpingectomy without complication. After finishing her postoperative orders and notes at 2 AM, you spent the rest of the night monitoring a patient with preterm labor at 27 weeks gestation.

After signing out the active patients to your partner at 6 AM, you proceeded to have breakfast and coffee. You had a patient with uterine fibroids scheduled for a total laparoscopic hysterectomy with bilateral salpingo-oopherectomy at 8 AM; a procedure that you frequently perform.

During the case, you encountered a large amount of bleeding secondary to aberrant vessels from multiple fibroids. After 15 minutes of poorly controlled hemorrhage, you finally controlled the bleeding and completed the hysterectomy without further incident. Before closing the abdomen you irrigated the pelvis and tried to locate the ureters. You identified the ureters and after waiting for 20 minutes you observed some peristalsis. You decided against doing a cystoscopy even though it is normally a part of your routine. At the end of the case, you realize you are extremely fatigued and decide to cancel your afternoon office hours.

During morning rounds the next day, your patient reported new-onset flank pain. Her abdomen was slightly tender on exam and her vital signs were stable. After reviewing her labs, you noted that her creatinine was increased from baseline. Subsequent CT urogram showed evidence of a ureteral injury.

You explained the findings to the patient, emphasizing that this is a complication that can be encountered in any gynecologic surgical procedure and one that you had mentioned as part of her consent process. A urologist was consulted to assist with management which included placement of a ureteral stent. While

in the nurses' station a few days later, you confided to a colleague that you thought this may not have happened if you hadn't been up all night, not realizing that the patient's son was standing behind you.

Three months later, you were served with a law suit citing gross negligence in causing the ureteral injury.

Case Discussion

Surgical complications can be life-changing events for the physician as well as the patient. For the patient, surgical complications can result in a more complicated mental and physical recovery and in some cases even death. On the other hand, for a surgeon, a surgical complication can lead to a loss of confidence in one's skills and potentially to a change in career. When this apprehension and guilt is further exacerbated by litigation, the impact on the practitioner may be devastating [8].

The 2009 Survey on Professional Liability conducted by ACOG found that 90.5% of respondents experienced at least one professional liability claim. On average there were 2.69 claims per obstetrician–gynecologist. The average age of the respondents was 48. This survey found that 62.1% of claims involved obstetric care, while 37.9% concerned gynecologic care. Although only a small percent of cases result in litigation, the emotional impact to individual physician defendant can be devastating. And although there is large amount of literature addressing the issue of malpractice, we had yet to amass a large amount of literature in regards to prevention of surgical complications.

Of the liability claims arising from gynecology care, 44% are related to major and minor surgical injuries [9]. The risk of surgical complications by attending physicians after performing nighttime procedures is increased when physicians have sleep opportunities of less than 6 hours [2]. Currently duty hour limits on physician work schedules apply only to physicians in training. Sleep deprivation adversely affects the performance of monotonous or routine tasks. Sleep deprivation is also associated with impairment of speech and advanced cognitive functioning. Nevertheless, senior physicians believe they can compensate for the effects of fatigue during critical situations and deny the effects of fatigue on performance [3]. The lack of regulation of duty hours for attending physicians is most likely related to the absence of a regulatory body governing the practice patterns of clinicians. The maximum number of continuous and cumulative hours that may be worked by pilots, air traffic controllers, and truck drivers are defined based on limited scientific evidence linking fatigue to significant adverse events. Are we any less responsible for patient safety than they are for passenger safety?

This case illustrates the potential for excellent physicians to alter their practice patterns when burdened by sleep deprivation and fatigue. Like pilots and others responsible for public safety, we know that evidence-based "check lists" and routines are valuable in maintaining standards and clinical excellence. A checklist can be a countermeasure in preventing errors of omission in the face of provider fatigue. We should always think twice when we abort a well-established clinical pattern. It should not happen in response to sleep deprivation or fatigue. Visualization of ureteral function at the conclusion of the case by opening the dome of the bladder or performing a cystoscopy was a routine for the physician in the example. Moreover, it was certainly indicated in this difficult case with bleeding often making visualization difficult. Apparently exhausted after prolonged visualization, the attending physician thought he saw ureteral peristalsis. Apparently because of his fatigue, he chose not to confirm normal ureteral function by cystoscopy. He therefore failed to recognize the ureteral injury until postoperative rounds the day following surgery.

Strategies and Conclusions

The Institute of Medicine report *To Err is Human* estimated that up to 100,000 people die each year in the United States as a result of medical error [10]. This chapter has highlighted the significant role that fatigue and sleep deprivation can play at all levels of obstetrical and gynecological practice, from a first-year resident to a seasoned attending.

So what can be done to prevent the effects of sleep deprivation and fatigue from harming our patients? The most effective countermeasure for sleep deprivation is naps. A 2- to 8-hour nap or sleep prior to 24 hours without sleep can improve vigilance and minimize sleepiness. Naps as short as 15 minutes but no longer than 2 hours can significantly ameliorate the performance decrements associated with fatigue and sleep deprivation. The time of the day most refractory to countermeasures is the circadian nadir, 2 AM to 9 AM [1]. To avoid drowsiness on awakening ("sleep inertia"), the nap should last for at least 40 minutes. Airline pilots who napped in their seats for 40 minutes

were more alert and performed better than those who did not nap [5].

The situation described in Case #1 is one that could have happened to any of us. Sleep deprivation, night float, a busy obstetrical floor and a desire to be self-sufficient all contributed to the poor outcome. Although there are some things over which we will never have control, we can and must do a better job of assessing our state of wakefulness and implementing strategies to reduce the effects of sleep deprivation. Helpful strategies to prevent fatigue involve schedule changes and back-up call. In formulating our work schedules, every practitioner needs to answer the following questions:

Questions (ACOG):

- Should I work a half day or a full day in the clinic after a night on call?
- Should I be at work for any length of time after a night on call?
- Should I perform surgery if I have been awake most of the previous night, or should the procedure be rescheduled?
- What back-up system is available if I recognize a worrisome level of fatigue?
- What adjustments should be made to my call schedule to avoid a worrisome level of fatigue?

In the article "Getting to Havarti," the author addresses "at risk behaviors" or "shortcuts" [11]. He states that because the system supports these behaviors and because there are rarely adverse consequences for taking such shortcuts and the incidence of adverse outcomes is low, we know that we will probably not have a problem most of the time. He additionally references an essay on *Just Cultures* from the Institute for Safe Medication Practices, which states:

Behavioral research shows that we are programmed to drift into unsafe habits, to lose perception of the risk attached to everyday behaviors, or mistakenly believe the risk to be justified. In general, workers are most concerned with the immediate and certain consequences of their behavior – saved time, for example – and undervalue delayed or uncertain consequences, such as patient harm. Their decisions about what is important on a daily list of tasks are based on the immediate desired outcomes. Over time, as perceptions of risk fade away and workers try to do more with less; they take shortcuts and drift away from behaviors they know are safer.

The reasons workers drift into unsafe behaviors are often rooted in the system. Safe behavioral choices may invoke criticism, and at-risk behaviors may invoke rewards ... Therein lies the problem. The rewards of at-risk behaviors can become so common that perception of their risk fades or is believed to be justified.

The overarching principle behind improving safety is recognition that 90% of patient injuries result from bad systems, not bad people [10]. By addressing the effects of sleep deprivation and fatigue with schedule modifications and back-up systems, we can all hopefully work together to change the system to improve patient safety. At the end of the day, physicians are the ones responsible for patient safety. We can only improve patient safety by changing the culture in which we work. Prevention, recognition, and amelioration of provider fatigue are an essential elements in this change.

References

1 Veasey S, Rosen R, Barzansky B, Rosen I, Owens J. Sleep loss and fatigue in residency training. *JAMA*. 2002;288(9):1116–1124.

2 ACOG Committee Opinion # 519: Fatigue and Patient Safety. March 2012.

3 Parshuram CS. The impact of fatigue on patient safety. *Ped Clin North Am*. 2006;53(6): 1135–1153.

4 Mountain SA, Quon BS, Dodek P, Sharpe R, Ayas NT. The impact of housestaff fatigue on occupational and patient safety. *Lung*. 2007;185(4):203–209.

5 Gaba DM, Howard SK. Fatigue among clinicians and the safety of patients. *N Engl J Med*. 2002;347:1249–1255.

6 Landrigan CP, Rothschild JM, Cronin JW, et al. Effect of reducing interns' work hours on serious medical errors in intensive care units. *N Engl J Med*. 2004;351:1838–1848.

7 Mitchell CD, Mooty CR, Dunn EL, Ramberger KC, Mangram AJ. Resident fatigue: is there a patient safety issue? *Am J Surg*. 2009;198(6):811–816.

8 Wu AW. Medical error: the second victim. The doctor who makes the mistake needs help too. *BMJ*. 2000;320(7237):726–727.

9 Klagholz BA, Strunk AL. ACOG Clinical Review: Overview of the 2009 ACOG Survey on Professional Liability. November–December 2009;1–13. www.acog.org/-/media/Clinical Review/clinicalReviewv14i6.pdf?dmc=1&ts=20180118T1859208109.

10 Pearlman MD, Gluck PA. Medical liability and patient safety: setting the proper course. *Obstet Gynecol*. 2005;105(5):941–943.

11 Veltman LL. Getting to Havarti: moving toward patient safety in obstetrics. *Obstet Gynecol*. 2007;110(5):1146–1150.

Chapter 17

Just Culture in Women's Health Services

Michael E. Barfield, Margaret Sturdivant, and Karen Frush

Overview

The patient safety movement, initiated over a decade ago after the publication of the Institute of Medicine (IOM) report "To Err is Human" [1] has led to great advancements in the science of safety and a deeper understanding of the humbling reality of patient harm. Physicians, nurses, and other healthcare professionals, although highly trained, well-intended and dedicated, work in a healthcare system that has become so highly complex and high-risk that they simply cannot be careful or vigilant enough to prevent all errors from occurring. In the traditional culture of medicine, the approach to errors often focused on identifying the "guilty person" or the healthcare provider at fault, rather than on broken processes and system errors. Indeed, many adverse events have been attributed to the failure of an individual clinician to perform, often to a level of perfection unattainable by any of us [2].

A major insight from the patient safety movement is the need for a cultural shift from a focus on individual performance to systems thinking, safety science, and human factors engineering, as noted by Lucian Leape [3]. Rather than focusing on mistakes, the more effective approach to improve patient safety is through safe and reliable system design which (1) identifies and eliminates conditions that lead to human error and violations, (2) catches or intercepts errors before they cause harm, or (3) mitigates the impact of those errors that penetrate layers of defenses and reach patients.

The shift from a culture of blame should not be misconstrued as a transition to a "blame-free" environment, but rather to a focus on accountability and an increased awareness of the impact of behavioral choices by healthcare professionals in the complex environment in which they work [4]. Healthcare providers have an awesome responsibility to keep patients safe while realizing their own vulnerability to error, as human beings.

This chapter will describe models of accountability and their application to the clinical setting.

Two case examples will be provided.

Background

To appreciate the importance of a fair and just culture in improving patient safety, one must first consider that healthcare is a human endeavor, and fallibility is a characteristic of being human. Thus, if patient safety was dependent upon healthcare professionals "doing the right thing every time," there would always be adverse events and harm due to our inherent fallibility. Safe systems must be designed to account for human errors and violations; that is, to prevent, catch and mitigate errors, and manage behavioral choices and violations.

Healthcare providers in women's services work in a highly complex, high-risk environment that sometimes "sets them up" for errors. This may be best understood by considering latent factors that often account for "holes in Swiss Cheese," as described by James Reason's model of organizational accidents [5]. Holes in the layers of defenses that protect patients from healthcare provider errors and violations may include such factors as poor equipment design or defective instruments, production pressures, high-stress/high-acuity clinical situations, inadequate staffing, poor teamwork and communication, and procedures or processes that seemingly necessitate a violation in order to get the job done [6]. In some organizations, these latent factors are recognized and addressed before harm occurs. Such organizations, referred to as high-reliability organizations (HROs), consistently function at safe levels despite operating in high-risk, highly complex environments [7]. HROs are characterized by systematic approaches to process improvement and strong safety cultures that support best safety practices, foster an environment of mutual respect, engender trust and effective communication among members of the healthcare team, and encourage reporting of and learning from errors and near-misses in order to prevent harm in the future [8].

A strong safety culture requires a shift from the traditional punitive approach to medical errors. As Lucian Leape testified before Congress in 2001, "The single greatest impediment to error prevention is that we punish people for making mistakes." As the patient safety movement began to take hold over the past decade, some patient safety advocates supported a radical shift from a "culture of blame" to a "blame-free" approach to adverse events. Other patient safety leaders countered, suggesting that because healthcare directly impacts peoples' lives, the appropriate shift is to a focus on accountability, especially when errors are due to neglect, recklessness or a deliberate deviation from or disregard for a safety practice.

A fair and just culture attempts to strike a balance between punitive and blame-free approaches to adverse events and medical errors [4]. Such a culture requires that leaders understand the basic concepts of human factors and human performance, especially as it relates to accident causation [9]. Human factors engineers believe that contributing factors to accident (adverse event) causation begin with leadership and management, as leaders and managers impact latent factors described by Reason, including the physical environment, operations and workflow, and the psycho-social environment and behavioral norms of clinicians on the unit. These factors then affect the performance of clinicians who, as humans, are subject to errors (mistakes, slips, lapses) and procedural violations [10]. Many times these errors are either insignificant or are intercepted, and no harm occurs. However, this is not always true.

From the perspective of human factors experts, *errors and violations* are behaviors that stray from practices required to maintain patient safety. *Slips and lapses* are unplanned deviations from that which was intended; *mistakes* are failures of intended actions to achieve desired goals; and *violations* are deliberate, but not necessarily reprehensible deviations from those practices deemed necessary to maintain the safe operation of a potentially hazardous system [6].

Human factors experts fundamentally believe that human errors are not the cause of patient harm, but the by-product of (human) providers trying to achieve success while working in an imperfect system that is often fast-paced, highly complex, and resource-constrained. Similarly, violations are not explanations

for adverse outcomes, as the overwhelming number of healthcare providers come to work to do the right thing. While violations are deliberate choices to deviate from rules and standards, they are often preceded by a long, slow drift in practice. The term "normalization of deviance" is sometimes used to describe a systemic migration of safe boundaries in which individuals repeatedly get away with a deviation from established standards and achieve their goal without any negative consequences [11]. Over time, the individual fails to see his or her actions as deviant. For example, many individuals drive approximately 5–10 mph over the speed limit, or just fast enough to pass the car in the "slow lane" of the freeway. This type of behavior seems "normal," as plenty of other drivers do the same thing.

At the time of an adverse event, it is easy for managers and senior leaders to point out "right and wrong choices" made by an employee or provider and blame those who "deviate" from a safe practice or are non-compliant with a hospital policy. Defining non-compliance, though, is not always straightforward. The expected level of compliance, and therefore the interpretation of non-compliance or violation, varies according to hospital or unit culture, which is influenced by leaders. A strong safety culture values transparency and best safety practices, and is shaped by leaders who support, expect, and model safety-sensitive behaviors. When expectations of behavioral norms and safety practices are clear, individuals can then be held accountable. On the other hand, when the rules and expectations vary from one professional group to another, or leaders model different behaviors than they promote, the expected level of compliance (and thus non-compliance) is much less clear. Leadership response to an adverse event should not be dependent on patient outcome, but too often, it is the degree of patient harm that determines the consequences for the involved clinician.

The factors that influence a person's propensity to violate are well-documented [12], and we can look again at the topic of driving habits to gain more understanding of these factors. When travelling on a freeway, many individuals drive 5–10 mph faster than the posted speed limit. When cars begin to pass, a common response is to speed up and travel at a higher rate of speed, equal to that of "everyone else" until some unstated maximum speed (the "danger zone") is reached. The conditions that shape these driving behaviors include low probability of being caught (for going "just a little over the speed limit"), lack of recognition of risk, group pressure, and copying the behavior of others [12]. These are human traits, and the same conditions exist in the clinical setting, influencing the behaviors of the healthcare professionals who work there.

Human fallibility is a part of healthcare, and effective leaders understand that healthcare providers cannot will themselves to be perfect. Several models of accountability that can help guide and manage behavioral choices of professionals are described below.

Models of Accountability

Patient safety experts commonly refer to two different "models of accountability": one described by James Reason and the other by David Marx.

Reason's model is best understood by first returning to the "Swiss cheese model of organizational accidents" referenced previously in this chapter [5]. Reason presented this model to illustrate that failures in a system, if aligned, could allow an adverse event, or accident, to occur. Each slice of cheese, representing a defense layer in the system, if intact, would prevent a possible accident from advancing. Defenses may be "hard stops," such as technical devices, or "soft stops," such as people or policies. Each defense layer, however, has weaknesses as illustrated by the "holes" in the Swiss cheese, and if the holes line up, a threat or potential harm is able to pass through and ultimately reach the patient. Having redundant checks or intact defense layers can create barriers, enabling the system to intercept the threat and prevent it from passing through to the patient [5].

Using Reason's model, it becomes clear that human error is only one weakness, or one hole in the Swiss cheese. The system must be designed with sufficient layers of defense to protect patients from providers' errors. When an adverse event occurs, it is nearly always the result of a faulty system, and thus blaming a single individual does little to prevent the same accident (or adverse event) from happening again in the future. Yet at the same time, healthcare providers bear great responsibility for their decisions and their behaviors, because patients' very lives are impacted, and potentially harmed, by these decisions and behavioral choices. Reason suggests that a safe culture is one in which healthcare professionals are clear about where the line must be drawn between acceptable and unacceptable behavior [12].

David Marx has described a similar culture, which he termed a "Just Culture." According to Marx, five skills are necessary for an organization to fully embrace a just culture:

(1) identifying values and setting expectations
(2) designing values-supportive systems
(3) helping humans make safe behavioral choices
(4) fostering reporting and learning systems
(5) being fair or "just" [13].

Each organization must define the behavioral expectations related to its primary values and outline specific duties of clinicians and employees. Marx has described three primary duties:

(1) the duty to produce an outcome
(2) the duty to follow a procedural rule and
(3) the duty to avoid causing unjustifiable risk or harm.

The duty to produce an outcome is under the control of the individual such as arriving to work at a predetermined time. The employer is not concerned with how the employee gets to the work setting. The employer is focused on the outcome, arriving on time. The duty to follow a procedural rule is a system that is controlled by the employer, such as defining the appropriate steps for a skill/task completion. The overarching duty to avoid causing unjustifiable risk or harm is our duty no matter what the task or issue at hand. As humans, we are expected to prioritize and balance the conflicting and overlapping duties with friends and families, patients, and employers. It is when a duty is breached that we must determine the level of accountability involved in the specific situation [13].

In a just culture, the organization is expected to define its underlying beliefs or principles for determining acceptable and unacceptable actions. The following principles should be considered:

- Humans make errors (slips and lapses)
- Humans drift from the procedural way of doing things
- We are surrounded by risk
- We are all accountable
- We must be consistent in applying our values
- We must measure our progress

One of the challenges in building a just culture is actually defining what is considered to be "justice" [14]. Decision trees or algorithms with standardized questions facilitate the reviewer in determining culpability for the event [14]. Two models that have been adopted widely across healthcare organizations to aid in the decision-making process are James Reason's Unsafe Acts Algorithm [12] and David Marx's Just Culture Algorithm [13].

The structured approach for investigating an event allows the organization to gather information that can be used to modify practices or redesign systems. After conducting the event investigation, it is critical to assess the behavioral elements of the person's actions. Was the event a result of inadvertent action (human error), or unintentional risk-taking (at-risk behavior), or intentional risk taking (reckless). The manager's decision in following the decision-making tree for a simple human error may result in consoling the individual while managing change in processes, procedures, training or design. For at-risk behavior, the manager may remove incentives for the at-risk behavior, create incentives for promoting healthy behavior, and increase situational awareness by coaching the individual(s). If intentional risk-taking behavior (recklessness) is determined, the employee will require remedial, administrative, or disciplinary action.

Following the investigation of an event, the assessment of behavioral choices of the clinicians or individuals involved is critical to maintaining a "Just Culture." Expectations must be made clear by the organization, and then all employees or clinicians, whatever their title, rank, or role, must be held accountable to the same behavioral expectations.

Making Safe Choices

Duke University Hospital (DUH), like many other academic institutions in the US, has always been dedicated to delivering high-quality care to patients and their families. After the publication of two IOM reports, *To Err is Human* in 2000 [1] and *Crossing the Quality Chasm* in 2002 [15], leaders at Duke recommitted themselves to improving patient safety and began a journey to increase the awareness of each person's role in providing safe care and creating a culture of safety. In 2007, DUH senior leaders sought an innovative way to empower frontline staff to enhance patient safety by understanding the importance of behavioral choices and system design through real event investigations. Leaders designed an experiential, one-day educational event in which multidisciplinary participants work in small groups and discuss local safety events. Participants were asked to identify and analyze risks taken by those involved, to review

and outline process failures, and to develop and assess potential solutions to enhance patient safety. The focus is on helping participants understand the behavioral factors (human error, at-risk, and reckless behaviors) involved, and clarifying the system's responsibility to create a safe culture. The multidisciplinary team members are encouraged to discuss issues related to role clarity, and they often gain a better understanding of the value of each member in detecting and mitigating risk and preventing harm in the future.

At the beginning of each session, a true story of a medical error resulting in harm is shared and serves to paint a vivid image to associate with the data. A brief introduction to the key concepts of a just culture and behavioral choices serves as the foundation for the training. An appreciation of behavioral choices is gained early from small group exercises describing risks taken in other activities, such as driving a car. Common themes for why a person may select a risk-taking behavior, such as the perception of "saving time," start to emerge among the participants. Following lively interactions, the group transitions to identifying risk-taking behaviors observed in the clinical setting, the incentives and the frequency of the occurrence. The participants are entrusted with details from specific events relative to their work area to conduct an analysis for a greater understanding of how human factors may have impacted the event, potential system concerns, and the appropriate response of leadership when considering the individuals' choices and personal accountability (console, coach, or discipline). At the conclusion of each case, participants discuss "lessons learned" and are informed of actions which resulted in improvements such as new policies, technology enhancements, or other system design enhancements.

One may decide to use this educational strategy for a large group or at the unit level to learn from safety events. The "Making Safe Choices" curriculum has expanded to include a course tailored for managers delving into the actual steps of the Just Culture algorithm and strategies for building personal accountability. In addition, customized sessions for specific patient populations, the receptionists, technicians, surgeons, nurses, and other members of the team have been developed to analyze how each person is accountable for their actions to promote a just and fair culture.

Case Examples

The following cases are based on real events with revisions to demonstrate how Just Culture principles can be applied to the Women's Services clinical setting.

Case #1

A young woman, 1 week postpartum, with an immunodeficiency and allergies to multiple medications including several antibiotics came to the Emergency Department late one afternoon with a fever and lower abdominal pain. She was placed in room 8. She had noticed an increase in blood-stained vaginal drainage over the past 2 days and this morning the discharge had started to become foul-smelling. Upon arrival to the ED she was found to be febrile and tachycardic but her blood pressure was in her normal range (118/62). IV access was obtained and IV fluids were started after blood was obtained and sent to the lab for appropriate studies. Due to her fever, the finding of lower abdominal tenderness on physical exam and her immunocompromised state, antibiotics were ordered by the ED physician.

The ED was very busy that day, and an older patient in the same care area began to seize, then suffered a cardiopulmonary arrest. Several nurses ran to the room to assist in resuscitation efforts. The care of the young woman in room 8 was handed off to a nurse who had recently arrived to start her shift. The nurse entered room 8, introduced herself and told the patient she had brought two medicines that had been ordered by the physician: one medicine for pain, and the other a penicillin-type antibiotic. The young woman, who was feeling worse as the day had gone on, spoke up and said, "Please don't give me any penicillin. I'm allergic to penicillin medications." The nurse paused briefly, but having picked up several patients who were in need of medications within the hour, stated, "OK, I'll go check the order for the antibiotic, but I'll give you your pain medicine first." The patient held out her arm with an IV in place, relieved to be getting some pain medicine for the increasing discomfort she was feeling. As the nurse began to infuse the medication, the patient realized her breathing had suddenly become more difficult and she cried out, "What medicine are you giving me?" "Relax," the nurse replied. "Sometimes patients feel a bit of a rush with IV morphine." "Morphine?? I can't have morphine," cried the patient. "I've had a bad reaction to morphine in the past. Please go get the doctor!" The nurse ran to get an ED physician, and when they returned to room 8, they found that the patient was breathing slowly and irregularly. The patient was successfully stabilized and admitted to the ICU for further care.

A root-cause analysis (RCA) was completed and revealed several contributing factors. Systems factors included staffing (a number of new nurses were working in the ED that day), production pressure, and equipment issues (one CT scanner was out of service).

Due to high patient volume, physical environment factors included the use of hallway beds, high noise level, and lack of space for private conversations with patients and families; patient acuity was also very high that day. Communication factors included multiple handoffs in care, and there were multiple patients in the ED who required translation services.

When reviewing behavioral choices of individual clinicians involved in the case, it became apparent that the nurse who administered the pain medication had identified the patient by room number (room 8), rather than by using a double identifier (checking the patient's name and medical record number on her ID bracelet). In the Just Culture framework, this choice would fall into the "risk-taking" category (even though the risk-taking was unintentional, and the nurse certainly meant no harm to the patient). This type of choice requires discussion and coaching, to help the employee understand the level of risk that is actually involved.

A patient safety leader in the ED met with the nurse, who had no past experience with a medication error or harmful patient event, to discuss the case. When asked how she usually identifies a patient before giving medications, the nurse acknowledged that she knew the policy states to use a double identifier. "Most times I do this. But that day in the ED was so busy, and there were a lot of really sick patients, and I picked up two patients side by side (rooms 8 and 9) who both needed pain medications and antibiotics. I took the medications into the room for the patient in room 9, and I just knew I was in room 9."

The nurse further described being somewhat distracted and feeling pressured by having to complete many time-sensitive tasks. Upon discussion and reflection, though, she acknowledged that she had drifted from the safe practice of checking a double identifier. She had given a few medications in the past to patients without checking the ID bracelet to confirm a double-identifier. She understood the policy and knew that it existed, but she had now acquired a whole new level of awareness and respect for following this safe practice with every single patient.

In coaching the nurse, the patient safety leader asked how "lessons learned" from this experience might be shared with other nurses and providers in the ED. The nurse paused and then stated that she would like to share the story at staff meeting. She felt sure that some of the other nurses in the ED had drifted from the safe practice of completing a double identifier before administering medications, and she wanted to share her experience so that they could gain increased awareness of the importance of this practice before another medication error took place.

Case #2

MG is a 24-year-old woman who is pregnant. She moved to the US from a small village in West Africa two years ago, and on the advice of her friends, she sought pre-natal care at her county health department at around 6 weeks. Ultrasound at 12 weeks gestation showed a healthy, normal fetus. She is encouraged to establish a relationship with a local obstetrician; however, her limited experience with the healthcare system in the US has taught her that doctor visits are expensive, not realizing that she will qualify for Medicaid. MG has rudimentary English skills and will have to continue to work during her pregnancy to ensure they have enough money to care for the baby. She elects to continue with checks at the health department until she delivers, when she plans to go to the large, local hospital. Some of her new friends have had babies in the US, and they have had uncomplicated pregnancies with this approach.

At 37 weeks, MG does not feel well. She has the familiar swelling in her feet and legs that she has grown to expect. However, the swelling is now affecting her hands and arms. She is concerned, but she is not having any pain or contractions. In her home country, one of the elder women of the village would come to visit her and likely give her some strong tea, but not here. It is a Sunday, and she decides that she will go to the health department after lunch on Monday to see if they can help her.

MG goes to the health department the following day. Her blood pressure is 160/90. The nurse then asks for a urine specimen and says that there is something "abnormal." The nurse asks MG who her obstetrician is because she wants to communicate this information. MG has not sought a doctor yet because of the expenses and feels guilty. She had looked at some of the doctors' names in a phone book left and recalls the name of one that had a very nice ad. She tells the nurse the name of the practice. Unfortunately the waiting room is quite busy, and the nurse assumes that MG understands the gravity of the situation. There is not a translator on site who speaks her particular language, and it will take "too long" to get one on the phone. On a piece of paper, the nurse writes a short note with a lot of numbers on it and hands the note back to MG. She tells her to take that to her doctor, and MG leaves the clinic. The nurse finishes documenting the visit and decides to give the doctors' office a call to alert them of MG's arrival. She speaks to one of the nurses there who says that their office has no record of MG. The nurse tries the phone number she has

on record for MG, but it was a prepaid cell phone which has expired.

Confused and uncertain, MG stares at the numbers on the paper. She doesn't feel well enough to go back to work so she goes home where her husband asks about her visit. MG says she is tired and wants to lie down for a while, but insists she'll be fine, and that he should go to work. Several hours later, MG awakens with a pounding headache and realizes that she has been bleeding, too. She is dizzy and confused, and she is having some pains in her abdomen. She does not have a phone and feels too weak to walk, so she tries to crawl to the front door hoping she can get the attention of one of her neighbors.

Later that night, her husband comes home from work and finds MG lying on the floor in the apartment. He wakes her up, and she tells him about the pain and the headache. Worried, he carries her to the car and drives to the hospital. They are checked through the metal detectors and x-ray machines and finally allowed to pass into a waiting room full of people. He helps MG to an empty chair and goes to the reception desk, where the clerk is quite busy. She asks him a few questions and, through his broken English, she determines that his wife has a headache. She gives him a clipboard with many papers on it, asking him to complete these and return to the desk. He dutifully proceeds to sit beside his wife while they try to negotiate the pages of questions about finances and medical history. He is frustrated because he forgot to bring the note from the nurse at the health department, which he thinks would help the doctors in the ED. They finish the paperwork and go back to the desk. MG is having more abdominal pain, and she is quite dizzy. The nurse calls her to the triage room, where MG's blood pressure is 182/104. The nurse calls for a transporter, and MG is wheeled out of the ED to go to the labor and delivery ward at 10 PM. As they arrive at L&D, the transporter notices that MG slumps down in the chair and begins shaking violently. MG is quickly taken back to a room, given magnesium, and attached to monitors. Her blood pressure slowly normalizes, and the delivery room team is successful in finding a faint fetal heartbeat. As treatment continues, MG begins to labor. She labors for several hours. Finally, at 6 AM the next morning, the infant is born with APGARs of 4, 6, 8. The infant is taken to the neonatal intensive care unit and receives oxygen therapy for the next several days. Ultimately, MG and Baby G do well and go home safely.

In this case, we can identify multiple opportunities for improvements in MG's care. At the beginning, we see a prenatal care system that is clearly overtaxed. For a normal pregnancy, MG's strategy may not be optimal, but it could be feasible. The Health Department nurse appropriately instructs the patient to contact an obstetrician's office; however, there is no mechanism in place to assure that this happens. While giving information to the patient that she can take to her provider is helpful, it does not appear the health department team checked with the patient to ensure that she understood the implications of her condition and the instructions to contact her doctor more quickly. It may have also been helpful at that point to have MG transported to the hospital for more formal evaluation. Once at the hospital, MG and her husband encountered many more obstacles before finally receiving appropriate care.

The Just Culture model of accountability suggests that patient safety requires a system of shared accountability in which leaders of healthcare institutions are accountable for designing safe systems and for encouraging and supporting safe choices of clinicians and staff. Each individual (clinicians and staff), in turn, is accountable for the quality of his/her choices – knowing that, as humans, one cannot will oneself to be perfect, but each individual can strive to make the best possible choices. Every employee is accountable for patient safety. Looking at MG's case from this perspective, it becomes apparent that there were many missed opportunities by all members of the healthcare team. Leaders and physicians from the hospital and from the Health Department need to establish effective communication systems and protocols to facilitate transfer of patients like MG, who may need a higher level of care than can be delivered at the clinic. Front desk staff and nurses may be the only healthcare team members who see a patient at the Health Department, so it is incumbent upon them to assure clear communication and follow-up, rather than assuming a patient understands. A teach-back is one example of a communication tool which may have worked well in this case, but each member of the healthcare team has a choice as to whether and when to use such tools.

Summary

Modern healthcare is a high-risk and highly complex industry, and healthcare providers, although very bright, hard-working and committed, are (simply) human beings, with human limitations. As the reality of unintended patient harm has become more clear over the past decade, patient safety leaders have advocated for systems-thinking and a transition in healthcare culture from the traditional culture of blame to a just and fair culture of accountability. As important

as "fixing defects" and building safety into the system is the responsibility of leaders to manage behavioral choices of clinicians and front-line providers. This requires leaders who provide clear expectations of behavioral choices, create an environment that encourages staff to speak up with safety concerns, and most importantly, leaders who model the very behaviors they expect of staff.

As we move into the second decade of enhanced attention to patient safety and culture continues to evolve, it will be imperative to adapt to the changing paradigms for patient care being modeled in undergraduate and graduate medical education. The 2007 American Association of Medical Colleges (AAMC) Presidential address highlighted important changes occurring at academic institutions across the nation with trends toward team-based approaches to patient care [16]. As the model shifts away from isolated, solo providers providing disjointed and often inconsistent care for patients to one in which multiple providers across specialties, age ranges, and training pedigrees function as a team delivering high-quality care, a shift in culture towards shared accountability and a focus on mitigating human error will enhance the overall experience for our patients, their loved ones, and the entire medical team.

Recognizing that "to err is human, and to drift is human," effective leaders understand the need for a transition from a culture of blame to a focus on accountability and an increased awareness of the impact of behavioral choices by healthcare professionals in the complex environment in which they work. Healthcare providers have an awesome responsibility to keep patients safe while realizing their own vulnerability to error, as human beings. Several models of accountability are available to help guide healthcare leaders and providers along this journey.

References

1 Kohn LT, Corrigan J, Donaldson MS. *To Err is Human: Building a Safer Health System*. Washington, DC: National Academy Press; 2000.

2 Leape, L. Error in medicine. *JAMA*. 1994;272(23):851–857.

3 Lucian Leape Institute at the National Patient Safety Foundation. The Patient Safety Imperative for Health Care Reform: Building Safe, Effective Health Care. Position Statement issued October, 2009. www.npsf. org/LLI (accessed January 1, 2014).

4   Wachter RM, Pronovost PJ. Balancing "no blame" with accountability in patient safety. *N Engl J Med.* 2009;361(14):1401–1406.

5   Reason J. *Human Error.* Cambridge: Cambridge University Press; 1990.

6   Bogner MS, ed. *Human Error in Medicine*: Hillsdale, NJ: Lawrence Erlbaum Associates; 1994.

7   Weick KE, Sutcliffe KM. *Managing the Unexpected: Resilient Performance in an Age of Uncertainty*, 2nd ed. San Francisco, CA: Jossey-Bass; 2007.

8   Petschonek S, Burlison J, Cross C, et al. Development of the Just Culture assessment tool: measuring the perceptions of healthcare professionals in hospitals. *J Patient Saf.* 2013;9(4):190–197.

9   Bonacum D, Frush K, Balik B, Conway J. The role of leadership. In: *The Essential Guide for Patient Safety Officers*. Oakbrook, IL: Joint Commission Resources; 2013: 1–12.

10 Gosbee JW, Gosbee LL, eds. *Human Human Factors Engineering to Improve Patient Safety*. Oakbrook, IL: Joint Commission Resources; 2005.

11 Vaughn D. *The Challenger Launch Decision: Risky Technology, Culture, and Deviance at NASA*. Chicago, IL: University of Chicago Press; 1996.

12 Reason J. *Managing the Risk of Organizational Accidents*. Aldershot: Ashgate; 1997.

13 Marx D. *Patient Safety and the "Just Culture": A Primer for Health Care executives.* New York, NY: Columbia University Press; 2001.

14 Dekker S. *The Field Guide to Understanding Human Error*. Burlington, VT. Ashgate; 2006.

15 *Crossing the Quality Chasm. A New Health System of the 21st Century*. Washington, DC: National Academy Press, 2001.

16 Kirch DG. Culture and the Courage to Change. AAMC President's Address; 2007.

Chapter 18

Medication Safety in Obstetrics and Gynecology

Roseann Richards and Angela Brenner

Patient Cases in Medication Safety

Magnesium – Patient Case

A 35-year-old G1P1 at 34 weeks is undergoing induction of labor for preeclampsia. Her nurse obtains two bags of Lactated Ringer's (LR) solution from stock and adds 40 g of magnesium sulfate to one bag for seizure prophylaxis. The nurse administers a 6-g bolus dose of magnesium sulfate and then starts a magnesium sulfate infusion at 2 g/hour as well as starting the maintenance solution of LR at 300 ml/hour. A few hours later, the patient reports feeling flushed and nauseated to her nurse and is assured by the nurse that these symptoms are expected. The patient is later found not breathing and without a pulse. *Findings:* An analysis found that the maintenance IV (300 ml/hour) contained 40 g of magnesium and the bag labeled as magnesium sulfate contained only LR. The admixture label had been placed on the wrong bag [1].

Oxytocin – Patient Case

A 28-year-old nulliparous woman at 41 weeks gestation age is admitted for a scheduled induction of labor. Orders for "Pitocin per protocol" are processed by the pharmacist and a vial of oxytocin is sent to the floor. The nurse mixes the vial with a liter of normal saline. The infusion is started at 1 mUnit/min and is increased by 2 mUnit/min every 20 minutes. After about 30 min the patient requests to ambulate. The patient's current status is noted and she is unhooked from the external monitor. The patient is reattached to the external monitor approximately 40 min later and maternal tachysystole and fetal bradycardia are observed.

Prostaglandin – Patient Case

A physician has finished the examination of the patient and has determined the need for induction of labor.

The chart cannot be located, so the nurse is given a verbal order to start "prostaglandin intravaginally q6h." The nurse recalls that the automated dispensing cabinet has misoprostol available on "override." A 100 μg misoprostol tablet is removed and is administered to the patient. The nurse is extremely busy and the verbal order is written in the chart after she administers the second dose. Shortly after the order has been sent to pharmacy, pharmacy calls to clarify the prostaglandin product, dose, and indication.

Findings: The recommended dosing is 25 μg, ¼ of the 100-μg tablet, for induction of labor. The patient has received a fourfold overdose for two doses.

For each case:

What major errors in the medication-use processes were involved in this case?

What safety measures could be implemented to prevent a similar incident from occurring in the future?

Medication errors, as well as medication-use processes, are key considerations in daily practice in healthcare following the report issued by the Institute for Safe Medication Practices (ISMP) in 1999, *To Err is Human: Building a Safer Health System* [2]. This report highlighted the complexity of the medication-use system and pushed for patient safety and error reduction within healthcare systems. Additionally, to help guide practitioners in obstetrics and gynecology, the American Congress of Obstetricians and Gynecologists (ACOG) issued a committee opinion in 2009 that recommends safety priorities by incorporating safe medical practices and improved communication among healthcare professionals and with patients [3].

The medication-use process is complex and can be divided into specific phases: prescribing, order processing, dispensing, administration, and monitoring [4]. These are key elements to patient safety and are

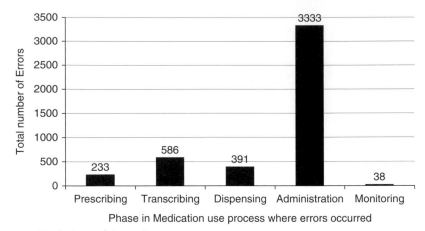

Figure 18.1 Errors occurred in all phases of the medication-use process.

(From Kfuri TA, Morlock L, Hicks RW, et al. Medication errors in obstetrics. *Clin Perinatol.* 2008;35:101–117.)

Table 18.1 Classification and examples of high alert medications.

High-alert classes/categories of medications	
Adrenergic agonist	Adrenergic antagonists
Antithrombotic agents	Inotropic medications, IV
Chemotherapeutic agents	Dextrose, hypertonic, ≥ 20%
Insulin	Parenteral nutrition
Moderate sedation agents	Hypertonic sodium chloride (> 0.9%)
Neuromuscular blocking agents	Parenteral nutrition
Epidural or intrathecal medication	Narcotics/opioids
Specific high-alert medications	
Methotrexate (oral and non-oncologic use)	Magnesium sulfate injection
Oxytocin, IV	Opium tincture
Potassium chloride for injection concentrate	Potassium phosphate injection
Promethazine, IV	Nitroprusside

Complete list available at: www.ismp.org/Tools/highalertmedications.pdf

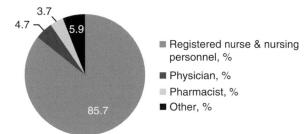

Figure 18.2 Level of staff associated with initial medication errors.

(From Kfuri TA, Morlock L, Hicks RW, et al. Medication errors in obstetrics. *Clin Perinatol.* 2008;35:101–117.)

evaluated when examining types and rates of errors. The ISMP has developed a guide that includes a list of medication classes and specific medications that are commonly associated with errors or those medications that when given in error can result in devastating effects to patients [5] (Table 18.1). This guide is designed to increase medication safety practices surrounding these products in an effort to reduce the risk of errors. Several of the listed high-alert medications

such as magnesium sulfate, oxytocin, and epidural medications are commonly used in daily practice in obstetrics and gynecology.

Several studies have evaluated medication error rates in the obstetric patient population. Kfuri et al. utilized a national, voluntary adverse event reporting program, MEDMARX®, to evaluate medication errors in labor and delivery areas, obstetric recovery rooms, and maternity wards [6]. Medication errors in obstetric and gynecology patients accounted for 4.8% of all errors reported to MEDMARX® from January 1, 2003, to December 21, 2005. It was consistently noted that errors occurred in all phases of the medication use process, but the vast majority (> 70%) were found to occur during the administration phase (Figure 18.1). Consistent with the findings of the origin of error, nursing staff was most frequently associated with medication errors (Figure 18.2). These trends were echoed in an article by the Pennsylvania Patient Safety Advisory [7]. In the data provided by Pennsylvania healthcare facilities from June 2004 to April 2009, administration errors including incorrect drug, dose, time, rate of infusion, route, and wrong patient accounted for approximately 40% of the medication errors reported in the labor and delivery population. These studies demonstrate the unique opportunities to reduce errors and improve patient safety. This chapter will examine the risk for medication errors in obstetrics and gynecology, focus on medications commonly used in this patient population and provide recommendations and models to improve medication safety.

Opportunities for Medication Errors in Obstetrics and Gynecology

Procurement and Product Selection

Procurement of medication and product selection are important components of the medication-use system to review when attempting to prevent or analyze medication errors. When available, premix or ready-to-use products should be utilized by the institution [8]. This practice reduces errors associated with preparation, labeling, and expiration dating that may be associated with sterile compounding. If a ready-to-use product is not available, medications requiring compounding should be prepared by pharmacy in a sterile environment instead of preparation or mixing on nursing units.

Lack of dosing and concentration standardization may also contribute to administration errors [9,10]. Standardized concentrations of key infusions in the obstetric population, such as magnesium sulfate and oxytocin, contribute to patient safety by limiting the need for infusion calculations, minimizing compounding errors, and providing the ability to fully utilize available technologies such as smart-infusion pump and medication barcode scanning. The implementation of standardized concentrations can also improve understanding between disciplines by providing common expectations regarding the medication or infusion.

Premixed or ready-to-use products have their own associated risks. These risks are often related to the packaging and labeling rather than the actual product itself. Look-alike premix packages, similar product lettering or similar over-wrap packaging has frequently led to incorrect product selection. To avoid these safety risks, these products should be stored in physically separate areas.

Prescribing

For an order to be considered complete, it must include a legible medication name, dose, route of administration, frequency or rate, and indication [11]. Computerized physician order entry (CPOE) can help to ensure the legibility and completeness of orders by requiring various information fields to be completed before the order can be processed. The avoidance of unapproved abbreviations and items such as leading or trailing zeros is important when writing orders [12,13] (Table 18.2). Finally, it is recommended that prior to ordering, the drug should be within the scope of practice of the prescriber and patient allergies should have been reviewed.

Table 18.2 The Joint Commission list of "do not use" abbreviations.

"Do not use" abbreviations		
Do not use	**Potential problem**	**Use instead**
U, u	Mistaken for "0" (zero), the number "4" or "cc"	Write "unit"
IU	Mistaken for IV (intravenous) or the number "10"	Write "International Unit"
Q.D.,QD, qd, q.d.	Mistaken for each other	Write "daily"
Q.O.D., QOD, qod	Period after the Q can be mistaken for "I" "O" can be mistaken for "I"	Write "every other day"
Trailing zero (X.0 mg) Lack of a leading zero (.X mg)	Decimal point may be missed	Write X mg Write 0.X mg
MS, MSO_4, $MgSO_4$	Confused for one another	Write "morphine sulfate" Write "magnesium sulfate"

Complete list available at: www.jointcommission.org/assets/1/18/Do_Not_Use_List.pdf and www.ismp.org/tools/errorproneabbreviations.pdf

Order Interpretation/Transcription

The medication order interpretation/transcription process has many inherent challenges. In paper-based systems, order interpretation accuracy is heavily dependent on order legibility, interpretation of abbreviations, knowledge of indications for which a medication is being prescribed, and understanding of how each newly prescribed medication interacts with and/or contributes to the overall medical plan. In the CPOE environment many of the same challenges exist, although the issues of legibility and abbreviation/notation interpretation are replaced by those of proper medication selection including dosage form choices. Furthermore, in the obstetrical setting the often fast-paced environment necessitates the use of verbal orders which add another layer of complexity to the order interpretation and transcription process [14]. The individual who received a verbal order must translate, transcribe, and then be certain to read back the order to the physician to verify that it is correct. A second practitioner should then interpret and verify that the orders are correctly entered into the computer system. This process involves multiple individuals to ensure that the end result is that which the physician intended.

Order sets can provide some structured guidance in the ordering process, and can be utilized in both the paper and computerized ordering environments. The improved safety gained by using this more standardized approach is only achievable if providers utilize the order sets as originally intended. Incomplete, reworked, or vague notations on standardized order sets can lead to as many or more errors in the interpretation process.

Dispensing

Medication dispensing has become increasingly complex over the years. Often multiple sources for the medication and multiple ways of dispensing a single agent exist in one facility. In both the pharmacy dispensing model and the automated dispensing cabinet approach, it is recommended that medications be stored alphabetically by generic name. As generic names can be very similar and look alike, sound-alike medications exist; therefore, it becomes a challenge to store these medications in a distinct manner.

Automated dispensing cabinets generally have medications appropriately listed alphabetically by generic name on the selection screen. Unfortunately, this can still lead to selection errors, particularly if the medications are not specific to the patient's medication profile (i.e., medications which can be retrieved on override). Lastly, although medications are intended to be ordered, stored, and identified by their generic names, providers are often in the habit of ordering these by the original branded name. This can lead to confusion, when medications are dispensed to practitioners who may not be as familiar with generic and brand name interchanges, and who also may be under pressure to provide the medications quickly.

To minimize the chances of errors in dispensing, it is important that a variety of checks and balances be put in place to make medication selection as clear as possible. Because the obstetric setting spans beyond the hospital and into procedural areas and outpatient settings, there are a variety of providers that may fill the dispensing role [15]. Ideally, all orders for medications would be reviewed by a pharmacist prior to being dispensed from the pharmacy or an automated dispensing cabinet. This check of the orders provides an opportunity to identify any ordering errors prior to dispensing and administration. All medications should be stored as safely as possible, with look-alike, sound-alike medications identified clearly. Techniques such as tall-man lettering have been employed for this purpose [16]. All medications recognized by the ISMP as high-risk should have additional labeling indicating the high-risk nature of the medication. For facilities utilizing automated dispensing cabinets, including a list of the cabinet contents with both the generic name and the "brand name" of those medications that are known well by both, can help to provide an additional reference in the interest of safety. Finally, if a medication presentation changes dramatically in appearance (i.e., a new dilution or syringe versus min-bag), communication should be provided to all staff that will be dispensing or receiving the product. Whenever possible, medications should be provided in the final form for administration with complete labeling.

Administration

The administration phase is likely the most critical and carries the most risk to the patient [5,6,17]. It is at this point where there are the fewest checks before the medication actually reaches the patient. The complexity in the number and types of available medications, the multiple indications, variations in dosing, and the variety of methods by which medications can be administered contribute to this risk. Additionally, the fast-paced environment of the labor and delivery unit can challenge the disciplined focus that is needed in the medication administration phase.

Because medication administration is an inherently high-risk task, measures must be taken to hardwire safety into medication administration processes. Systems, such as profiled automated dispensing cabinets, can be implemented to enhance safety [18]. Profiled automated dispensing cabinets require that medication orders be reviewed and entered by a pharmacist for a specific patient prior to allowing the withdrawal of the medication and subsequent administration. Allowing medications to be on "override" and able to be dispensed and administered to any patient with or without an order is a more error-prone practice. If medications need to be available on override for emergency use, those medications should have specific warnings and/or storage alerts to aid in proper medication selection. Furthermore, if the medications are considered "high-risk" in general or in the obstetrical setting, more robust labeling and stop/check measures should be included.

There are a variety of additional technologies designed to hardwire safety in the medication administration phase. Smart-infusion pumps are a method to reduce intravenous (IV) medication administration errors by providing comprehensive, customizable medication lists that are specific to particular areas of care and include soft and hard stops for minimum and maximum doses and infusion rates. These administration "guardrails" can be further customized by medication and associated indication when additional safety checks are deemed useful (i.e., oxytocin used for induction of labor has a far lower rate than that used for prevention of postpartum bleeding) [19]. Barcode medication administration is another electronic system that has been shown to reduce medication errors by hardwiring some of the verification steps of the medication administration process [20]. Additionally, the selection and clear labeling of IV tubing and IV connection sites can minimize wrong-site administration errors. Finally, all providers should have a solid working knowledge of a medication and its use prior to administration.

Creating a Culture of Safety

Every institution must stress the importance of patient safety as a core component of training. Quality and improvement efforts should be transparent and ongoing. As more payers look at performance and safety measures, medication safety has taken center stage [21]. Institutions have a variety of available resources to aid in optimizing medication safety. Reports such as the ISMP Quarterly Action Report are useful for looking at trends in medication safety and errors, reviewing general suggestions for improvements, and promoting the commitment to a routine review of medication errors and the specific impact on the individual institution [22]. As important as it is to proactively prevent errors from occurring, it is also of great importance to create a culture that encourages reporting of errors without fear of judgment or serious personal repercussions. Error reporting should be viewed as an opportunity to improve and perfect systems and processes, as opposed to looking at individual performance failures. A variety of constructive tools can be utilized to systematically review all steps of the medication use process, identify potential process failure points, and to aid in initiating improvements.

Drugs in Pregnancy

The Food and Drug Administration (FDA) of the United States currently classifies prescription medications for use during pregnancy into five categories based on teratogenic potential: A, B, C, D, and X [23] (Table 18.3). The FDA is considering new labeling requirements to replace the current classification

Table 18.3 FDA classification of drug use in pregnancy.

Pregnancy categories	
Category	Definition
A	No risk to the fetus in well-controlled human trials
B	No risk to the fetus in animal studies, but there are no adequate studies in humans or animal studies have shown some risk to the fetus, but studies in humans have not shown harm
C	Adverse effects in animal studies, but there are inadequate human studies
D	Shown to cause fetal harm in human studies
X	Fetal harm in either animal or human studies, and the risk of use outweighs any potential benefits

system. The new labeling would include more scientific data and more specific information beyond teratogenic potential related to use in pregnant women.

In general, medications should only be used during pregnancy when absolutely necessary. For most medications, there simply is not enough data on safety in pregnancy. Some women require prescription medication to treat chronic medical conditions, and will need to work with their physicians to find the most appropriate medication for use during pregnancy. Examples of medications for chronic conditions that are known to cause fetal harm include medications for blood pressure such as angiotensin-converting enzyme inhibitors (ACEIs), for the treatment of seizures such as valproic acid and phenytoin, and for treatment of depression such as paroxetine [24]. Pregnant women should not start or stop a medication without first speaking with their doctor.

Prenatal vitamins are safe and important to take during pregnancy. Herbal medicines have not been tested for safety during pregnancy and patients should be advised to avoid. Over-the-counter medications should also be avoided during pregnancy unless necessary. Data on the safety of herbal and over-the-counter medications is often inconsistent, sparse, or even nonexistent. For pain relief, acetaminophen alone is a relatively safe choice. Non-steroidal anti-inflammatory agents such as aspirin, ibuprofen, and naproxen may be cautiously used during the first and second trimesters, but they are not recommended for use in the third trimester due to the potential for premature closure of the fetal ductus arteriosus. Antihistamines such as diphenhydramine may be used cautiously, but decongestants such as pseudoephedrine and phenylephrine can affect blood flow to the placenta and should not be taken during pregnancy [24]. Because over-the-counter products are often formulated with multiple ingredients, extreme care must be used in selecting a safe product for use in pregnancy. In all cases, patients should always consult with their physician or pharmacist before using an over-the-counter medication. Physicians and pharmacists can consult references such as Clinical Pharmacology, Micromedex, and the Lexi-Comp Drug Information Handbook, as well as more specific resources such as Drugs in Pregnancy and Lactation, LactMed, and Reprotox for guidance in selecting the most appropriate medications for use during pregnancy.

Medications Used in Obstetrics

Oxytocin

Oxytocin, used for the induction of labor and management of postpartum hemorrhage, is the most commonly used medication during the labor and delivery process. It has been reported that approximately 30% of women will receive oxytocin while in labor [25]. Oxytocin is considered a high-risk medication by the IMSP based on its association with significant adverse events which have led to both fetal and/or maternal harm when administered in error. Adverse events include cardiac arrhythmias, uterine hypertonicity, uterine rupture, and subarachnoid hemorrhage. Fetal adverse reactions include cardiac arrhythmias, neonatal seizures, hypoxia leading to permanent brain damage, and possibly death [26].

The risk associated with oxytocin stems from the pharmacokinetic properties of this drug. The half-life of oxytocin ranges from 3 to 10 minutes, resulting in a time to steady state of approximately 40 minutes [27,28]. To ensure appropriate prescribing and administration, knowledge of this medication is vital due to the wide range of effects noted within the therapeutic index. During induction of labor, oxytocin should be started at a predefined dose and titrated in small dosing increments every 30–60 minutes with the goal of using the lowest dose to achieve uterine contractions that are of normal intensity, frequency, and duration, as opposed to a predetermined maximum infusion rate. This will reduce potential risks to both mother and fetus. The practice of increasing the oxytocin infusion every 15–30 minutes should be avoided. Based on the pharmacokinetic properties of the drug, rapid titration (i.e., every 15–30 minutes) has been associated with negative effects on fetal status including oxygen saturation and fetal heart rate patterns [29]. Additionally, due to the associated maternal and fetal risks associated with oxytocin, it should only be used for medical rather than elective induction of labor [26].

Key Medication Safety Recommendations

• Standardized order sets

The order set should include predefined initial rate and titration parameters, standardized monitoring parameters. Guidance for nursing staff should include when to "call MD" and "point of care" instructions as how to adjust the infusion for adverse events such as uterine tachysystole and fetal heart rate abnormalities.

- Standardized concentration

  Ready-to-use or premix products should be utilized. If a premix product is not available, all medications requiring compounding should be prepared by pharmacy. Whether it is a premix product or pharmacy compounded product, utilization of a standard concentration, such as oxytocin 30 units/500 ml, should be implemented to decrease the risk of ordering and infusion errors.

- Smart-pump infusion technology should be used with all medication infusions

  Initial programming of these infusion pumps should include specific drug libraries and safety guardrails.

Magnesium Sulfate

IV magnesium sulfate is used for a variety of indications, but is most commonly used in the obstetric population as the prophylactic anticonvulsant of choice for preeclampsia and eclampsia. During intrapartum hypertension management, magnesium sulfate is routinely used along with antihypertensives, such as labetalol, hydralazine, or nifedipine.

Loading doses of 4–6 g of magnesium sulfate are administered followed by an infusion of 1–2 g/h. These dosing regimens for preeclampsia/eclampsia are significantly higher than those used for other indications such as hypomagnesemia, cardiac arrhythmia, and status asthmaticus. With higher dosing comes an increased risk for toxicities and adverse events. Because of this increased risk and rates of errors associated with prescribing and administration, magnesium sulfate has been listed as a high-alert medication by the ISMP. Signs and symptoms of magnesium toxicity include flushing, hypersomnolence, muscle weakness, loss of deep tendon reflexes, pulmonary edema, central nervous system depression, and respiratory depression [30].

Key Medication Safety Recommendations

- Standardized order sets

  The order set should include predefined bolus doses and infusion rates, monitoring parameters. Guidance for nursing staff should include a defined frequency for clinical assessment (i.e., every 1 hour), specific signs and symptoms

of magnesium toxicity as well as when and how to respond to these, when to "call MD." Additionally the antidote, calcium gluconate, with appropriate dosing should be included on the order set.

- Standardized concentration

  Ready-to-use or premix products should be utilized. If a premix product is not available, all medications requiring compounding should be prepared by pharmacy. Whether it is a premix product or pharmacy compounded product, utilization of a standardized concentration, such as Magnesium sulfate 20 g/500 ml bag, should be implemented to decrease the risk of ordering and infusion errors.

- Product selection and administration guidance

  Separate premix products for initial bolus dose and infusion are recommended. Bolusing from the maintenance magnesium infusion is not recommended.

- Smart-pump infusion technology should be used with all medication infusions

  Initial programming of these infusion pumps should include specific drug libraries and safety guardrails.

Prostaglandins

Prostaglandins are used in the obstetric population for multiple indications including cervical ripening, induction of labor, medical management of early pregnancy failure, as well as postpartum hemorrhage. This class of medication's similar names, indications, number of dosing options and routes of administration contribute to the potential errors associated with prostaglandin use in the obstetric population (Table 18.4a). Incorrect administration or doses of prostaglandin therapy have been associated with uterine tachysytole, uterine rupture, fetal bradycardia associated with hypoxia, hypotension, and death [31]. Because misoprostol can be given orally, sublingual, vaginally, or rectally, the route of administration is selected based on the route's pharmacokinetic and pharmacodynamics and the desired response based on indication (Table 18.4b).

Key Medication Safety Recommendations

- Standardized order sets

  Separate standardized order sets should be available and used for each indication.

Table 18.4a Prostaglandins commonly used in Obstetrics.

Name	Dosing range*	Available dosage forms (routes)	Indications
Misoprostol	25 µg to 1000 µg	100 µg, 200 µg (PO, SL, PR, intravaginally)	Cervical ripening or induction of labor
			Postpartum hemorrhage
			Termination of pregnancy
Dinoprostone	0.5 mg to 20 mg	0.5 mg/3 g gel 10 mg vaginal insert 20 mg vaginal suppository (intravaginally)	Cervical ripening or induction of labor
			Postpartum hemorrhage
			Termination of pregnancy
Carboprost tromethamine	250 mg	250 mg/ml injection (IM)	Postpartum hemorrhage

* Dose dependent on indication, route, and product.

Table 18.4b Administration of misoprostol.

Indication	Route	Dosing (rationale)
Induction of labor	Vaginal**	25 µg (1/4 of a 100 mg tab) q 3–6 hr (Higher doses ≥ 50 µg have been associated with increased rates of tachysystolic uterine contractions)
	Oral	50 µg q 4 hr (Oral route has been shown to be less successful than the vaginal route)
Postpartum hemorrhage	Rectal**	800–1,000 µg (High uterine activity and few side effects)
	Oral	600 µg (High uterine activity but increase side effects compared to rectal)
	Sublingual	800 µg (High uterine activity but increase side effects compared to rectal)
	Vaginal	Vaginal administration not recommended due to concerns of the tablet washing out with ongoing bleeding
Termination of pregnancy	Oral**	Incomplete abortion: 600 µg orally
	Sublingual	Incomplete abortion: 400 µg sublingually is a potential alternative, research is limited. Missed abortion: 600 µg sublingually; may be repeated q 3 hours for two doses
	Vaginal**	Missed abortion: misoprostol, 800 µg vaginally

** Preferred route based indication [32,33].

- Limit available "override" capabilities of automated dispensing cabinets.

  If deemed necessary to have as an override medication for emergency use, limit the number of strengths and products available with this function.

- Medications should be provided in the final form with complete labeling.

  Provision of commonly used strengths, such as 25 µg tablets (¼ of the 100 µg) would reduce the potential for errors associated with the administration of an incorrect dose and any error that may occur while manipulating the product to achieve the desired dose.

Methotrexate

Methotrexate use in obstetrics is limited to treatment of early ectopic pregnancy when detected by ultrasound and no contraindications exist. Ideal candidates are hemodynamically stable, have pretreatment hCG levels less than 5,000 mIU/ml, have tubal size of less than 3–4 cm, no fetal cardiac activity, and are able to comply with post-treatment monitoring. The doses used to medically manage an ectopic pregnancy (50 mg/m^2) are very low compared to those used for other indications (i.e., malignancies). Methotrexate is considered a high-risk medication by the ISMP due to its potential to cause significant patient harm if it is used in error. Patients with renal insufficiency or baseline hematologic or hepatic abnormalities can have significant complications. Therefore, extreme caution must be used when selecting patients who can safely receive this medication. Patients with clinically important abnormalities in hematologic, renal, or liver function studies, patients who are hemodynamically unstable, those with symptoms of potential ectopic rupture, and those with immunodeficiencies, active pulmonary disease, or peptic ulcer disease should not receive methotrexate. Additionally, patients with an hCG of greater than 5,000 mIU/ml are more likely to experience treatment failure [34].

Key Medication Safety Recommendations

- Standardized order sets

  Methotrexate order set for use in obstetrics include indication, dosing recommendations, as well as a checklist of contraindications that would exclude its use in this population.

- Implement a double-check process for the medication

  A pharmacist should review all orders for methotrexate use in obstetric patients prior to dispensing the medication. Prior to methotrexate administration, nursing should perform a double-check of the medication against the orders to confirm accuracy.

- Medications should be provided in the final form with complete labeling

  All doses of methotrexate should be prepared and dispensed ONLY from the pharmacy.

Antibiotics

Antibiotics are frequently used in the obstetrical setting. Specifically, antibiotics are used to both prevent and treat infection in the mother and to prevent infection in the baby during labor and delivery. The American Congress of Obstetricians and Gynecologists (ACOG) released a practice bulletin

in 2011 addressing the use of antibiotics during labor and delivery [35]. Intrapartum prophylactic antibiotics are used for women whose group B streptococci (GBS) culture results are unknown and whose risks include gestation < 37 weeks, prolonged rupture of membranes ≥18 hours, or maternal temperature of ≥ 100.4°F. In cases where GBS culture is positive or those patients who have previously delivered an infant with invasive GBS disease, antibiotic prophylaxis is recommended [36]. The types of antibiotics used range from narrow-spectrum choices such as penicillin and broaden to include ampicillin and cefazolin. Clindamycin or erythromycin is used for those patients who are allergic to penicillin and are at high risk for anaphylaxis. Vancomycin may also be chosen for patients whose GBS isolates are resistant to clindamycin or erythromycin or when susceptibility is unknown.

The risks of using antibiotics in labor and delivery include missed allergies in the mother and the emergence of resistant organisms in both mother and neonate. Often, in the process of managing labor and preparing for delivery, allergies may be addressed incompletely or even missed prior to the initiation of antibiotics. It is important to elicit complete and accurate information regarding the nature of the allergy in order to provide the optimal antibiotic from a safety and efficacy standpoint. Patients who report mild to moderate allergic reactions to penicillins (i.e., rash, itching) often tolerate the first-generation cephalosporins (i.e., cefazolin) without complications. Therefore, unless the patient reports a history of a serious allergic reaction to the penicillins (i.e., difficulty breathing, swelling of the lips/face, anaphylaxis) it is most prudent to use a narrow-spectrum antibiotic for GBS prophylaxis. Although empiric therapy is generally limited to short courses of antibiotics, increasing resistance of GBS isolates is a concerning trend.

Key Medication Safety Recommendations

- Allergy screen

  All patients MUST be screened for allergies and be fitted with an up-to-date allergy band prior to the administration of antibiotics or other medications.

- Standardized order sets

  Antibiotic orders for use in obstetric patients should follow the recommended guidelines for use (narrow to broad spectrum) and include indication, dosing recommendation, intended length of therapy, and alternatives for use when allergies are suspected or confirmed.

- Smart-pump infusion technology

  Antibiotics that are not administered by IV push should be administered via a smart-infusion pump to assure safe administration.

- Medications should be provided in the final form with complete labeling

  Antibiotics that require preparation beyond simple vial activation should be prepared by pharmacy.

Patient Cases in Medication Safety Review

Magnesium – Patient Case

A 35-year-old G1P1 at 34 weeks is undergoing induction of labor for preeclampsia. Her nurse obtains two bags of Lactated Ringer's (LR) solution from stock and adds 40 g of magnesium sulfate to one bag for seizure prophylaxis. The nurse administers a 6-g bolus dose of magnesium sulfate and then starts a magnesium sulfate infusion at 2 g/hour as well as starting the maintenance solution of LR at 300 ml/hour. A few hours later, the patient reports feeling flushed and nauseated to her nurse and is assured by the nurse that these symptoms are expected. The patient is later found not breathing and without a pulse. *Findings:* An analysis found that the maintenance IV (300 ml/hour) contained 40 g of magnesium and the bag labeled as magnesium sulfate contained only LR. The admixture label had been placed on the wrong bag [1].

What major errors in the medication-use processes were involved in this case?

Dispensing, Administration, Monitoring

What safety measures could be implemented to prevent a similar incident from occurring in the future?

Dispensing: *Magnesium sulfate infusion should be dispensed as a premix or ready-to use product when available. If a premix product is not available, all medication preparations should be prepared in a sterile environment and dispensed with proper labeling by the pharmacy department. Premixed products may have reduced the risk of "look-alike" that occurred with the 2 – 1 liter LR bags. If emergency product preparation or compounding is performed on a nursing unit, it is recommended*

to always prepare one product at a time to completion prior to starting or labeling the next pharmaceutical product to reduce the risk of mislabeling the product.

Administration: *Bolus doses of magnesium should be infused as a separate preparation. Following the bolus, a separate magnesium infusion should be started. This reduces the potential of continuing the increased infusion rate used during the bolus. When administering IV medications other than IV push, smart-pump technology should be utilized.*

Monitoring: *In this event, the signs and symptoms of magnesium toxicity were not recognized. The employment of an order set that contains monitoring parameters and guidance as to when to notify the MD or use an antidote may have helped direct the care of the patient.*

Oxytocin – Patient Case

A 28-year-old nulliparous woman at 41 weeks gestation age is admitted for a scheduled induction of labor. Orders for "Pitocin per protocol" are processed by the pharmacist and a vial of oxytocin is sent to the floor. The nurse mixes the vial with a liter of normal saline. The infusion is started at 1 mUnit/min and is increased by 2 mUnit/min every 20 minutes. After about 30 minutes the patient requests to ambulate. The patient's current status is noted and she is unhooked from the external monitor. The patient is reattached to the external monitor approximately 40 minutes later and maternal tachysystole and fetal bradycardia are observed.

What major errors in the medication-use processes were involved in this case?

Prescribing, Order Processing, Dispensing, Monitoring

What safety measures could be implemented to prevent a similar incident from occurring in the future?

Prescribing: *Generic orders such as "per protocol" should be avoided or attached to a specific order set or protocol. A protocol, should be written in a way such as to direct care and avoid "prescribing" or the option of choice/preference [11].*

Order processing: *Pharmacy should have clarified "Pitocin per protocol" and included the actual protocol to provide guidance for the various disciplines and to ensure that everyone is clear as to the intent of the orders.*

Dispensing: *Pharmacy providing a vial for admixing on the nursing unit is not a safe practice. Admixing* products on the nursing units should be reserved for emergency situations only [11]. A standardized concentration and, if available, a ready-to-use premix product should be selected and dispensed.

Monitoring: *Drug knowledge is important when administering any medication, particularly titratable drips in which monitoring parameters dictate when and how the medication is adjusted. Protocols for ongoing monitoring as well as order sets should be implemented to provide guidance and mitigation for deficiencies in drug knowledge.*

Prostaglandin – Patient Case

A physician has finished the exam of the patient and has determined the need for induction of labor. The chart cannot be located, so the nurse is given a verbal order to start "prostaglandin intravaginally q6h." The nurse recalls that the automated dispensing cabinet has misoprostol available on "override." A 100-µg misoprostol tablet is removed and is administered to the patient. The nurse is extremely busy and the verbal order is written in the chart after she administers the second dose. Shortly after the order has been sent to pharmacy, pharmacy calls to clarify the prostaglandin product, dose, and indication.

Findings: The recommended dosing is 25 µg, ¼ of the 100-µg tablet, for induction of labor. The patient has received a fourfold overdose for two doses.

What errors in the medication-use processes were involved in this case?
Prescribing, Order Processing, Dispensing, Administration

What safety measures could be implemented to prevent a similar incident from occurring in the future?

Prescribing: *A complete order should always contain: medication name, dose, route, frequency, and indication. CPOE can help aid in the inclusion of these criteria by having "required" fields that must be filled in when entering an order. CPOE systems also reduce the need for verbal orders secondary to the lack of availability of the patient's chart.*

Order processing: *If a telephone or verbal order is received it should be immediately written down and read back to the prescriber to ensure it is correctly transcribed. If an emergency medication is needed before it is verified by pharmacy, a second-check from an additional practitioner should be utilized and appropriate references reviewed to verify the correct dosing, route, and frequency for the prescribed indication.*

Dispensing: *If possible, medications should be provided in the final form with complete labeling although misoprostol is not currently available in a 25 µg tablet, consideration should be made to providing packaged 25 µg per ¼ tablets to help limit the need to alter or prepare. The availability of medications within the "override" function should be limited to truly emergency medications with limited strengths or concentrations. This should limit the bypass the safety processes that are required to check and verify orders prior to administration.*

Administration: *The medication dose, route, and frequency should always be verified prior to administration; if any of these components are missing, the order should be clarified.*

References

1 Simpson KR, Knox GE. Obstetrical accidents involving IV magnesium sulfate. *Am J Maternal Child Nurs.* 2004;29:161–171.

2 Institute of Medicine. *To Err Is Human: Building a Safer Health System.* Washington, DC: National Academy of Press; 2000.

3 ACOG Committee Opinion No. 447. Patient safety in obstetrics and gynecology. *Obstet Gynecol.* 2009;114:1424–1427.

4 Cohen, M. *Medication Errors*, 2nd ed. Washington, DC: American Pharmacist Association; 2007.

5 Institute for Safe Medication Practices. ISMP's list of high-alert medications. www.ismp.org/Tools/highalertmedications.pdf, updated 2012 (accessed April 1, 2013).

6 Kfuri TA, Morlock L, Hicks RW, et al. Medication errors in obstetrics. *Clin Perinatol.* 2008;35:101–117.

7 Pa Patient Saf Advis 2009 Dec 16, 6[Suppl 1]:1–6.

8 Institute for Safe medication Practices. Proceedings from the ISMP Sterile Preparation Compounding Safety Summit: Guidelines for SAFE Preparation of Sterile compounds. www.ismp.org/Tools/guidelines/IVSummit/IVCGuidelines.pdf, updated 2013 (accessed April 1, 2013).

9 Cullen DJ, Sweitzer BJ, Bates DW, Burdick E, Edmondson A, Leape LL. Preventable adverse drug events in hospitalized patients: a comparative study of intensive care and general care units. *Crit Care Med.* 1997;25:1289–1297.

10 Parshuram C, Ng G, Ho T, et al. Discrepancies between ordered and delivered concentrations of opiate infusions in critical care. *Crit Care Med.* 2003;31:2483–2487.

11 Joint Commission Medication Management Standards E-dition Version 5.0 Build 0.3, 2013. https://e-dition.jcrinc.com/MainContent.aspx (accessed April 1, 2013).

12 The Joint Commission. Official "Do not use" list. www.jointcommission.org/assets/1/18/Do_Not_Use_List.pdf, updated June 2012 (accessed April 1, 2013).

13 Institute for Safe Medication Practices. ISMP's List of Error-Prone Abbreviations, Symbols, and Dose Designations. http://ismp.org/Tools/errorproneabbreviations.pdf, updated 2013 (accessed April 1, 2013).

14 Fidler SA, Barger DM. Patient Safety: Medication Safety in Obstetrics. ASHRM FORUM Q3 2011.

15 Ciarkowski S, Stalburg C. Medication safety in obstetrics and gynecology. *Clin Obstet Gynecol.* 2010; 53(3):482–499.

16 Institute of Safe Medication Practices. FDA and ISMP Lists of Look-Alike Drug Names with Recommended Tall Man Letters. http://ismp.org/Tools/tallmanletters.pdf, updated 2011 (accessed April 13, 2013).

17 American College of Obstetricians and Gynecologists. Patient Safety in Obstetrics and Gynecology. ACOG Committee Opinion No. 447. *Obstet Gynecol.* 2009;114:1424–1427.

18 American Society of Health-System Pharmacists. ASHP guidelines on the safe use of automated dispensing devices. *Am J Health-Syst Pharm.* 2010;67:483–490.

19 Rothschild JM, Keohane CA, Cook EF, et al. A controlled trial of smart infusion pumps to improve medication safety in critically ill patients. *Crit Care Med.* 2005;33:533–540.

20 Poon EG, Keohane CA, Yoon CS, et al. Effect of bar-code technology on the safety of medication administration. *N Engl J Med.* 2010;362:1698–1707.

21 Lindenauer PK, Remus D, Roman S, et al. Public reporting and pay for performance in hospital quality improvement. *N Engl J Med.* 2007;356:486–496.

22 Institute for Safe Medication Practices. ISMP's Quarterly Action Agenda. http://ismp.org/Newsletters/acutecare/actionagendas.asp, updated 2013 (accessed April 14, 2013).

23 Food and Drug Administration. FDA Pregnancy Categories. http://depts.washington.edu/druginfo/Formulary/Pregnancy.pdf (accessed April 10, 2013).

24 Briggs GG, Freeman RK, Yaffe SJ. *Drugs in Pregnancy and Lactation: A Reference Guide to Fetal and Neonatal Risk*, 9th edition. Philadelphia, PA: Lippincott Williams & Wilkins; 2011.

25 Oscarsson ME, Amer-Wahlin I, Rydhstroem H, Kallen K. Outcome in obstetric care related to oxytocin use. A population-based study. *Acta Obstet Gynecol Scand.* 2006;85:1094–1098.

26 *Lexi-comp's Drug Information Handbook*, 21st ed. Hudson, OH: American Pharmacists Association; 2012: 1272–1273.

27 Amico JA, Seitchik J, Robinson AG. Studies of oxytocin in plasma of women during hypocontractile labor. *J Clin Endocrinol Metab.* 1984;58:274–279.

28 Seitchik J, Amico J, Robinson AG, Castillo M. Oxytocin augmentation of dysfunctional labor. IV. Oxytocin pharmacokinetics. *Am J Obstet Gynecol.* 1984;150:225–228.

29 Simpson K, James D. Effects of oxytocin induced uterine hyperstimulation during labor on fetal oxygen status and fetal heart rate patterns. *Obstet Gynecol.* 2008;199:34.e1–34.e5.

30 *Lexi-comp's Drug Information Handbook*, 21st edition. Hudson, OH: American Pharmacists Association; 2012: 1047–1049.

31 Up-to-Date. Adverse events of prostaglandins. www.uptodate.com.libproxy.lib.unc.edu/contents/search-comp (accessed April 2, 2013).

32 Chong Y, Chua S, Shen L, et al. Does the route of administration of misoprostol make a difference? The uterotonic effect and side effects of misoprostol given by different routes after vaginal delivery. *Eur J Obstet Gynecol Reprod Biol.* 2004;113:191–198.

33 *Lexi-comp's Drug Information Handbook*, 21st edition. Hudson, OH: American Pharmacists Association; 2012: 1141–1142.

34 *Lexi-comp's Drug Information Handbook*, 21st edition. Hudson, OH: American Pharmacists Association; 2012: 1098–1102.

35 ACOG Committee Opinion No. 485. Prevention of early-onset group B streptococcal disease in newborns. *Obstet Gynecol.* 2011;117(4):1019–1027. www.acog.org/~/media/Committee%20Opinions/Committee%20on%20Obstetric%20Practice/co485.pdf?dmc=1&ts=20130415T1508315558 (accessed April 4, 2013).

36 Verani JR, McGee L, Schrag SJ. Prevention of perinatal group B streptococcal disease – revised guidelines from CDC, 2010. Division of Bacterial Diseases, National Center for Immunization and Respiratory Diseases, Centers for Disease Control and Prevention (CDC). *MMWR Recomm Rep.* 2010;59(RR–10):1–36.

Chapter 19

Improving Patient Safety Through Team Training

Christian M. Pettker and Edmund F. Funai

Introduction

Although expected to work in teams, nurses, physicians, and other allied health professionals are often trained in distinct silos and styles. Healthcare education rarely incorporates interdisciplinary approaches; nursing students and medical students hardly cross paths until they reach the offices or the hospital floors. At these times, often in the most critical moments, the distinctions in training manifest as critical gaps in collaborative and communication skills. Nurses often use a narrative and descriptive style of communication and documentation, while physicians take an evidence and factual approach largely based on the "SOAP" mnemonic: subjective, objective, assessment, and plan. The result is a workforce that works in groups – as individuals working synchronously but independently with distinct goals – rather than in teams. To paraphrase Eduardo Salas, a leading social scientist who specializes in human factors research: medical training is efficient at creating teams of experts, but fails at training expert teams [1].

A system with a workforce operating in silos is bound to fail when latent errors surface or when the inherent fallibility of humans and technology manifests. Individuals who are not trained to communicate with each other cannot respond rapidly or efficiently to mitigate error. This background illuminates why poor collaboration is a leading cause of medical errors. According to The Joint Commission, communication is the leading root cause of sentinel events, involved in over 60% of cases [2]. A 2004 Joint Commission sentinel event report echoed these findings for obstetrics [3]. Of 47 perinatal deaths, the leading contributor to these adverse events was poor communication in over 70% of cases.

In light of this, team training, also known as crew resource management (CRM), has become a prominent part of post-graduate healthcare education and instruction in many institutions. In fact, this same Joint Commission sentinel event report recommends: "Since most perinatal injury is related to communication and organizational culture issues … recommend team training in perinatal areas to teach staff to work together and communicate more effectively" [3]. Advocates for CRM include major oversight and leadership organizations in healthcare and Ob/Gyn, including: The Joint Commission (TJC or JCAHO), the Institute of Medicine (IOM), the Institute for Healthcare Improvement (IHI), the Agency for Healthcare Research and Quality (AHRQ), the Accreditation Council for Graduate Medical Education (ACGME), and the American College of Obstetricians and Gynecologists (ACOG).

The case for team training in obstetrics is highlighted by a widely referenced report from Beth Israel Deaconess Medical Center in Boston [4]. An induction of labor in a nulliparous patient resulted in a stillbirth, hysterectomy, and a course that included massive transfusions, a critical care unit admission, and a prolonged hospitalization. The case is notable for uterine tachysystole, abnormal fetal heart rate patterns without expedient remedies, and delayed diagnoses and interventions. The report offered remarkable event review, a unique morbidity and mortality assessment that included narratives from the providers and the patient that exposed the systemic barriers that exacerbated each error and latency contributing to injury. The case involved several "failures in terms of communication and planning," including "four errors in judgment" and "six system failures." Among these, inadequate performance cross-monitoring, ineffective conflict-resolution, poor situational awareness, and failed high-workload management stood out. What is clear in review of the case is that an inability to communicate and collaborate allowed the team to fail the patient. No one person was to blame and no specific individual practiced recklessly or with incompetence. Rather, the team failed to prevent each oversight and misdirection from resulting in such tragic consequences, even when some individuals knew that things were not going right.

Background, Definition, and Fundamentals of Team Training

CRM is a set of instructional methods that improve teamwork and make optimum use of available resources and equipment, with the goal of promoting safety and enhancing efficiency. CRM, then known as cockpit resource management, originated in the aviation industry in the 1970s, when it was recognized that approximately 70% of aircraft-related fatalities were the result of human errors and poor teamwork [5]. Investigators began to understand that a number of accidents occurred even though a member of the flight crew knew something was not right, because he or she did not feel empowered or comfortable to speak up. It became clear that the traditional paradigm of the pilot having sole individual responsibility for flight safety was vulnerable, and thus aviation experts advocated programs of shared responsibility and enhanced communication. Application of CRM principles and training in commercial aviation has provided substantial improvements in safety culture and is thought to have influenced the significant safety improvements in this industry during the 1980s and 1990s [5]. Since then, effective teamwork has become an essential component of high-reliability organizations, institutions that operate without error in high-risk environments over long periods of time.

The call to arms for team training in medicine came in 1999, with the Institute of Medicine report, *To Err is Human* [6]. While this report is best known for providing an estimate for the burden in mortality of mistakes and errors in healthcare, it more importantly proscribed many of the remedies to fix this problem. A major point of the IOM report was that the majority of errors in medicine are the result of system failures, rather than substandard performance of individual caregivers. The IOM envisioned interdisciplinary team-training programs as part of the establishment of organizational safety systems, as a way of supporting dedicated and skilled individuals who are still prone to error and mistakes [7].

To understand how to train individuals to work in teams, the concept of a team must be broken down. An Agency for Healthcare Research and Quality (AHRQ) commissioned report helps outline the concept of

teams [7]. Teams consist of two or more individuals, and these individuals have specific roles and perform specific tasks but interact to achieve a common goal. Teams possess specialized knowledge and skills and often must function under conditions of high workload. Teams make decisions, and often these decisions must be made by consensus. Finally, teams demonstrate a collective action that is interdependent; that is, teamwork requires individual team members to make adjustments, either sequentially or simultaneously, during tasks in order to accomplish the team goals.

Teamwork is the process by which the team, responding to various environmental inputs, carries out the tasks to achieve the goal or outcome. *Effective* teamwork requires that individuals are willing to work together and can effectively communicate their individual and group goals, roles, and abilities [7]. Creation of a team structure does not ensure effective teamwork; functional relationships must take precedence. Furthermore, team members do not have to necessarily work together consistently; the use of a shared set of teamwork skills is more important than day-to-day familiarity.

The foundation required for building team training should not be underestimated; major institutional commitment is essential. Salas and colleagues have identified seven "evidence-based" factors required for success in preparing, implementing, and sustaining a team-training program [8]:

(1) align team training objectives and safety aims with organizational goals
(2) provide organizational support for the team training initiative
(3) get frontline care leaders on board
(4) prepare the environment and trainees for team training
(5) determine required resources and time commitment and ensure their availability
(6) facilitate application of trained teamwork skills on the job
(7) measure the effectiveness of the team training program.

The success of a team training program depends on leadership understanding and mapping these organizational factors.

In summary, CRM seeks to train workers to develop habits of teams, such as having a clear and valued vision, developing trust and confidence in each other, understanding leadership and following, and adoption of clear communication tools.

The Evidence for Medical Team Training

Before embarking on a team training program, individuals within the workforce often want to see the evidence justifying the time and energy they are about to spend. Anecdotes, such as the Beth Israel Deaconess event in the introduction, are powerful examples, but objective proof can provide more convincing reasons to workers with scientific backgrounds. Studies in medical team training are just beginning to appear in the literature, and the science of medical team improvement is in development. However, this is not an indication of an absence of supporting evidence. A recent review of CRM in acute hospital settings looked at the general literature connecting team training to improved clinical outcomes [9]. Most studies provided a "low quality of evidence," with much being qualitative and involving pre- and post-intervention surveys. However, nearly all published studies showed qualitative improvements in teamwork culture and climate.

Medical teams which lack evidence of strong qualities of teamwork are at higher risk for errors. For example, using a standardized tool to directly observe and assess teamwork behaviors, one group from the Kaiser health system observed that surgical units demonstrating strong team performance showed lower 30-day mortality and complication rates than weaker performing teams [10].

One of the more important quantitative studies investigated the impact of team training on surgical mortality within the Veterans Health Administration [11]. This retrospective health services cohort study involved a total of 108 VHA facilities, with 74 implementing CRM. There was an 18% reduction in mortality over time in the CRM-trained facilities, versus a 7% reduction mortality in the others, demonstrating a 50% improved risk-adjusted mortality associated with team training. In obstetrics, the only randomized trial for team training to date failed to demonstrate improvements in clinical adverse outcomes, as measured by the obstetrical adverse outcome index [12]. However, team-trained institutions did see improved cesarean decision-to-incision times (21.2 vs. 33.3 minutes ($p = 0.03$)).

Other study designs also provide consistent evidence. A prospective observational study of formal team training (MedTeams™) in nine community and academic emergency departments demonstrated concurrent improvements in the quality of team behaviors and the clinical error rate (decreased from 30.9%

to 4.4% ($p = 0.039$)) [13]. In the field of obstetrics, the team at Beth Israel Deaconess demonstrated improvements in the frequency and severity of clinical adverse events, along with improvements in staff safety culture, in response to a comprehensive CRM program [14].

Team training has been used in conjunction with simulation in obstetric settings in several centers. A meta-analysis that included four randomized trials and four cohort studies showed improvements in several clinical outcomes (5-minute Apgars, hypoxic–ischemic encephalopathy) as well as teamwork culture and climate (knowledge, skills, communication, and team performance) [15–18].

CRM has been an important part of larger quality-assurance initiatives in several centers. The obstetrics team at Yale implemented a comprehensive safety program that included team training as well as a patient safety nurse, vast array of new protocols and guidelines, an adverse event reporting tool, electronic fetal monitoring, and a 24-hour supervision system staffed by Maternal–Fetal Medicine specialists [19]. Far from a controlled study, this unit observed concurrent improvements in both obstetrical adverse outcomes and teamwork culture/climate [20].

Team Training Strategies and Tools

As Atul Gawande points out, medicine is a team sport, without the benefit of a coach [21]. The task for team training is to supply this coaching in order to teach team and teamwork concepts to workers and equip those users with tools to effectively work together. These workers often come from diverse educational and cultural backgrounds, have distinct communication styles, sometimes have short-term relationships with each other, and may have distinct goals that conflict with each other at work. However, the overarching goal of a collaborative approach to provide quality and safe patient care is emphasized to bring people together. Training typically consists of didactic lectures, video review, and team-building exercises, which may include role-playing or simulation work.

Several paradigms and courses for team training are available (including MedTeams®, Medical Team Management, and Dynamic Outcomes Management©, now named Lifewings®), although one, TeamSTEPPS® (Team Strategies and Tools to Enhance Performance and Patient Safety), being available in the public domain, is arguably the most widely available and used. Developed jointly by the Department of Defense and the AHRQ from a consensus conference of medical, human factors, and safety experts convened in 2003, TeamSTEPPS emphasizes four core skills: leadership, situation monitoring, mutual support, and communication [22].

The basic concepts taught in CRM courses like TeamSTEPPS® include demonstrating a mutual willingness to work together, replacement of hierarchical relationships with mutual decision-making, providing avenues for real-time performance feedback during work situations, and teaching tools for conflict resolution and communication. Specific tools that are often discussed include:

1. *Team huddles*: For example, our unit uses multiple huddles throughout the day, including a morning report including midwives and physicians, a post-report labor and delivery "board meeting" of team leadership to assess the team status and resource status, patient bedside huddles or rounds, and a midnight huddle including leadership from all obstetric units to reassess team and resource status.
2. *Briefings/debriefings*: Pre-event briefings can develop a shared mental model for care and anticipate problems, and a post-event debriefing can develop an appropriate handoff for the next stage of care and educate the team on goals for success for the future.

3. *SBAR* (situation–background–assessment–recommendation): A handoff tool for precise communication of care pathways.
4. *Two-challenge rule*: A conflict-resolution tool to communicate a staff members' level of concern. If a team member requests clarification or explanation of a treatment, and meets an unsatisfactory result, after two attempts a more assertive strategy or a superior in the chain of command should be invoked.
5. *Check-backs*: A closed loop communication tool to verify information exchange where a verbal order or command is written down and read back before it is carried out.
6. *Call-outs*: Call-outs are communication tools used for emergencies, such as a code of shoulder dystocia, where a designated person communicates important information (such as who is in charge or who else is being called) to an entire team simultaneously.
7. The *"CUS"* words of Concerned, Uncomfortable, and Scared used to communicate levels of concern. Using the terms in that order specifies an escalation of concern and should trigger the listener to respect the other team member's discomfort with a particular situation.
8. *Chain of command* (Figure 19.1, example from Yale-New Haven Hospital): A readily available

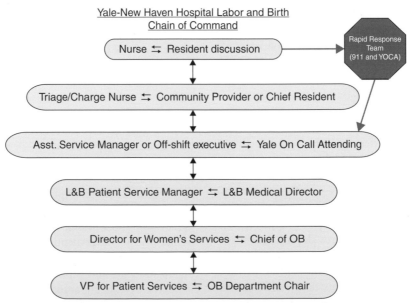

Figure 19.1 Example of a chain of command. Note the nursing/provider dyad on each level, reducing traditional concepts of hierarchy and encouraging interdisciplinary discussions at each level.

chain of command demonstrates to workers who are available to manage resolution when team conflict arises. The most effective chains of command include contact information for individuals at each level, to promote a sense of accessibility, and a nursing/provider dyad at each level, to reduce the silos and encourage open discussions between pairs.

Implementation is often preceded by pre-training assessments of the site and current culture as well as training of a cadre of coaches amongst the staff who champion the effort [22].

While implementation of a team training program is a formidable undertaking, sustaining the principles in practice is probably the biggest challenge. Leadership must be committed to asking staff what team training principles they incorporated any time a complaint or concern is discussed after an event.

In fact, we post and supply our staff with laminated cards with the basic principles of CRM (Figure 19.2) for reference and reminding. Continuous assessment of the teamwork culture, through surveys (below), is another critical element for sustainment.

Simulation training can be an important adjunct to a team training program. While many simulation efforts are aimed at teaching knowledge and skills related to specific conditions or scenarios (e.g., eclampsia, shoulder dystocia, hemorrhage), they can also focus on teamwork training skills. A team should decide to work on one or the other when initiating a simulation program. Simulations can occur *in situ*, on a labor and delivery unit, such as during a time of low workload. Unannounced *in situ* simulation events, however, can test a unit's preparedness and provide important feedback to a team for troubleshooting or systems improvement. Off-site simulation centers allow for a more controlled atmosphere for practice

Team Training Communication Tools	
CUS	Identify level of concern "I'm **c**oncerned" "I'm **u**ncomfortable" "This is a **s**afety concern" "I'm **s**cared" } Stop the Line
SBAR	Focus the communication **S**ituation - Current clinical situation / What is going on with the patient? **B**ackground - What is the pertinent clinical background or context? **A**ssessment - What do you think is the problem? **R**ecommendation - What would you like done?
Two Challenge Rule	Refocus the discussion when an initial assertion is ignored Restate and voice concern at least **two times** to ensure it is heard
Call-Out	Strategy used to communicate important or critical information • Informs all team members simultaneously during emergent situations • Helps team members anticipate next steps • Direct responsibility to a specific individual responsible for the task
Check Back	Closing the loop to ensure that information conveyed is understood by the receiver • Sender initiates message • Receiver accepts message and provides feedback – "Write it down & read it back" • Sender re-confirms message or clarifies if needed
Chain of Command	Escalation of concern until resolution realized • Incorporates nursing and medical representation at all levels • Initiate when: 　- Above procedures of resolution have not been effective 　- There is need to proceed to a higher authority for discussions or decisions regarding: 　　◦ Patient care or safety 　　◦ Operational issues

Figure 19.2a,b Example of a laminated card, describing the core concepts and tools of crew resource management (side 1 and side 2).

Team Training Key Concepts	
Team Structure	Team size, membership, leadership, composition, identification, and distribution Team includes every staff member that influences patient care; licensed and non-licensed staff have equal responsibility for patient safety
Team Leadership	Ability to: • Organize the team • Articulate clear goals • Empower team members to speak up • Make decisions • Role model desired behavior • Skillful at conflict resolution

Team Events
        BRIEF
 	
        HUDDLE
        DEBRIEF
	
	Planning: session to discuss team formation; assign roles; establish expectations; anticipate outcomes and contingencies
	Problem Solving: ad hoc planning ; assessing the need to adjust the plan
	Process Improvement: after action review; informational exchange to improve Team performance and effectiveness

Situation Monitoring	An individual skill: Continual scanning and assessing what's going on around you
Situation Awareness	An individual outcome: Knowing what's going on around you
Cross Monitoring	A Team skill: Watching each other's back; provides a team safety net
Shared Mental Model	A Team outcome: All team members are on the same page

Mutual Support
        Feedback
 	
        Task Assistance
	
	Information given for the purpose of improving team performance and patient Safety
	Mutual support; assistance is actively sought and offered

Communication	Process by which information is clearly and accurately exchanged by team members

Figure 19.2a,b *(Cont.)*

and learning and often incorporate high-fidelity simulation technologies, but require substantial preparation and resources. For team training, off-site simulation allows for video taping so that behaviors and interactions can be reviewed. Demonstrating its perceived importance for education and improvement, ACOG and the Society for Maternal–Fetal Medicine are developing programs to assist units in implementing simulation programs [23].

Often, before initiating a team training program, it is important to make a baseline assessment of the teamwork culture, which can be compared over time. Inducing a perception of change is not enough; documenting and producing evidence of change is usually necessary. Many comprehensive safety programs often start with a safety assessment survey [20]. Teamwork culture and climate can be assessed through two types of validated survey tools, AHRQ's Hospital Survey on Patient Safety Culture or the Safety Attitude Questionnaire (SAQ). Both are anonymous surveys that can be handed out to staff to assess general perceptions of safety, error mitigation, and collaboration, with specific sections devoted to teamwork. The former has the advantage that, being developed and maintained by a government institution, it has open access and results can be compared to accumulated national standards reported to AHRQ. The latter assesses teamwork in one of its six categories and, as validated from aviation, emphasizes that differences of 10% or more, over time or between staff groups, are clinically significant and overall scores showing 80% agreement or more are the targets for change. In fact, to date, the SAQ is the only safety climate survey that has demonstrated links between improvements safety and teamwork culture and improvements in patient outcomes [24].

Conclusion

The arguments for team training are persuasive, and begin with the fundamental understanding that medical and nursing education do not train individuals to work in teams, but they are expected to and their performance is enhanced when they do this well.

Integrating team training into medical and nursing schools will be a huge step forward in improving collaboration and team skills. Yet until then, structured team training programs will be required, to the point of being mandated by the major medical oversight and regulatory bodies.

Barriers to implementation will exist but are not formidable. Institutional inertia is overcome with enthusiasm and commitment from key leadership, with further backup from employment mandates or medical staff membership requirements. Appointment of key trainers and content experts with further specialized training, such as unit leadership and even a patient safety nurse selected for their approachability and availability, can provide further support. Finally, tailoring the team training program to the specifics of the unit and the type of medical care given, as in obstetrics, can make effective general principles more applicable and palatable.

The cost of implementation, both in the time to train the workforce and the investment in training resources, is substantial and should not be underestimated. However, the cost in human life and suffering on behalf of even one patient who may be affected by a poorly functioning team under stress, surely justifies any calculable expense.

References

1 Salas E, Cannon-Bowers JA, Johnston JH. How can you turn a team of experts into an expert team?: Emerging training strategies. In Zsambok CE, Klein GA, eds. *Naturalistic Decision Making*. Mahwah, NJ: Lawrence Erlbaum Associates; 1997.

2 JCAHO. Sentinel Event Statistics, 2011. www.jointcommission.org/SentinelEvents/Statistics/ (cited February 1, 2012).

3 JCAHO. Sentinel Event Alert #30, 2004. www.jointcommission.org/sentinel_event_alert_issue_30_preventing_infant_death_and_injury_during_delivery/ (cited February 1, 2012).

4 Sachs BP. A 38-year-old woman with fetal loss and hysterectomy. *JAMA*. 2005;294(7):833–840.

5 Helmreich RL, Merritt AC, Wilhelm JA. The evolution of Crew Resource Management training in commercial aviation. *Int J Aviat Psychol*. 1999;9(1):19–32.

6 Kohn L, Corrigan J, Donaldson M, eds. *To Err is Human: Building a Safer Health System*. Washington, DC: National Academy Press; 2000.

7 Baker DP, Gustafson S, Beaubien JM, Salas E, Barach P. Medical team training programs in health care. In Henriksen K, Battles JB, Marks ES, Lewin DI, eds. *Advances in Patient Safety: From Research to Implementation, Volume 4: Programs, Tools and Products*. Rockville, MD: AHRQ; 2005.

8 Salas E, Almeida SA, Salisbury M, et al. What are the critical success factors for team training in health care? *Joint Comm J Qual Patient Saf*. 2009;35(8):398–405.

9 Buljac-Samardzic M, Dekker-van Doorn CM, van Wijngaarden JD, van Wijk KP. Interventions to improve team effectiveness: a systematic review. *Health Policy*. 2009;94(3):183–195.

10 Mazzocco K, Petitti DB, Fong KT, et al. Surgical team behaviors and patient outcomes. *Am J Surg*. 2009;197(5):678–685.

11 Neily J, Mills PD, Young-Xu Y, et al. Association between implementation of a medical team training program and surgical mortality. *JAMA*. 2010;304(15):1693–1700.

12 Nielsen PE, Goldman MB, Mann S, et al. Effects of teamwork training on adverse outcomes and process of care in labor and delivery: a randomized controlled trial. *Obstet Gynecol*. 2007;109(1):48–55.

13 Morey JC, Simon R, Jay GD, et al. Error reduction and performance improvement in the emergency department through formal teamwork training: evaluation results of the MedTeams project. *Health Serv Res*. 2002;37(6):1553–1581.

14 Pratt SD, Mann S, Salisbury M, et al. Impact of CRM-based training on obstetric outcomes and clinicians' patient safety attitudes. *Joint Comm J Qual Patient Saf*. 2007;33(12):720–725.

15 Merien AE, van de Ven J, Mol BW, Houterman S, Oei SG. Multidisciplinary team training in a simulation setting for acute obstetric emergencies: a systematic review. *Obstet Gynecol*. 2010;115(5):1021–1031.

16 Deering S, Poggi S, Macedonia C, Gherman R, Satin AJ. Improving resident competency in the management of shoulder dystocia with simulation training. *Obstet Gynecol*. 2004;103(6):1224–1228.

17 Draycott T, Sibanda T, Owen L, et al. Does training in obstetric emergencies improve neonatal outcome? *BJOG*. 2006;113(2):177–182.

18 Draycott TJ, Crofts JF, Ash JP, et al. Improving neonatal outcome through practical shoulder dystocia training. *Obstet Gynecol*. 2008;112(1):14–20.

19 Pettker CM, Thung SF, Norwitz ER, et al. Impact of a comprehensive patient safety strategy on

obstetric adverse events. *Am J Obstet Gynecol.* 2009;200(5):492 e1–8.

20 Pettker CM, Thung SF, Raab CA, et al. A comprehensive obstetrics patient safety program improves safety climate and culture. *Am J Obstet Gynecol.* 2011;204(3):216 e1–6.

21 Gawande A. *Better: A Surgeon's Notes on Performance.* New York, NY: Metropolitan; 2007.

22 King H, Battles J, Baker D, et al. TeamSTEPPS: Team strategies and tools to enhance performance and patient safety. In: Henriksen K, Battles J, Keyes M, Grady M, eds. *Advances in Patient Safety: New Directions and Alternative Approaches, Vol 3 Performance and Tools.* Rockville, MD: Agency for Healthcare Research and Quality; 2008.

23 Argani CH, Eichelberger M, Deering S, Satin AJ. The case for simulation as part of a comprehensive patient safety program. *Am J Obstet Gynecol.* 2012;206(6):451–455.

24 Colla JB, Bracken AC, Kinney LM, Weeks WB. Measuring patient safety climate: a review of surveys. *Qual Saf Healthc.* 2005;14(5):364–366.

A Systems-based Approach to Shoulder Dystocia Safety

William A. Grobman

Case

Dr. X was called at home when her patient, SD, arrived at the hospital in spontaneous labor at 39 weeks of gestation. SD was a G1P0 with a BMI of 32 kg/m² whose medical history was unremarkable and whose antepartum care had been uncomplicated. On admission, she was 3 cm dilated and completely effaced, with the vertex at 0 station. Fetal weight was estimated to be 3,900 g by physical exam and a prior ultrasound, and her pelvis was considered gynecoid and adequate. After three hours she spontaneously ruptured her membranes and was 6 cm dilated; she received an epidural for analgesia. Two hours thereafter, she was completely dilated. Her second stage was uneventful and lasted for 90 minutes. Upon delivery of the head, Dr. X used traction typically used at vaginal delivery to enable delivery of the anterior shoulder, which did not deliver. After approximately 45 seconds, the doctor asked the nurse to pull the patient's legs back, assuming a shoulder dystocia was occurring. The physician proceeded to attempt rotational maneuvers and delivery of the posterior arm, but neither was successful and she asked the nurse to call for additional assistance. The nurse called out to her charge nurse, who, after paging anesthesia and another attending physician on the premises, came to the room with a third nurse who was available to help. The three nurses assisted the physician with the McRoberts maneuver and with application of suprapubic pressure, as the physician continued to attempt delivery of the posterior arm. The shoulder dystocia was resolved at approximately 2–3 minutes after delivery of the fetal head (and as additional physicians were arriving in the room). The birth weight was 3,625 g and Apgars were 3 at 1 minute and 8 at 5 minutes. There was no apparent neonatal trauma. The nurse asked Dr. X if she would like pediatrics to be called. Dr. X asked her to do so, and the pediatrician subsequently confirmed the absence of neonatal trauma.

Discussion

Shoulder dystocia is an obstetric emergency that has been reported in 0.2%–3% of all vaginal deliveries [1]. Clinically, a shoulder dystocia is most often diagnosed when the typical gentle downward traction on the fetal head that is used to deliver the anterior shoulder is not sufficient to enact this delivery, although sometimes it is diagnosed when ancillary obstetric maneuvers are required to effect delivery of the fetal shoulders. Some have suggested that time from delivery of the fetal head to the shoulders could be used to indicate the occurrence of a shoulder dystocia, but no consensus has been achieved with regard to the time interval that would underpin such a standard [2].

Multiple factors have been reported to be associated with shoulder dystocias. For many of these factors, though, the associations are neither independent nor consistently demonstrated [3]. Even when a factor has been shown to be independently and consistently associated with the occurrence of shoulder dystocia, the predictive value of such factors has been poor [4,5]. For example, the frequency of shoulder dystocia increases as birth weight increases [6]. Nevertheless, approximately 40%–60% of shoulder dystocias occur in infants weighing less than 4,000 g [5]. The predictive value of a factor such as birth weight is also undercut by the fact that birth weight cannot be known with certainty until after a shoulder dystocia is diagnosed and delivery has occurred. While birth weight can be estimated from fetal weight, the tools to allow estimation of fetal weight are imperfect. Ultrasonography has been shown to have low sensitivity and poor predictive value for birth weight thresholds such as those greater than 4,000 or 4,500 g [7]. In fact, the accuracy of ultrasound has been shown to be no better than that provided by clinical palpation (Leopold maneuvers) or that of a parous woman's assessment of her own fetus' weight [8]. Correspondingly, strategies incorporating estimated fetal weight in an effort to reduce the incidence of shoulder dystocia have not been shown to be effective in practice. For example, induction of labor due to suspected or impending fetal "macrosomia" has not been shown to improve health outcomes. In one prospective study, non-diabetic women with an ultrasonographic fetal weight estimation of 4,000–4,500 g were randomly assigned to either induction of labor or expectant management. The frequency of shoulder dystocia was similar in the two groups [9]. Likewise, prophylactic cesarean delivery has not been consistently demonstrated to result in a reduction of shoulder dystocia without incurring significant increases in cesarean delivery and its associated complications [10,11]. The decision analysis by Rouse et al. demonstrated that a policy of cesarean delivery for estimated weight over 4,500 g would result in 3,695 cesarean deliveries at a cost of $8.7 million for each brachial plexus injury prevented. Further, there is little account of the additional operative morbidities that would be encountered by both mother and fetus with a policy of preemptive cesarean.

Once shoulder dystocia is recognized, for example, due to the lack of delivery of an anterior shoulder after typical gentle downward traction on the fetal head, alleviating maneuvers should be utilized. However, there is no consensus on which particular maneuver is best to use initially or which particular sequence of maneuvers is preferred. Many providers initially employ the McRoberts maneuver (abduction and hyperflexion of the maternal thighs upon the abdomen), suprapubic pressure or both because of ease of implementation, relatively high success rate (approximately 40%–60%), and involvement of only maternal manipulation [5]. Techniques that involve fetal manipulation may also be helpful. One such technique is a rotational maneuver, in which the operator rotates the fetus to an oblique rather than anterior–posterior axis, thereby allowing disimpaction of the anterior shoulder from the symphysis pubis. Another technique is the delivery of the posterior arm. To perform this maneuver, the provider should apply pressure at the antecubital fossa to flex the fetal forearm and then sweep the arm across the fetus' chest, with ultimate delivery of the arm over the perineum.

Based on the aforementioned description of shoulder dystocia and the approach to its care, several characteristics are evident that make it a particular challenge to manage effectively:

1. Relative infrequency – Although a well-known obstetrical event that most providers will experience some time during their careers, shoulder dystocia occurs with a frequency such that even a relatively busy provider – for example, a provider attending 100 deliveries a year – may experience and need to respond to a shoulder dystocia once every year or so.
2. Criterion for diagnosis – Lacking an objective criterion for diagnosis, shoulder dystocia may not be understood simultaneously to have occurred by all members of the care team who are present.
3. Unpredictability – Although there are many factors that have been identified to be associated with shoulder dystocias, many women who have these factors will not experience a shoulder dystocia, and many shoulder dystocias will occur in the absence of these factors. Put another way, the predictive accuracy of currently identified "risk" factors for shoulder dystocia is low. Consequently, healthcare providers cannot reliably know when a shoulder dystocia will occur.
4. Need for coordinated actions of an ad-hoc provider team – The care team at the delivery (attending physician or midwife, nurses, anesthesiologists, resident physicians) will have been formed on the day of the delivery, and all members may not have worked together before, let alone have worked together before in a case involving a shoulder dystocia. Yet, the use of maneuvers meant to resolve a shoulder dystocia may require multiple members of the care team to be involved in a coordinated fashion.

Given these potential barriers, investigators have attempted to enhance care during a shoulder dystocia by utilizing protocols and simulation training.

Tools to Enhance Communication and Team Response

Protocols and Checklists

There is evidence from different aspects of medical care that protocols (i.e., items selected for completion to lead the user to a predetermined outcome) and checklists (i.e., a list of action items or criteria arranged in a systematic manner, allowing the user to record the presence/absence of the action items listed to ensure that all are considered or completed) can improve outcomes. Pronovost et al. have demonstrated how the introduction of checklists reduced catheter-related blood stream infections in the Intensive Care

Unit (ICU) [12]. In that study, checklists detailing five key actions required during any central catheter placement were introduced in 108 ICUs throughout the state of Michigan. By three months after checklist implementation, the incidence of catheter-related bloodstream infections had significantly declined (incidence rate ratio 0.62, 95% confidence interval 0.47–0.81). This decline continued to be evident through 18 months of study (incidence rate ratio 0.34, 95% confidence interval 0.23–0.50). In the realm of obstetrics, the potential benefits of checklist use have been shown for preeclampsia [13]. After establishing a set of best practices for preeclampsia management, Menzies et al. introduced these practices at British Columbia Women's Hospital [14]. After the standardized approach was put into place, there was an 86% reduction in the composite endpoint of maternal adverse outcomes (5.1% to 0.7%, P < .001). Adverse perinatal outcomes also were reduced, although this finding did not reach statistical significance (OR 0.65, 95% confidence interval 0.37–1.16).

Prior to developing their shoulder dystocia protocol, Grobman et al. explored the components of communication that providers believe are important for a team to incorporate during a shoulder dystocia [15]. In that study, 27 providers, drawn from the multidisciplinary team that contributes to obstetric care on a labor and delivery unit, were interviewed during a two-month period by a single individual. Interviewees, and nurses in particular, noted that the team of obstetric providers was not always collectively and simultaneously aware that a shoulder dystocia was occurring and had been diagnosed. Once the care team was alerted to the occurrence of a shoulder dystocia, providers commented that they believed it was important to be able to efficiently summon assistance and additional personnel. Providers also noted that when additional staff did arrive, there was the potential for lack of role clarity. This was particularly noted with regard to nursing staff who needed to perform multiple actions (including calling other staff, performing maneuvers, obtaining other requested resources, and documenting activities). Physician respondents, in particular, noted that during a shoulder dystocia their concentration was so focused on alleviating the dystocia that they could lose track of the duration, which they felt was important to know so that optimal management decisions could be made.

Subsequent to the interviews, Grobman et al. developed a shoulder dystocia protocol that incorporated specific solutions to the concerns that had been voiced. The first component of this protocol, the unambiguous announcement by the delivery provider that a "shoulder dystocia is present," triggers the remaining steps in the protocol. Once announced, the roles and actions of the team members are delineated. The delivery provider then focuses on directing the alleviating maneuvers, while the patient's primary nurse directs the actions of her nursing colleagues. This primary nurse also summons other relevant staff (including nurses, anesthesiologists, additional obstetricians, and pediatricians) through a single emergency call system. During the dystocia, a nurse is charged with calling out, in 30-second intervals, the length of time that has elapsed after delivery of the fetal head. To facilitate this action and the accuracy of the response, the primary nurse routinely (i.e., at all deliveries) marks the fetal monitoring strip at the time of the delivery of the head. The entirety of the protocol is presented in Figure 20.1.

Simulation

Simulation refers to the recreation of an actual event that has previously occurred or could potentially occur [16]. Simulation may be used to enhance patient safety because an action or procedure can be repeated without ever exposing providers or patients to harm. Simulation of events is therefore an opportunity for healthcare workers to prepare and train for interventions. Although simulation may have benefits for any type of obstetric procedure (e.g., vaginal delivery), it has often been studied in the context of obstetric emergencies such as shoulder dystocia and eclampsia. In these occurrences, simulation may be helpful not only for individuals at the start of their career, but also for experienced professionals, who must maintain the skills needed during unpredictable and uncommon events.

Simulation and Protocols in the Context of Shoulder Dystocia

Studies have illustrated that simulation may enhance several aspects of shoulder dystocia management, including performance of the maneuvers, communication among team members, and documentation. Deering and colleagues demonstrated, in a randomized trial, that residents who were assigned to train for a shoulder dystocia using a birth simulator were significantly more likely to utilize maneuvers in

OB Provider

- Announce Shoulder Dystocia

- Communicate with patient / family

- Direct Nurses to perform maneuvers, as appropriate
  – McRoberts
  – Suprapubic pressure

- Perform secondary maneuvers, as necessary
  – Rotational
  – Deliver posterior arm

Triggers
→
RN response

L&D Nurses

- Nurse announces her "lead"

- Employ **TEAM** approach:

  Time
    - Note delivery of head using fetal monitor event marker
    - Call out 30 second intervals

  Emergency call light button
    - "We have a shoulder in LOR # and need a nurse and a resident to assist."

  Activate shoulder dystocia page

  Perform **M**aneuvers

- Upon arrival, 3rd Nurse retrieves worksheet and acts as Documenter:
  – Observe & record key information

Figure 20.1 Shoulder dystocia protocol used by Grobman et al. [15].

a timely and correct fashion in a subsequent simulation than residents who did not undergo initial simulation training [13]. Furthermore, residents who underwent training scored higher on measures of overall performance and preparedness, as judged by a blinded observer. Goffman et al. studied outcomes after simulation training of both resident and attending physicians [17]. In this study, participants underwent a simulation of a shoulder dystocia followed by a debriefing that included: (1) a brief lecture about shoulder dystocia; (2) a review of the basic maneuvers and a basic algorithm for management of shoulder dystocia; (3) a discussion of approaches that optimize team performance during an emergency; (4) a review of the key components of documentation; (5) a review of the digital recording of the simulations; and (6) a discussion of provider performance. During a subsequent shoulder dystocia simulation, providers demonstrated significant improvements in use of maneuvers, communication, and overall performance. Crofts et al. obtained similar results in their multi-center comparison of pre- and post-simulation outcomes [18]. In this study, the investigators additionally randomized participants to partake in either a high-fidelity simulation (i.e., using a mannequin with a high degree of biofidelity) or a low-fidelity simulation (e.g., using a simple doll-like mannequin). Performance during a simulated shoulder dystocia subsequent to the simulation training was then evaluated in both groups. Although some measures of performance (e.g., total applied force) were improved to a greater extent in those participants who had undergone high-fidelity simulation

training, many other measures (e.g., peak force, use of maneuvers) were similar between the two groups. Nevertheless, because actual clinical outcomes were not evaluated, it cannot be known from these studies whether a simulation program will necessarily result in fewer brachial plexus palsies among parturients.

There is some evidence, albeit limited, that a program of shoulder dystocia simulation may be associated with fewer transient brachial plexus palsies. In one observational study in the UK, Draycott et al. studied the outcomes associated with the introduction of a mandatory shoulder dystocia simulation for personnel on a labor and delivery unit. The frequency of transient brachial plexus palsy associated with a shoulder dystocia significantly decreased after providers underwent simulation training (7.4% to 2.3%, RR 0.31, 95% CI 0.13–0.72) [19]. In contrast, MacKenzie and colleagues, in another study from the UK, were unable to demonstrate a decrease in even transient brachial plexus palsies after introduction of a training program. Although they found that management of shoulder dystocia improved after training, the frequency of brachial plexus palsy at the time of shoulder dystocia actually increased [20].

The results of two investigations of transient brachial plexus palsy in the United States have been more consistent with the results of Draycott et al. Inglis et al. studied the frequency of brachial plexus palsy at their institution over 9 years [21]. During this time, a shoulder dystocia protocol and training with a simulated shoulder dystocia were introduced. The frequency of brachial plexus palsy associated with shoulder dystocia, which was 30% at baseline, decreased to 10.7% after implementation of the protocol and simulation program ($P < .01$).

In another study, the protocol developed by Grobman et al. was introduced at multidisciplinary sessions to all labor and delivery staff through a low-fidelity simulation that involved only simulation of the team response, with an actress portraying a patient, and no repetition of maneuvers or delivery using a model pelvis. After introduction of this protocol, there was a decline in the frequency of brachial plexus palsies diagnosed at delivery (10.1% to 2.6%, $P = .03$) and at neonatal discharge (7.6% to 1.3%, $P = .04$) [15].

Despite the evidence that shoulder dystocia protocols and simulations may be associated with a reduction in the frequency of transient brachial plexus palsies, there is, at present, a lack of information about the consequence with regard to permanent brachial plexus palsies. For example, after the introduction of their simulation program, Draycott et al. did not discern a significant difference in brachial plexus palsies that persisted either at six months (RR 0.28, 95% CI 0.07–1.1) or at 12 months (RR 0.41, 95% CI 0.1–1.77) [19]. Inglis et al. and Grobman et al. did not collect data even for this length of time, and thus it is unknown whether their protocols were associated with any alteration in the frequency of permanent brachial plexus palsies [15,21].

The effect of protocols and simulations on long-term outcomes associated with shoulder dystocia therefore remains uncertain. Indeed, optimizing the approach to shoulder dystocia management will require research into several aspects of systems-based care for this obstetric emergency. For example, it remains uncertain whether there is any difference in terms of subsequent team performance after simulations in a simulation laboratory as opposed to on the clinical unit (i.e., labor and delivery) where the actual shoulder dystocias will occur. Similarly, after simulation training is performed, the length of time that elapses before enhanced skills degrade is not well understood.

References

1 American College of Obstetricians and Gynecologists. Shoulder dystocia. ACOG Practice Bulletin No. 40. *Obstet Gynecol*. 2002;100:1045–1050.

2 Beall MH, Spong C, McKay J, Ross MG. Objective definition of shoulder dystocia: a prospective evaluation. *Am J Obstet Gynecol*. 1998;179:934–937.

3 Dildy GA, Clark SL. Shoulder dystocia: risk identification. *Clin Obstet Gynecol*. 2000;43:265–282.

4 Grobman WA, Stamilio DM. Methods of clinical prediction. *Am J Obstet Gynecol*. 2006;194:888–894.

5 Gherman RB. Shoulder dystocia: an evidence-based evaluation of the obstetric nightmare. *Clin Obstet Gynecol*. 2002;45:345–362.

6 Nesbitt TS, Gilbert WM, Herrchen B. Shoulder dystocia and associated risk factors with macrosomic infants born in California. *Am J Obstet Gynecol*. 1998;179:476–480.

7 Chauhan SP, Grobman WA, Gherman RA, et al. Suspicion and treatment of the macrosomic fetus: a review. *Am J Obstet Gynecol*. 2005;193:332–346.

8 American College of Obstetricians and Gynecologists. *Fetal Macrosomia*. ACOG Practice Bulletin 22. Washington, DC: ACOG; 2000.

9 Gonen O, Rosen DJ, Dolfin Z, Tepper R, Markow S, Fejgin MD. Induction of labor versus expectant management in macrosomia: a randomized study. *Obstet Gynecol*. 1997;89:913–917.

10 Gonen R, Bader D, Ajami M. Effects of a policy of elective cesarean delivery in cases of suspected fetal macrosomia on the incidence of brachial plexus injury and the rate of cesarean delivery. *Am J Obstet Gynecol*. 2000;183:1296–1300.

11 Rouse DJ, Owen J, Goldenberg RL, Cliver SP. The effectiveness and costs of elective cesarean delivery for fetal macrosomia diagnosed by ultrasound. *JAMA*. 1996;276:1480–1486.

12 Pronovost P, Needham D, Berenholtz S. An intervention to decrease catheter-related bloodstream infections in the ICU. *N Engl J Med*. 2006;355:2725–2732.

13 Deering S, Poggi S, Macedonia C, Gherman R, Satin AJ. Improving resident competency in the management of shoulder dystocia with simulation training. *Obstet Gynecol*. 2004;103:1224–1228.

14 Menzies J, Magee LA, Li J, et al. Instituting surveillance guidelines and adverse outcomes in preeclampsia. *Obstet Gynecol*. 2007;110:121–127.

15 Grobman WA, Miller D, Burke C, Hornbogen A, Tam K, Costello R. Outcomes associated with introduction of a shoulder dystocia protocol. *Am J Obstet Gynecol*. 2011;205;513–517.

16 Hunt EA, Shilkofski NA, Atavroudis TA, Nelson KL. Simulation: translation to improved team performance. *Anesthesiol Clin*. 2007;25:301–319.

17 Goffman D, Heo H, Pardanani S, Merkatz IR, Bernstein PS. Improving shoulder dystocia management among resident and attending physicians

using simulations. *Am J Obstet Gynecol*. 2008;199:294.
e1–294.e5.

18 Crofts JF, Bartlett C, Ellis D, Hunt LP, Fox R, Draycott
TJ. Training for shoulder dystocia: a trial of simulation
using low-fidelity and high-fidelity mannequins. *Obstet
Gynecol*. 2006;108:1477–1485.

19 Draycott TJ, Crofts JF, Ash JP, et al. Improving
neonatal outcome through practical shoulder dystocia
training. *Obstet Gynecol*. 2008;112:14–20.

20 MacKenzie IZ, Shah M, Lean K, Dutton S,
Newdick H, Tucker DE. Management of
shoulder dystocia. Trends in incidence and
maternal and neonatal mortality. *Obstet Gynecol*.
2007;110:1059–1068.

21 Inglis SR, Feier N, Chetiyaar JB, et al. Effects
of shoulder dystocia training on the incidence
of brachial plexus injury. *Am J Obstet Gynecol*.
2011;204:322.e1–6.

Creating a Learning Culture
Debriefing and Root-cause Analysis

Nancy Chescheir

Healthcare is primarily delivered by teams of individuals. When there are poor outcomes or near-misses, it is important to take appropriate steps to try to prevent similar incidents in the future, to learn together as a team, and to identify individual team members who may be suffering distress due to the incident. Because maternal mortality in the US and other developed countries has become quite rare, quality improvement through debriefing maternal near-miss events affords a substantial opportunity to make systematic improvements that would be missed if only mortality cases were debriefed. While such post-event meetings can take several forms, a debrief occurs in the immediate time frame after the event and is typically very focused while a root-cause analysis is done days to weeks after the event and is a deeper evaluation of the event and contributory factors.

Case Scenario

A 27-year-old patient at 38 weeks gestation arrived on a Friday night with contractions occurring every 5 minutes for the last 2 hours. This is her third baby and she received her care at a local health department that uses paper medical records. She has been unable to attend her last three weekly appointments. The ward secretary was flustered because L&D was full. She looked through the file of prenatal records from the Health Department but could not locate the patient's records.

The patient noted that she had one prior cesarean for a breech at 28 weeks and one vaginal birth preceding that delivery. These were done elsewhere. The nurse in triage documented vital signs with a blood pressure of 130/80, pulse of 78 between contractions, normal respiratory rate and temperature. Pain score was 5/10 with contractions. External monitoring confirmed regular contractions every 5 minutes and there was a category 2 tracing with variable decelerations. Laboratory studies were sent. There were two cesareans being done. The patient was not evaluated by a physician for 35 minutes.

When the doctor arrived, the patient was complaining of constant pain at 9/10. Her blood pressure was 100/60. The nurse started oxygen by mask and there was an 18-gauge IV with normal saline infusing at 200 cm³/hour. The nurse inserted a Foley catheter. Vaginal exam showed no presenting part palpable with moderate bloody show. The fetal monitor strip was category 3 at that time. An emergency cesarean section was called for presumed uterine rupture but no operating room was available. The anesthesiologist reviewed the laboratory studies and noted that the type and screen was positive and her hemoglobin was 8 mg/dl. When requested, the blood bank reported that it would take 90 minutes to get blood crossmatched because they were short-staffed and there was a positive antibody screen.

The infant was delivered 45 minutes later. At laparotomy, the infant's arm and leg were protruding through the ruptured prior hysterotomy scar and there were 1.5 liters of blood in the maternal abdomen. Apgar scores were 3 at 1 minute and 5 at 5 minutes. Arterial cord blood shows a base excess of 15 and a pH of 6.9. The infant was taken to the Newborn intensive Care Unit (NICU) after being intubated. He was placed on the head cooling protocol. The mother, who was under general anesthesia, became hypotensive during the surgery. Fluid resuscitation was performed and 2 units of O-negative blood was administered until type-specific, cross-matched blood became available. She required cesarean hysterectomy because of uncontrolled bleeding. Postoperatively she was admitted to the Intensive Care Unit. At the end of the shift, the entire team was exhausted, frustrated, and distraught. They wanted to know how such an event could be avoided in the future.

Organizations with a strong learning culture incorporate quality-improvement steps to analyze suboptimal events after they happen in order to identify ways that future patients can be spared bad outcomes. Effectively analyzing a sentinel event, or a near-miss event, is an important systems-based quality-improvement function in order to acknowledge excellence; develop team and individual knowledge, skills, and attitudes; and identify processes that can be improved in order to prevent safety problems in the future.

Many quality-improvement and patient safety concepts are derived from manufacturing quality control. Having a common vocabulary and a shared mental model of the process and its purpose are key.

Common Definitions

Near-miss: A condition that did not result in injury, illness or damage, but had the potential to do so [1].

Severe acute maternal morbidity (SAMM) or "maternal near-miss": A severe health condition during pregnancy, childbirth or postpartum which the patient experiences and survives [1].

Critical incident: Deviation from expected course with potential for adverse outcomes [2]; events that are highly unusual or unusually successful or unsuccessful [3].

Second victim: A healthcare provider involved in an unanticipated adverse patient event, medical error, and/or a patient-related injury who becomes victimized in the sense that she or he is traumatized by the event [4].

Debriefing: A process that allows members of the healthcare team to actively reflect upon the events. What went well? Where are there opportunities for improvement? Debriefing allows individuals and teams to actively reflect upon their experience, to identify and share the mental models that led to the behaviors or cognitive processes used in the event, and, to build or enhance new mental models to be used in the future [5].

Root-cause analysis: A "formalized investigation, used extensively in engineering and industry, which uses a standard problem-solving approached focused on identifying and understanding the underlying causes of an event as well as potential events that were intercepted" [6].

Debriefing

Recurring and critical incident debriefs are important models to understand and incorporate into clinical practice. Both are forward-focused, describing processes that promote learning and performance improvement.

Recurring debriefs are those that are scheduled to occur at specific times, such as at the end of each surgical case, shift, daily, or weekly. Recurring debriefs are not stimulated by an adverse events, but rather they are scheduled opportunities for the healthcare team to reflect on what is going well, what could be improved, and what steps can be taken to make those improvements. Such debriefs are critical for creation of a learning environment and for teams to develop a sense of trust amongst themselves [3].

Critical incident debriefs, on the other hand, are unscheduled. Ideally, these occur as soon as possible after an adverse or near-miss event and may last less than five minutes. The entire team should be present and a facilitator or leader should identify and review the nature of the problem and relevant issues. The facilitator should allow team members to discuss various decisions that were made. Discussion should then address things that could have been differently, and potential for remediation, training or process change. In this way the team can be guided to introspection and self-correction [3].

Several important characteristics of the debriefing process are summarized in Table 21.1.

Analysis of sentinel events in obstetrics, as with other inpatient care services, show that communication failures and poor team functioning are major contributors

Table 21.1 Characteristics of successful debriefs [3,5,7].

1. The debrief structure should be formalized. Use of a checklist enhances this structure

2. Goal should be self-reflection, learning, and team development but not disciplinary

3. All members of the team should be given the opportunity and encouragement to participate

4. Environment should be non-judgmental, yet honest and open

5. One focus should be to identify team members at risk for stress, fear, self-doubt, and feelings of personal failure and allow for support for them

6. Focus on a few critical performance issues and provide feedback to all team members

7. Record team recommendations for future system changes or for team and individual learning

8. Create an environment for learning and change – a quiet or isolated location; sitting or standing in a circle helps diffuse the traditional medical hierarchy

to the adverse outcomes [8]. As hospitalists and laborists increasingly form the core of inpatient teams, and with physicians coalescing into larger groups, schedules are becoming more shift-based – healthcare teams are continually forming and regrouping [9]. These transient teams often lack a shared history. For instance, Riley et al. [9] estimated that there were 318 million possible combinations of nurses, obstetrical, anesthesia, and pediatric physicians and staff in a typical labor and delivery unit. Clinical cases resulting in an adverse event and near-miss may include several teams. It is important that the debriefing process includes members from all the relevant teams.

These short, focused, and forward-looking critical incident reviews should allow the team to answer the question "What do we know now that we did not know before?" [3].

Root-cause Analysis (RCA)

There are times when a substantially more in-depth analysis of an adverse or near-miss event is necessary. Unit or hospital leadership may call for an in-depth review if the facts suggest multiple or important process failures, if there was a significant degree of patient harm, or if the staff sequelae seems unusually great. One of the most common types of in-depth analysis that is done in healthcare is the root-cause analysis (RCA). Its goal is to determine *why* an event happened, not just *what* or *how* it occurred [10]. Since 1997, The Joint Commission (TJC) requires that an RCA be performed and reported for all sentinel events. Further, TJC requires that hospitals develop and implement an action plan based on the results from the RCA.

According to the Agency for Healthcare Research and Quality (AHRQ), the central purpose of an RCA is to identify underlying problems that increase the likelihood of errors, while avoiding the trap of focusing on individual mistakes [11]. As is well known, most medical errors and adverse events are the result of system deficiencies, not individual errors. Human error is a given – it will happen. Systems should be developed to minimize human errors from occurring and to reduce the risk of those errors that do occur from causing patient harm [12]. While an individual error may be identified as part of an RCA, the goal is to develop systems that will prevent such errors from causing harm.

Participants in an RCA try to identify all of the different errors and circumstances related to a specific patient harm or near-miss. Errors are commonly

described as active errors and latent errors [13]. Active errors occur at the direct interface with the patient or the so-called "sharp end" of the interaction of the patient with her providers and the healthcare system, broadly defined. Active errors that involve failure of behavior or lapse of concentration due to fatigue, distractions due to noise are sometimes referred to as "slips" and can be reduced by the use of check lists, standard orders sets and protocols. Mistakes occur at the sharp end thus are active errors, commonly related to knowledge or training deficits. Latent errors are system deficiencies that allow patient harm to happen but usually don't actively cause harm to happen. These occur at the so-called "blunt end" of care. Examples of this type of error include national drug shortages, personnel shortages, and computer failures. Latent errors typically involve hospital management, policies, devices, and regulations, and some of the factors that lead to latent errors are listed in Table 21.2 [14].

For a RCA, a multidisciplinary team is appointed, determined in part by the specifics of the event. The RCA team generally follows a prespecified process. Initially, they go through a process of data collection, reconstructing the event through record review, and participant interviews. The team then analyzes the sequence of events leading to the adverse or near-miss event to identify active and latent errors in order to prevent future harms, primarily by eliminating the latent errors [11]. The following are typical questions that should be addressed by an RCA:

1. What happened?
2. What normally happens?
3. What do policies and procedures require?
4. Why did it happen?
5. How was the organization managing the risk before the event?

The goal of RCAs is to determine all the contributory factors of an event in order to suggest preventive

Table 21.2 Factors leading to latent errors (from [14]).

Institutional or regulatory errors
Organization and management issues
Work environment
Team environment
Staffing
Task-related issues
Patient characteristics

steps for the future. Critical to this process is explicating the difference between what normally happens and what the policies and procedures suggest should happen. A latent error may cause a healthcare team to work around the problem rather than dealing with it directly. An RCA should look beyond this work-around to identify and correct the underlying latent error. Following this analysis, the RCA team is charged with making recommendations to the unit, hospital or healthcare system for systematic process improvements based on their findings. Every hospital in the United States accredited by TJC is required to use RCA for analysis of sentinel events. Many also use this technique for analysis of near-miss events.

RCA is a useful method to identify various types of errors in order to inform improved quality in the future. It is imperfect, however, with various possible shortcomings listed in Table 21.3.

A second systematic approach to systems improvement, also borrowed from manufacturing quality improvement, is the Failure Mode Effect Analysis (FMEA). FMEA is prospective and seeks to identify error-prone situations before there is an adverse event as opposed to the retrospective RCA [14]. Targets for FMEA are high-risk, high-volume, problem-prone processes. For instance, if a department has identified risks associated with the outpatient surgery program and desires to mitigate these risks, they may conduct an FMEA. Initially, an FMEA should identify each step in any given process. As an example, the steps in the process of outpatient surgery include: (1) identification of patients who are candidates, (2) scheduling of surgery, (3) preparing the patient for surgery, (4) transition from the preoperative area to the operating room, (5) transition from the operating room to the post-anesthesia care unit, and (6) discharge procedures and

Table 21.3 Possible shortcomings of root-cause analyses.

- Failure to address behavioral issues
- Failure to identify deep-seated latent failures
- Failure to evaluate human factors
- Failure to seek outside knowledge
- Failure to link causes to proposed interventions
- Selecting weak interventions, i.e., "staff education" and "downstream double checks"
- Failure to measure results of interventions
- Focus too narrow or too broad
- Unjust punitive actions (Just Culture)

follow-up. During an FMEA, the possible ways each step can fail will be identified. In addition, the FMEA team estimates the potential degree of harm to patient for each failure. The "criticality index" is the product of the likelihood that an individual failure will occur times the consequences of that failure. The more likely that a failure will occur; the greater the resultant patient harm, the higher is the criticality index. The "criticality index" thus allows the department to prioritize their improvement efforts to focus on the flawed processes most likely to cause significant patient harm.

Returning to the clinical scenario presented at the beginning of this chapter, the case described is appropriate for both a critical incident debriefing and an RCA. Once the mother is stable in the ICU, the team should return to L&D and request a debrief, to include the ward secretary, triage nurse, charge nurse, physicians from all involved specialties, learners such as residents and students involved in the care, and operating room staff. The leader should gather the participants in a quiet room and, using a checklist to guide the process, should review the clinical scenario and identify the key issues to be addressed. In the case described, the leader might acknowledge that the team had been extremely busy during the shift. The purpose of the debriefing is not to affix blame but to understand the system failures. The leader should then present a brief summary of the case. This case involved a patient about whom little was known because there were no records available. Shortly after arrival, she experienced a uterine rupture and was taken as quickly as possible, but outside the "30 minute" decision to incision framework due to the need to clean the operating room. The triage nurse had the patient ready for surgery once a room was available. The team had acted as quickly as they could and still had poor outcomes. After this summary, the leader should ask for thoughts from the team about what went well and what didn't go well. Any obvious system failures should be identified. Acknowledging the emotional impact of a poor outcome on the providers, the leader should offer individual counseling and support. Recall that the critical incident debriefing can only focus on a few processes. Recommendations for improvement, based on the debrief, should be recorded and communicated to management. Specific issues in this case might include:

1. The transfer of prenatal records from outside prenatal care systems to L&D and their storage and retrieval process in L&D.

2. The policy around back-up operating rooms for L&D if all of the unit's ORs are in use or dirty.

These critical incident debriefs are not the setting in which solutions to these problems should be sought.

Several weeks later, the results of an RCA for this case may have surfaced the following summary of causal factors and recommendations.

Causal factor 1: Patient records were not available when she presented.

A number of *contributing factors* may have been related to non-availability of the patient's records. Her admission occurred after hours on a weekend when the health department could not be contacted. Labor and delivery was very busy and the ward secretary could not find available records. The patient had not attended her last three visits and this may have contributed to failure at the Health Department to send the records on schedule. The patient's inability to attend her last three scheduled appointments may have been due to stressors in her life that will contribute to her coping with the current situation, including a sick child, transportation problems, or domestic violence. The *recommendations* from the RCA panel related to this causal factor may include a review of the procedure for obtaining the records from outside clinics and filing them or scanning them into the EMR; recommendations to the health department to review and enforce their "no show" policy; procedures to follow for the ward secretary when the unit is so busy that she or he needs additional help; recommendations for all of the offices at which patients who deliver in the hospital receive care use the same electronic medical record.

Causal factor 2: Patient with prior classical cesarean section should have been delivered by unit protocol by 37 weeks to avoid uterine rupture.

Contributing factors here may have included failure on the part of the health department personnel to obtain the history of the prior cesarean section, to document it or to recognize it as a potential problem. The patient may not have provided that history or may not have known the type of prior surgery she had. She should have been referred earlier in pregnancy for a consultation about the need to do a repeat cesarean in the early term period. The clinic schedule may have been full or slots unavailable when the patient could arrange time and transportation. *Recommendations* could include a review of the protocols with all health departments as well as a didactic presentation that

would reinforce the importance of early referral; review of access for patient visits; review documentation processes.

Causal factor 3: There was a relatively long delay before a physician initially saw the patient and then a further delay beyond the 30 minute "decision to incision" window for emergency cesarean births.

Contributing factors included the very high census in labor and delivery at the time the patient presented, the number of operative deliveries that were occurring at the time; the physician on call from home was not called to come in to help; there is no protocol for using the main OR when the L&D ORs are not available; there was a lack of knowledge by the clinical team regarding the evolving clinical picture; the delivery volume has increased 25% in the last 3 years and the L&D space and staffing are now insufficient. *Recommendations* from the RCA may have included reinforcement for all including physicians and nurses to be able to call back-up help when things are busy; assignment of a multidisciplinary committee to develop a hospital protocol to use the main operating room when emergencies occur without a clean L&D operating room; developing a learning module for nurses and doctors on uterine rupture; ask the planning office to consider a need for expanded L&D facilities including operating rooms.

Causal factor 4: Delay in transfusion with acute anemia

Contributing factors included a preoperative anemia in a patient with a previously known positive RBC antibody screen; delay at the blood bank due to staffing issues and an excessive overtime after several staff left for higher pay at the Red Cross. *Recommendations* would include the same ones for promoting a planned delivery at 37 weeks, in addition to documentation in her records to obtain cross match upon arrival to L&D due to the known positive antibody screen; salary review for retention of staff; incentive pay to avoid call-outs.

The focus of the RCA is not accusatory but rather based on problem-solving. In this example, the RCA team identified as many underlying contributors to the poor outcome as possible. Inclusion of the full richness and nuance of the circumstances yielded recommendations ranging from the health department work flow, protocol development, staffing, budgets, provider education, use of electronic medical records, and use of "on call" physicians.

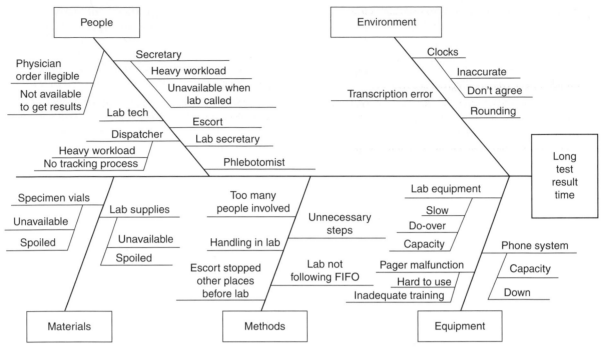

Figure 21.1 The "fishbone" diagram is a useful way of framing the approach to root-cause analysis.
(Reproduced by permission of Institute for Healthcare Improvement).

Summary

Professionals who work within a culture in a hospital or office that is focused on best outcomes will take advantage of near-miss or adverse events to identify ways of improving the quality of care going forward. The majority of such events result from multiple system failures. These failures can be used to inform system change, not individual blame, by using critical incident debriefing and RCA. Thus, patient care can be improved through better teamwork and better processes throughout the organization.

References

1   Say L, Souza JP, Pattinson RC, WHO Working Group on Maternal Mortality and Morbidity Classifications. Maternal near miss – towards a standard tool for monitoring quality of maternal health care. *Best Pract Res Clin Obstet Gynaecol*. 2009;23(3):287–296.

2   Manser T. Managing the aftermath of critical incidents: meeting the needs of health-care providers and patients. *Best Pract Res Clin Anaesthesiol*. 2011;25(2): 169–179.

3   Salas E, Klein C, King H, et al. Debriefing medical teams: 12 evidence-based best practices and tips. *Joint Comm J Qual Patient Saf*. 2008;34(9):518–527.

4   Scott SD, Hirschinger LE, Cox KR, McCoig M, Brandt J, Hall L. The natural history of recovery for the health care provider "second victim" after adverse patient events. *Qual Saf Health Care*. 2009;18(5):325–330.

5   Zigmong JJ, Kappus LJ, Sudikoff SN. The 3D model of debriefing: defusing, discovering and deepening. *Semin Perinatol*. 2011;35:52–58.

6   Hughes RG. Tools and strategies for quality improvement and patient safety. In: Hughes RG, ed. *Patient Safety and Quality: An Evidence-based Handbook for Nurses*. Rockville, MD: Agency for Healthcare Research and Quality; 2008. Chapter 44. Available from: www.ncbi.nlm.nih.gov/books/NBK2682/

7   Ahmed M, Sevdails N, Paige J, Paragi-Gururaja R, Nestel D, Arora S. Identifying best practice guidelines for debriefing in surgery: a tri-continental study. *Am J Surg*. 2012;203;523–529.

8   *Preventing Infant Death and Injury During Delivery*. Sentinel Event Alert; Issue 30. Oakbrook Terrace, IL: The Joint Commission; 2004. Available at: www.jointcommission.org/SentinelEvents/SentinelEventAlert/sea_30.htm

9   Riley W, Hansen H, Gürses AP, Davis S, Miller K, Priester R. The nature, characteristics and patterns of perinatal critical events teams. In: Henriksen K, Battles JB, Keyes MA, Grady ML, eds. *Advances*

in Patient Safety: New Directions and Alternative Approaches, Volume 3: Performance and Tools. Rockville, MD: Agency for Healthcare Research and Quality; 2008.

10 Rooney JJ, Vanden Heuval LN. Root cause analysis for beginners. *Quality Progress.* 2004;45–53.

11 AHRQ Patient Safety Network Root Cause Analysis. www.psnet.ahrq.gov/primer.aspx?primerID=10

12 Hor Su-yin, Iedema R, Williams K, White L, Kennedy P, Day AS. Multiple accountabilities in incident reporting and management. *Qual Health Res.* 2010;20(8):1091–1100.

13 Gluck PA. Patient safety in obstetrics and gynecology: improving outcomes, reducing risks medical error theory. *Obstet Gynecol Clin.* 2008;35(1):11–17.

14 Web M&M. Morbidity and Mortality Rounds on the Web. Patient safety primers-systems approach. AHRQ. http://webMM.ahrq.gov/primer.aspx?primerID=21 (accessed June 4, 2013).

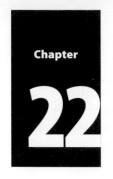

22

Safe Patient Handoffs

Diana Behling and Bonnie Dattel

Case Presentation

An 18-year-old Gravida1 woman with Class C Diabetes Mellitus was admitted for induction of labor at 39 weeks gestation. Her pregnancy had been complicated initially by poor diabetic control; however, as pregnancy progressed, blood sugars were in the target range and her most recent HbA1c was 6.2%. She had an unfavorable cervix for induction with a Bishop's score of 0. Membranes were intact. Estimated Fetal Weight (EFW) was 3,300 g, and Group B *Streptococcus* culture was negative. On admission her blood sugar was 110 mg/dl and urine ketones were negative.

On hospital day one cervical ripening by cervidil was initiated, and after 12 hours an oxytocin induction was started. Fetal heart rate tracing remained Category I throughout the day.

At 5 PM the resident team changed. Sign out occurred on Labor and Delivery in the resident office among the resident team. The off-going day attending gave sign out separately to the oncoming night attending – his first night of call since joining the faculty.

At 10 PM the attending called the intern and told her that the patient should have the induction stopped so that she could eat, shower, and rest. The intern relayed the information to her third-year resident who then relayed that information to the chief resident. The chief resident informed the nurse that her patient was to rest and restart the induction the next morning. The patient was removed from the monitor, the oxytocin stopped, and the intravenous line was capped. The patient showered and ate, taking her usual insulin dosage. She then slept through the night.

The following morning, at 0800 the day shift nurse entered the room and placed the patient on the fetal monitor. She was unable to obtain a fetal heart rate and a bedside ultrasound was performed by the day team resident that revealed a fetal heart rate of 80 beats per minute. The oncoming attending brought the patient to the operating room for an emergency cesarean delivery which was performed in less then 10 minutes.

At delivery a 3,200 g female infant was born with APGARS of 0/1/1. Neonatal resuscitation was performed and the newborn was transferred to the NICU. Arterial cord pH was 6.78. The newborn expired shortly after birth. The patient was brought to the recovery room where she was found to be in diabetic ketoacidosis (DKA).

Handoff

A handoff is an interactive process of transferring patient-specific information from one caregiver to another or from one team of caregivers to another for the purpose of ensuring the continuity and safety of the patient's care [1]

Since the publication of the Institute of Medicine report *To Err Is Human*, hospitals nationally have worked to make healthcare safer [2]. During the same time period, in July 2003, the Accreditation Council for Graduate Medical Education (ACGME) set limits for resident duty hours [3]. It is generally accepted that although restrictions to resident duty hours were intended to promote patient safety by preventing sleep deprivation, they have had an unintended result of discontinuity of care via an increased number of handoffs in the acute care setting [4]. At one residency program, work-hour reform was found to increase the number of sign-outs by 40%, with each resident now engaging in patient care handoffs 300 times a month [5]. In a study that investigated reduced resident duty hours in New York State, researchers found that the presumed increase in discontinuity resulted in delayed test ordering and an increased number of hospital complications [6]. Studies have also linked resident discontinuity with longer length of stay, increased laboratory testing, and more frequent medication errors [5,7].

According to a Joint Commission evaluation of root-cause analyses, communication problems caused almost 70% of sentinel events in accredited healthcare organizations (Figure 22.1) [8].

Researchers exploring the nature and causes of human errors in the intensive care setting found that verbal communication between physicians and nurses was cited as a factor in 37% of errors. A review of four insurers in three regions including 444 surgical claims found that "systems factors" contributed in 82% of cases, communication breakdowns in 25% of cases, inadequate handoffs or personnel changes in 11%, RN–MD communication, inability to reach attending surgeon, or failure to establish clear lines of responsibility (9%) [9]. Singh et al. reported handover failures are a significant source of medical failures and account for 20% of malpractice claims in the United States [10]. Kluger and Bullock reported that 14% of 419 adverse events in the recovery room were because of communication failures in the handover process [11]. One study of 889 malpractice claims found that information transfer breakdowns at the handoff contributed to errors in 19% of the cases involving medical trainees and 13% of the cases involving non-trainees [10].

Recognizing the importance of information transfer at these numerous transition times, The Joint Commission (TJC) issued the 2006 National Patient Safety Goal 2E: "Implement a standardized approach to 'hand off' communications, including an opportunity to ask and respond to questions" [12]. The elements of performance measured by the Joint Commission in an organization's handoff process include:

1. Interactive communication that allows for the opportunity for questioning between the giver and receiver of patient information.

2. Up-to-date information regarding the patient's condition, care, treatment, medications, services and any recent or anticipated changes.

3. A method to verify the received information, including repeat-back or read-back techniques.

4. An opportunity for the receiver of the handoff information to review relevant patient historical data, which may include previous care, treatment or services.

5. Interruptions during handoffs are limited to minimize the possibility that information fails to be conveyed or is forgotten [13].

Ineffective handoffs can have serious consequences, including adverse events, delays in medical diagnoses and treatment, additional and potentially unnecessary procedures and tests, lower team and patient satisfaction, higher costs, longer hospital stays, more hospital admissions, and less effective training for healthcare providers.

An overriding risk is that clinical judgments will be made for the patient with missing or inaccurate data. Vulnerability results from the fact that errors or omissions in the information communicated through the handoff often become "fact" for the next person or team using the information [14]. Consequences can include failure to identify patients whose condition is becoming critical, inefficient prioritization and allocation of resources to patients, duplication of services, tests, procedures, and deviation from a previously established plan of care [15].

Despite the requirement for "effective" handoff, most nurses and physicians receive little to no formal education in communication techniques [16]. In one investigation, few internal medicine residency

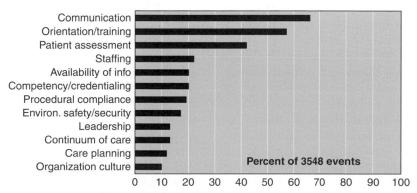

Figure 22.1 Root causes of sentinel events (all categories; 1995–2005).

programs across the United States reported having a comprehensive sign-out system in place, and a only minority reported that they conducted lectures or held workshops on handoff skills [16]. For instance in a survey of New York State residency programs, 60% reported no formal curriculum in sign out skills [16]. According to The Joint Commission Journal on Quality and Patient Safety, no single tool has been proven to be most reliable and effective, and regulation proscribes no specific way to meet the effective handoff standard.

The handoff process itself is ill-defined in literature and in practice, and it covers multiple clinical team events. Informal handoffs occur throughout the shift, as providers adjust to unit volume, acuity and milieu, exchanging information and temporary responsibility as staff leave and return to a unit for various tasks. For example; "Listen for a call for delivery on LDR 8 while I go and do a circ," and "I need to run to the ER. Can you write admission orders on the patient in Triage A." These informal transfers are often done on the fly, without defined structure or a clear sense of beginning and end, and with some assumption as to what the receiver of the handoff actually understands about the patient. More formal handoffs, also known as "sign-out," occur at the end of duty hours. They can be a written or verbal transfer of patient care information between individuals or groups of care providers clearly defining the end of duty. The process includes a formal transfer of responsibility for the patient from one team to the next. Lastly, handoffs occur between providers as patients are transferred geographically hospital to hospital, from primary to tertiary levels of care.

Mukherjee described the resident sign-out process as "a precarious exchange" and "one of the most poorly examined transactions in medicine" [17]. Each time a handoff occurs, the possibility for miscommunication arises. In the tertiary setting the complexities of the patients are compounded by the simultaneous existence of the learning environment and educational process of the medical students and residents. Training background, ethnic and cultural heritage, social relationships, and work ethic all play a role in how individuals relay information to others. Varied cultural, educational and gender characteristics are superimposed on a hierarchical structure for work and communication. Teams frequently change, and the same team will work together for limited periods before changing to move on to the next rotation. In a program with 16 residents, 8 attendings, 60 nurses,

and a variety of technical and support staff, the team combinations are endless. In our own survey at the tertiary facility, 7% of nurses agree: "There is effective communication between physicians across shifts," and 17% of physicians agree: "There is effective communication between nurses across shifts." These results offer insight into how each team perceives the effectiveness of the other, and forms the basis of a vibrant RN–MD Liaison Committee to undertake interprofessional work on these and other unit-based issues.

The process of handoff may be dependent upon local customs handed down from year to year. Handoffs are often riddled with omitted or inaccurate information that could be critical to patient care, such as code status or allergies, resulting in uncertainty in the covering residents' decisions for patients [18]. The problem is compounded by the dynamic environment with process improvement likened to fixing an engine that's running.

Discussion of Case

This case illustrates several of the pitfalls of patient handoffs that can result in adverse events.

Environment

Labor & Delivery is a unique and complex environment, functionally operating in a spectrum of specialty areas, including emergency room, postanesthesia recovery room, labor room, operating room, antepartum, postpartum, adult intensive care, neonatal intensive care, newborn nursery, and anesthesiology all in one unit, while caring for two patients simultaneously – the maternal–fetal pair. Low-risk patients can, with little warning, become acutely ill requiring rapid assessment, emergency mobilization of the team and immediate intervention. Meanwhile, patients also present with myriad obstetric and medical comorbidities further complicated by the presence of one or more fetuses.

Ideally, handoffs would occur in a quiet environment, with few distractions. The L&D unit is often challenged to provide such conditions. In the case above, the end of duty resident to resident handoff began in the resident lounge as is often the tradition. The handoff process continued beyond the office as the team attended to patient needs prior to completion of the handoff, communication occurring in the active unit, the formality and attention to the passing of information diminished by the environment of beeping machines, ringing telephones, and personnel distractions. The nature of the handoff became more "on the fly" versus a formal, controlled exchange of information.

Method of Communication

The chain of communication contributed to the adverse events in the case. After formal sign out, the new faculty member relayed an order to the least experienced individual of the team, who then relayed what she heard to her "next in command" who in turn reported the order to her "chief." The chief resident then gave the "order" to the nurse. Four handoffs of what each sender and receiver perceived to be the message. This is similar to the game of telephone where each person whispers the same information to the next person in line. At the end of the line the words and the intent are completely different than what the initiating individual stated.

In this case, the faculty sign-out occurred independent of the residents' process. This practice resulted in an incomplete transmission of information and is greatly impacted by the style and attention of the individuals involved. It also eliminates a team mentality or shared mental model, and leaves other providers out of the communication loop.

Finally, the order for "rest" was given over the telephone rather than in person which may have impeded any questioning of the order from more experienced personnel.

Language

When questioned, the shaken new faculty member had no idea that his "suggestion" to allow the patient to rest would have led to interruption of standard orders and care for diabetic mothers and their fetuses on Labor and Delivery. At his prior institution that language was routinely meant to stop the oxytocin only, and to continue other orders while allowing the patient to rest prior to proceeding with the induction.

This error in communication underscores the need to use standard medical terminology rather than colloquialisms. The message had been to let the patient "rest," which was open to a variety of interpretations. Had the clear concise medical order to stop the oxytocin been given, there would have been little room for different interpretation.

Documentation

Documentation in the process of patient handoff is a key feature as it allows all providers to clearly see the plan of care and ask for clarification if necessary. In this instance,

no orders were changed in the patient's record. The standard Labor and Delivery orders for laboring diabetic patients remained in effect. No plan of care was documented stating that only the Pitocin was to be stopped. Had appropriate documentation taken place a plan of care would have been written in the patient's medical record and orders specifying exactly what was to occur during this "rest" would have left little room for error.

Hierarchical Culture

Traditionally in medicine, in residency programs and many Labor and Delivery suites, a hierarchal culture exists, undermining any true culture of safety. In such environments, questions about specific plans or their rationale are often perceived as challenges to the authority or stature of more senior providers, thwarting a key strategy in patient safety. The hierarchy within the managing team precluded the questions being asked that could have altered the course of tragic events. Exactly what does "rest" mean?

No one wanted to challenge the new faculty member despite the fact that his recommendation was contrary to established Labor and Delivery protocols. He was not well known to them, and it was his first night on call after all. The handoff went through three levels of residents and an experienced nurse, and not one person felt comfortable enough to question the order or ask for clarification. This culture of hierarchy or deference contributed to errors that lead to this poor outcome and is the crux of so many adverse events. This difficulty of communicating against an authority gradient was certainly compounded by the lack of an effective handoff from the start of the shift, with a failure to have clarity regarding the plan of care, failure to allow time for questions and discussion, and a failure in leadership on the part of the attending in not engaging his team on his first night of call.

Finally, the patient was not included in this process. Information regarding her plan of care was delivered through individuals rather than her care team which prevented yet another possible question of the plan of care that could have resulted in a better outcome.

Strategies for Improvement

Both the giver and receiver of patient information have important responsibilities for ensuring effective handoffs, and each party must be comfortable with the information exchange. The handoff is not a quick "down and dirty" exchange of a few facts, but a coordinated effort among two professionals or groups of professionals [19]. Examples of best practice are available in looking at high-reliability organizations (HRO) using principles of crew resource management (CRM) such as nuclear power, aviation, aircraft carrier flight decks, and automobile racing pit crews. The picture of an effective handoff emerges as a structure that is evidence-based, simple, easy to implement, conveys relevant information in a time-limited way, and can be acculturated into everyday practice.

A key principle in building effective handoff strategies is rooted in identifying and managing the handoff as a patient safety device. Inadequate handoff can be the cause of events of harm, a failure of information exchange. Well-designed handoffs may be an important opportunity for recovery, correction, and intervention before events become harmful to the patient. A look at shift change in the emergency department recognized that while handoff is poorly studied, despite its importance, handoff at shift change is a source of potential failure and also a potential source of recovery [20]. This is no small distinction, the source of recovery as these pick-ups during handoffs may be the thing that prevents and event from evolving into an actual event of harm.

Environment

Work on L&D is often task-oriented and non-linear, with bedside providers frequently physically and mentally multitasking. There are many interruptions and distractions as the volume, acuity, and flow of patients can be chaotic and unpredictable. The aviation industry has tackled this issue by creating a distraction-free cockpit where the captain and crew engage only in flight-related conversation. This requirement evolved as it became apparent that a number of accidents and near-misses were related to distracting conversations among the flight deck and cabin personnel.

At the very least, an effort to identify a quiet location for report is key to allowing handoff participants to attend to the matters at hand. Likewise, elimination of all non-clinical distractions such as cell-phones, iPads, and the like go far to provide the type of environment for effective handoff. In support of a distraction-free handoff, solutions must consider that patient care needs continue during handoff periods. A structure that allows for a team member to be available for emerging patient needs is important in assuring that the handoff does not lead to neglect of other clinical issues.

Method of Communication

All communication involves the transfer of information between a source and a destination. Studies show that speakers systematically overestimate how well their messages are understood by listeners [21] and that people in general believe that their thoughts are transparent to others [22]. Senders assume that receiver has the same knowledge as they do. These assumptions may worsen with the personal familiarity of the receiver.

In the implementation phase of any handoff improvement initiative, there must be a consideration of the principles of effective communication. Well-established concepts include:

- Active listening
- Open-ended questions
- Reflective statements
- Identifying emotional cues
- Empathic responding
- Get the person's attention
- Effective eye contact
- Express concern
- Use a standardized communication technique
- Use a standardized communication tool/checklist
- Re-assert as necessary
- Escalate if necessary

A variety of structured communication techniques are found in the literature (see Table 22.1).

Documentation

Researchers have begun to look at the role of documentation to support a safe and efficient handoff process. In many L&D suites homegrown spreadsheets are used by residents to pass vital information. The spreadsheets can be inaccurate, incomplete, and are often non-standardized for service [28]. Much time is spent managing the tool rather than managing the patient. Valuable time is expended updating the spreadsheet by cross-referencing personal notes, anecdotal recall of events of the day, followed by the time actually giving–receiving the handoff. Consider also how soon anxiety builds around preparing the sheet for the next shift, and the diversion of critical resources from patient care to a cumbersome administrative task.

Table 22.1 Structured communication techniques.

Technique	Features
ISBAR [23] I – Introduction: I am S – Situation: What's going on B – Background: Brief, relevant history A – Assessment: What I think is happening R – Recommendation: What you are asking them to do	• Initially developed by the military to standardize communication during situational briefings • Structured tool to help overcome steep hierarchy and different communication styles • Creates common expectations so people don't feel "out of line" • Gives a full picture, reduces ambiguity • Synthesis of information and redundancy
"I PASS THE BATON" [24] I – Introduction: Introduce yourself, your role in the team P – Patient: Name: identifiers, age, sex location A – Assessment: "The problem" procedure, etc. so far in the process S – Situation: Current status/circumstances, uncertainty, recent changes S – Safety concerns: Critical lab values/reports; threats, pitfalls and alerts B – Background: Comorbidities, previous episodes, current meds, family A – Actions: What are the actions to be taken and brief rational T – Timing: Level of urgency, explicit timing, prioritization of actions O – Ownership: Who is responsible (person/team) including patient/family N – Next: What happens next? Anticipated changes? Contingencies	• Technique is recommended by the Department of Defense's Patient Safety Program to provide an optimal structure to improve communication during transitions in care • Should include opportunities to confirm receipt, ask questions, clarify information, and verify that the information, is understood • Designed to assist with both simple and complex handoffs
"5-Ps" [25] Use the 5 Ps: • Patient • Plan • Purpose • Problems • Precautions	• Ensures proper information is passed during patient transfers or provider shifts change • Developed to streamline the transfer of responsibility among caregivers and patient information
US Forest Service Fire Chiefs "Sense-making" [26] • Here's what I think we face. • Here's what I think we should do. • Here's why. • Here's what we should keep our eye on. • Talk to me (tell me if you do not understand, cannot do it, or see something I do not)	• Focus on "sense-making" • Fosters clarification, questions and communication from lesser-experienced members of the team • Sense-making consists of five major tasks: observe, question, act, reassess, and communicate
"PACE" [27] P – Patient/Problem A – Assessment/Actions C – Continuing [treatments]/changes E – Evaluation	• Focuses on problems and dynamics of the patient condition in the present time and anticipating the future needs

Evidence supports the use of electronic tools and "sign-out" forms in improving the handoff process and reducing preventable adverse events [29,30]. End-of-shift transfers of information utilized in high-reliability industries [31] may offer helpful models for the patient handoff, and guide efforts to devise methods of combining hospital IT data with resident-entered details to improve handoffs [32].

Culture

Healthcare cultures, including those on maternity units, operating suites, offices, and beyond significantly influence the effectiveness of handoffs. This may be further magnified in the academic setting, where patient care and educational priorities may occasionally be at odds. Further, overly steep hierarchies, which can be present in any environment but are commonly considered in the academic stereotype, can do more to undermine a culture of safety than any other influence. Some hierarchies are less obvious or severe, but still influential in the safety culture. Indeed, medical students, interns, residents, fellows and attending combine to form an interesting practice milieu described by Philibert et al. (Table 22.2) [33].

Compounding the problems of this hierarchy are the resident's individual emotional intelligence and ability to communicate against the authority gradient, and our general human tendency to "fake it 'til you make it" so as to not appear stupid or unknowing. The team's ability to effectively develop a shared mental model of the L&D unit during the handoff process via productive communication techniques using emotional intelligence, and interpersonal factors such as trust, is key to the development of a safe care delivery model where errors are identified and managed effectively before patient harm can occur. Failures in these areas may result in a series of possible errors:

- Not knowing critical information, resulting in feeling unhelpful and loss of credibility with care team or family
- "Not knowing patient well" and having to look up information when the patient is deteriorating
- Omission of or delay in tests, therapeutic interventions or discharge ("To do list errors of omission")

- Duplication of tests and therapies resulting in waste ("To do list errors of commission")
- "Failure to rescue" (failing to notice a patient is deteriorating)
- Wrong intervention for the patient (e.g., wrong treatment or medication due to outdated or erroneous information, coding patient who is DNR) [33]

Handoff communication is best understood as a dialogue between health professionals – an interaction that fosters empathy, equity, and common ground, in addition to transferring necessary information. Through ongoing, professional give and take, one party must paint a picture and the other must see it, understand it, act on it, and, ultimately, communicate it to someone else. Furthermore, both handoff parties should recognize and anticipate potential differences in handoff communication expectations. Those expectations can influence what is said in a handoff (content) and how messages are communicated (style) [34].

HIPAA

Healthcare providers have become familiar with the structure of communication that is compliant with the Health Insurance Portability and Accountability Act of 1996 (HIPAA). HIPAA regulations were designed to:

(1) Protect individuals' rights to privacy and confidentiality, and
(2) Assure the security of electronic transfer of personal information.

Most clinicians take all reasonable steps to protect a patient's personal health information (PHI) by making sure that individuals without the "need to know" do not overhear conversations about PHI. Clinicians

Table 22.2 Problems with different healthcare cultures (from [28]).

The intern	• Is "green" with limited knowledge of the specialty and little ability, especially at the outset of the year, to discern the important from the unimportant. They are beginning their journey from novice to expert and may have a tendency to report everything in lieu of forgetting something • Effect of level of training: pronounced from 1st to 2nd year, negligible after (handoff is learned somewhere in the first year)
Mid years resident	• As residency progresses: "Nothing in the handoff is important, I get my information from a fresh look at the patient" (the Consult Effect) • May be impacted by a false sense of mastery over subject matter until they have an error or near-miss of their own
The Senior Resident	• Integrated information from the outgoing resident AND the patient are important • At more advanced levels information is evaluated based on whether it comes from a "trusted source" (assessment based on prior interactions) • Sense of wariness has returned

are taught to refrain from conducting discussion about PHI in elevators or cafeteria and to limit its entry in to the medical record to physicians directly in their charge.

Often residents develop their own computer-based methods for managing patient information required for the handoff process. While Word documents and Excel spreadsheets may be a step-up from handwritten notes, the potential for transcription error and HIPAA concerns make them less than ideal.

The information entered into these homegrown systems can be inaccurate, which creates the potential for serious medical errors. Important privacy concerns loom because large amounts of protected health information reside in files and on disks that may not be password-protected, are given to the "team" at shift handoff, and with little chain of responsibility for the proper disposal of outdated or "used" report sheets. A far better alternative is to consider the use of the actual medical record and working with IT to develop tools that can live in the medical record. With the adoption of electronic medical records, there is opportunity to develop handoff tools that populate directly from the record.

Education

> It is naïve to bring together a highly diverse group of people and expect that, by calling them a team, they will in fact behave as a team. It is ironic indeed to realize that a football team spends 40 hours a week practicing teamwork for the two hours on Sunday afternoon when their teamwork really counts. Teams in organizations seldom spend two hours per year practicing when their ability to function as a team counts 40 hours per week! [35]

In the educational environment of a residency program, a most basic element in considering the handoff process is how a provider learns to hand off. Currently no practical strategies meaningfully and consistently connect knowledge of handoff "science" and strategy to everyday teaching of residents. Few curricula include education on effective sign out. Few programs provide any real-time structured assessment of handoff techniques in use, let alone constructive critique for improvement. The handoff process is often learned on the job by direct observation and/or direct instruction on "this is how we hand off" [7,15].

Teaching strategies related to communication have been considered in the literature with recommendations including didactic lectures, small group

experiential learning via simulation and role play including debrief and critique for improvement with subsequent practice [36]. Teaching the handoff is more than the mechanics of the process and must include development of understanding of the expectations and values underlying its purpose in the management of patient care [37]. In the last year the GME put forth requirements related to handoff education. The ACGME standards note that effective transitions of care are essential for resident education in order to enhance patient safety:

- Evaluate the importance of handoff communication in transitions of care
- Appraise transitions of care improvement initiatives
- Apply intervention strategies for improving handoff communication and transitions of care
- Discuss methods and processes to improve transitions of care among and between residents
- Enhance structured handoff processes and resident competency in handoffs [38].

Through the educational process resident physicians may be armed with the knowledge regarding communication techniques and pitfalls in support of more effective and safe transitions in patient care.

Recommendations

Improving communication between healthcare providers in the process of transferring patient care is crucial for patient safety. The handoff is a teaching and a learning moment in a communication that is an active process for both the giver and the receiver. Clearly defining a construct for what information needs to be passed, the mode of transfer of information and responsibility, and a means of evaluating effectiveness are key to further the likelihood of optimal patient outcomes by design and not chance (see Table 22.3).

Conclusions/summary

Improvement in the transfer of patient care is critical to provide a safe environment for the patient. This process involves changes in the mindset and habit of how clinicians interact on a daily basis. The process has evolved from the "old days" where one physician covered only his/her patients in their entire hospital stay. Driven by concerns for patient safety, new work hours preclude healthcare providers working continuously, but such restrictions added a new element: that

Table 22.3 Evaluating effectiveness as the key to further the likelihood of optimal patient outcomes by design and not chance.

	Suggestions/considerations
Data points	• Patient name • Medical record number/location (room, unit) • Pertinent history • Trends of pertinent laboratory values • Trend of labor curve • Trend of vital signs including identification and possible cause of aberrant vital signs such as tachycardia, fever, decreased blood pressure and low oxygen saturation
Process	• Identify sickest patient(s) • Anticipating changes in patient condition with specific intervention • Clarity about the patient's current condition, including severity of illness • Anticipate potential problems and potential solutions • Alert to incoming information (e.g., lab results, consultant recommendations), and what action, if any, needs to be taken • What may go wrong and what to do about it • What has or has not worked before (e.g., on 2 g Magnesium Sulfate and has required intermittent Labetolol ivp to control BP) • Have enough time for interactive questions at the end • Plan time for assignment of duties • Give directions with rationale to avoid ambiguity. Don't say "check Hgb," say "she had a 1500 ebl and needs a Hgb at 0800"
Environment	• Conduct in a quiet, distraction-free place at a designated time • May consider handoff in the patient room so the plan of care is clear to all involved, including the patient • Include all members of the care team
Language	• Standard medical terminology and abbreviations • NICHD terminology for fetal heart rate • Feedback from patient and other members of the team
Method of Communication	• Consider standard SBAR • Face-to-face communication allows for direct interaction and questions • Summary of the plan of care • Routine time and place for sign out/handoff • Encourage questions about the plan of care • Use IF… THEN statements (i.e., if hgb less than 6 then transfuse prbc) • "Read back" all to-do items – closed-loop communication
Documentation	• Pertinent patient information-demographics, history, acute problems, allergies, lab results (i.e., GBS status) • A clear, concise plan of care should be documented • Linking handoff to hospital electronic medical record (EMR) may decrease chances of inaccurate data, transcription errors • Limit repeated selecting, copying and pasting text from past EMR notes into current notes or "handoff sheets" to prevent dissemination of inaccuracies • Too much attention on written handoff tool obscures what is going on now. The chart is used to keep track of everything about the patient
Culture	• Encourage a culture where all questions are answered • All members should feel equal in discussions during patient handoff
Confidentiality	• HIPAA compliance at all times during discussions especially in open clinical areas • HIPAA compliance in all electronic communication, homegrown Excel and Word data sheets, texts, emails

of the patient handoff. An organized and thoughtful approach to managing change, particularly in the handoff tradition in Labor & Delivery or any clinical setting, would be wise to consider Kotter's 8-Step approach to leading change:

- Establish urgency amongst the team, highlight the risk to all involved
- Form a powerful guiding coalition based on consideration of best practice
- Create a vision for the team of the future state
- Communicate the vision to all stakeholders
- Empower others to act on the vision
- Plan for short-term wins through observational compliance rating
- Consolidate improvements, revise initial plan based on user feedback
- Institutionalize new approach in education and practice with deviations disallowed [39].

The process of implementing an effective handoff tool is a cultural transformation with many years of tradition and culture to "undo." To be effective the focus must be not only on the mechanics, but also include a look at the social structure as well. Strong cultural structure will work against innovation unless those issues are part of the change process. Ideally, with time and attention, the process of the safe patient handoff should become second nature.

There is a need for ongoing research into the impact of structured communication on patient outcomes in healthcare. The implementation of the outlined criteria for the safe transfer of patient care between providers may help to decrease errors that result in adverse patient events and allow for the achievement of a safe patient environment. In the process, patient satisfaction may also increase due to continuity of the plan of care, the knowledge that there is a "team" of healthcare professionals caring for them, and their participation in the process.

References

1 Wallace TE. *Preventing Fatalities – Effective Critical Communication Handoffs*. Palo Alto, CA: Joint Commission Resources Inc.; 2005.

2 Leape LL, Berwick DM. Five years after *To Err Is Human*: what have we learned? *JAMA*. 2005;293:2384–2390.

3 Accreditation Council for Graduate Medical Education. Resident Duty Hours and the Working Environment. Available at: www.acgme.org/acWebsite/dutyHours/dh_Lang703.pdf (accessed April 24, 2012).

4 Fletcher KE, Saint S, Mangrulkar RS. Balancing continuity of care with residents' limited work hours: defining the implications. *Acad Med*. 2005;80:39–43.

5 Vidyarthi AR, Arora V, Schnipper JL, Wall SD, Wachter RM. Managing discontinuity in academic medical centers: strategies for a safe and effective resident sign-out. *J Hosp Med*. 2006:1:257–266.

6 Laine C, Goldman L, Soukup JR, Hayes JG. The impact of a regulation restricting medical house staff working hours on the quality of patient care. *JAMA*. 1993;269:374–378.

7 Arora V, Johnson J, Lovinger D, Humphreys HJ, Meltzer DO. Communication failures in patient sign-out and suggestions for improvement: a critical incident analysis. *Qual Saf Health Care*. 2005;14:401–407.

8 Collation of sentinel event-related data reported to The Joint Commission (1995–2005). Available from www.jointcommission.org/SentinelEvents/Statistics/ The Joint Commission. Improving handoff communications: Meeting National Patient Safety Goal 2 E. Joint Perspect Patient Safety. 2006;6:9–15.

9 Rogers Jr. SO, Gawande AA, Kwaan M, et al. Analysis of surgical errors in closed malpractice claims at 4 liability insurers. *Surgery*. 2006;140:25–33.

10 Singh H, Thomas EJ, Petersen LA, et al. Medical errors involving trainees: a study of closed malpractice claims from 5 insurers. *Arch Intern Med*. 2007;167:2030–2036.

11 Kluger MT, Bullock MF. Recovery room incidents: a review of 419 reports from the Anaesthetic Incident Monitoring Study (AIMS). *Anaesthesia*. 2002;57:1060–1066.

12 Solet DJ, Norvell JM, Rutan GH, Frankel RM. Lost in translation: challenges and opportunities in physician-to-physician communication during patient handoffs. *Acad Med*. 2005;80:1094–1099.

13 The Joint Commission. National Patient Safety Goals: History Tracking Report 2009–2008. Available at: www.jointcommission.org/PatientSafety/NationalPatientSafetyGoals/09_hap_npsgs.htm

14 Reason JT, Carthey J, de Leval MR. Diagnosing "vulnerable system syndrome": an essential prerequisite to effective risk management. *Qual Saf Health Care*. 2001;10(Suppl II):ii21–25.

15 Philibert I, Leach DC. Re-framing continuity of care for this century. *Qual Saf Health Care*. 2005;14:394–396.

16 Horwitz LI, Krumholz HM, Green ML, Huit SJ. Transfers of patient care between house staff on

internal medicine wards: a national survey. *Arch Intern Med.* 2006;166:1173–1177.

17 Mukherjee S. Becoming a physician: a precarious exchange. *N Engl J Med.* 2004;351(18):1822–1824.

18 Sutcliffe KM, Lewton E, Rosenthal MM. Communication failures: an insidious contributor to medical mishaps. *Acad Med.* 2004;79(2):186–194.

19 The Joint Commission. Perspectives on Patient Safety, October 2010, Volume 10, Issue 10.

20 Wears R, Roth E, Patterson E, Perry S. Shift Change Signovers as a Double-Edged Sword: Technical Work Studies in Emergency Medicine. Society for Academic Emergency Medicine, Annual Meeting. New York, NY; May 25, 2005. Available at www.saem.org/meetings/05hand/wears.ppt

21 Keysar B, Henly AS. Speakers' overestimation of their effectiveness. *Psychol Sci.* 2002;13(3):207–212.

22 Gilovich T, Savitsky K, Medvec VH. The illusion of transparency: biased assessments of others' ability to read our emotional states. *J Pers Soc Psychol.* 1998;75(2):332–346.

23 Q&A: implementing the SBAR technique. *Joint Comm Perspect Patient Saf.* 2006;6:8,12.

24 Department of Defense Patient Safety Program. Healthcare Communications Toolkit to Improve Transitions in Care. 2008.

25 Yates G. Sentara Healthcare. Panel 1 – Promising Quality Improvement Initiatives: Reports From the Field. AHRQ Summit – Improving Health Care Quality for All Americans: Celebrating Success, Measuring Progress, Moving Forward; 2004.

26 Weick K. *Sensemaking in Organizations.* Thousand Oaks, CA: Sage; 1995.

27 Schroeder SJ. Picking up the PACE: a new template for shift report. *Nursing.* 2006;36:22–23.

28 Wayne JD, Tyagi R, Reinhardt G, et al. Simple standardized patient handoff system that increases accuracy and completeness. *Journ Surg Educ.* 2008;65: 476–485.

29 Parker J, Coiera E. Improving clinical communication: a view from psychology. *JAMIA.* 2000;7(5):453–461.

30 Petersen LA, Orav EJ, Teich JM, et al. Using a computerized sign-out program to improve continuity of inpatient care and prevent adverse events. *Jt Comm J Qual Improv.* 1998;24:77–87.

31 Patterson ES, Roth EM Woods DD, et al. Handoff strategies in settings with high consequences for failure: lessons for health care operations. *Int J Qual Health Care.* 2004;16:125–132.

32 Van Eaton EG, Horvath KD, Lober WB, et al. Organizing the transfer of patient care information: the development of a computerized resident sign-out system. *Surgery.* 2004;136:5–13.

33 Wohlauer MV, Arora VM, Horwitz LI, Bass EJ, Mahar SE, Philibert I. The patient handoff: a comprehensive curricular blueprint for resident education to improve continuity of care. *Acad Med.* 2012;87(4):411–418.

34 Gibson SC, Ham JJ, Apker J, Mallak LA, Johnson NA. Communication, communication, communication: the art of the handoff. *Ann Emerg Med.* 2010;55(2):181–183.

35 Wise, H. The primary-care health team. *Arch Intern Med.* 1972;130:438–444.

36 Rosenbaum ME, Ferguson KJ, Lobas JG. Teaching medical students and residents skills for delivering bad news: a review of strategies. *Acad Med.* 2004;79(2):107–117.

37 Gardner H, Csikszentmihalyi M, Damon W. *Good Work: When Excellence and Ethics Meet.* New York, NY: Basic Books; 2001.

38 GME Today. Achieving Effective Transitions of Care 2012 PRIME Education, Inc. www.gmetoday.org/graduate-medical-education/current-residents/GME14-Achieving-Effective-Transitions-of-Care

39 Kotter JP. Leading change: why transformation efforts fail. *Harv Bus Rev.* March 1995;73(2):3.

Using Clinical Scenarios to Teach Patient Safety

Dotun Ogunyemi, Bruce B. Ettinger, and Steve Rad

Using the Healthcare Matrix to Teach the ACGME Competenices, IOM Aims, and Patient Safety

Clinical Case Scenario: Spontaneous Uterine Rupture in a Jehovah's Witness Patient

1430:

A 38-year-old Gravida 3 Para 0 at 41 weeks gestation was admitted to labor and delivery unit with spontaneous rupture of membranes and early labor. She reported a gush of fluid at 0100 with clear fluid. Her prenatal care was uneventful and her Group B Streptococcal culture was negative. During intake, the patient informed the nurse that she was a Jehovah's Witness, and she declined any blood products.

1900:

Vaginal examination revealed a cervix 4 cm dilated, 80% effaced, and the vertex was at −1 station. Fetal heart rate was normal, but uterine contractions were inadequate; therefore, Pitocin was started and epidural anesthesia was initiated.

0546:

The fetus had a prolonged heart rate deceleration to 60 beats per minute for 6 minutes. Pitocin was turned off, and Terbutaline was given. Vaginal examination showed that the cervix was 9 cm dilated, 100% effaced, and the vertex was at +1 station. The attending obstetrician was present in the patient's room.

0552:

The cervix was completely dilated, and she started to push. The charge nurse noted late decelerations with pushing (Figure 23.1) on the monitors at the nurse's station and went into the patient's room. The charge nurse suggested to the obstetrician to have her only push on alternate contractions. Obstetrician continues to push with patient.

0640:

The junior resident and chief resident approach MFM fellow to review concerning fetal heart rate patterns.

0645:

The MFM fellow discussed the case with the obstetrician who wanted the patient to continue to push because he thinks delivery is imminent. The residents and MFM fellow asked the MFM faculty to come to the unit.

0700:

MFM faculty asked the obstetrician to step outside the room for further discussion.

Obstetrician refused to leave the room because the delivery might be imminent, and he is concerned for his patient.

0705:

Obstetrician decides to perform an emergency cesarean delivery.

0716:

At laparotomy, an extensive uterine rupture extending along the left lateral uterine wall from the cervix to the fundus was noted. A cesarean–hysterectomy was performed due to the extent of the uterine rupture. The attending obstetrician and anesthesiologists were notified by the nurse that the patient was a Jehovah's Witness. A gynecologic oncologist was present to assist in the cesarean–hysterectomy.

0830:

A live female infant who was partially extruded into the abdominal cavity was delivered with a birth weight of 3,280 g and Apgar scores of 1 at one minute and 3 at five minutes. Infant umbilical cord gases:

Arterial pH 6.8, pCO_2 110, pO_2 20 base excess −19.5 Venous pH 6.8, pCO_2 127, pO_2 23, base excess −33.

The infant was intubated and taken to NICU.

Intraoperative hemoglobin/hematocrit was 6.0 mg/dl/17.8% (preoperatively it was 11.8/33.8). Patient

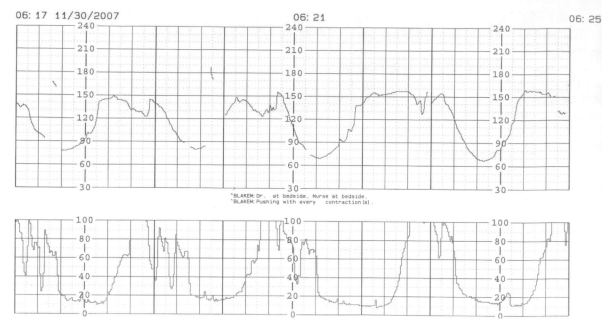

Figure 23.1 Fetal heart rate pattern in the second stage of labor for case with spontaneous uterine rupture in a Jehovah's Witness patient who refused blood product transfusion.

declined transfusion of packed red blood cells and any other blood products. Estimated blood loss at this time was approximately 1,500 ml. The anesthesiologist held multiple conversations with the husband regarding transfusions and different blood product options, all of which were declined.

0910:
End of surgery: an abdominal x-ray was performed to r/o retained foreign object.

1000:
Patient was transferred to the Surgical Intensive Care Unit (SICU).

Maternal Course
Hemoglobin/hematocrit reached a nadir of 4.9 mg/dl/ 14% on the second postoperative day and was 5.5/15.4 on the fourth postoperative day. The patient was counseled on transfusions and risk of myocardial ischemia and death due to severe anemia, but she still declined transfusion. She underwent a slow recovery and was ultimately discharged home in stable condition.

Neonatal Course
1. Respiratory failure – requiring mechanical ventilation for 1.5 weeks
2. Pneumothorax – requiring bilateral, tube thoracostomy insertion

3. Renal failure – oligouria/anuria, peak creatinine 7.1 mg/dl
4. Hepatic failure – with transaminase elevations and poor liver synthetic capacity
5. Coagulopathy – requiring fresh frozen plasma, platelet administration, and packed red blood cell administration

Infant female died on day 27 life.

Preliminary postmortem findings: Severe cerebral anoxia, pulmonary atelectasis, and renal ischemia.

Discussion

In 2005, Doris C. Quinn and John W. Bingham developed an educational tool called the Patient Healthcare Matrix at Vanderbilt University Medical Center [1,2]. The matrix juxtaposes the six Institute of Medicine (IOM) aims and the six ACGME competencies. Complex patient care can be assessed and reviewed in terms of the ACGME competencies and IOM aims.

A selected resident chooses a clinical case based on concerns, interest or questions about the clinical management or outcome. The resident reviews the case and develops a draft matrix under faculty supervision. A multidisciplinary team is invited based on the chosen case. The matrix is presented at conference and a consensus action plan for implementation is generated after discussion. An example of a healthcare matrix session is shown in Table 23.1. In this example involving a case with abnormal fetal heart rate patterns (Figure 23.1), uterine rupture and neonatal mortality, the residents learn about issues with documentation, communication, and teamwork. An action plan is developed and implemented [3].

Using a Field Case to Teach Regulatory Oversight and Compliance for Patient Safety and Quality of Care

Clinical Case Scenario: Postpartum HELLP Syndrome and Intracranial Hemorrhage

0120:

A 28-year-old primigravida at 37 weeks gestation in early labor was admitted to a Level II facility. Prenatal care records documented persistent unexplained mild proteinuria, a 40-pound weight gain, and possible fetal growth restriction from 34 weeks gestation. Blood pressure ranged between 90/50 and 116/70 in the prenatal records, but was 133/86 on admission.

0330:

The on-call obstetrician, who did not know the patient, gave telephone orders for oxytocin augmentation.

0410:

Her nurse notified the on-call obstetrician that the patient's blood pressure was 140–152/80–97, and that the patient reported seeing spots on the day prior to admission. The on-call obstetrician gave orders for laboratory studies.

0648:

The patient had a spontaneous vaginal delivery of a female infant weighing 2,010 g (4 lbs 7 oz.). The on-call obstetrician performed the delivery.

1215:

The nurse notified the on-call obstetrician of the patient's increasingly severe abdominal pain (8/10), vomiting, agitation, and blood pressure of 175/85. The obstetrician was in another delivery at the time and gave telephone orders for oral analgesics.

1430:

The nurse urgently paged the on-call obstetrician because of the patient's blood pressure and symptoms.

The on-call obstetrician was in a cesarean delivery and requested an internal medicine consultation. The consultant evaluated the patient and ordered a complete blood count, abdominal x-ray, and analgesics. The patient was started on a liquid diet.

1605:

The laboratory reported thrombocytopenia to the nursing staff, but there was no evidence of physician notification.

1637:

The patient suffered a grand mal seizure. Her blood pressure was 146/99. She was treated with intravenous magnesium sulfate by an Emergency Department physician and transferred to the Intensive Care Unit (ICU).

1740:

The on-call obstetrician saw the patient at 1740 and transferred care to the critical care physician.

1800–1930:

Gross hematuria was documented and drowsiness noted.

0001–0409:

At midnight, the patient was unresponsive, and decerebrate status was noted at 0330. CT of the head revealed extensive intracranial bleeding. A review of all laboratory studies supported the diagnosis of HELLP Syndrome.

0610:

Brain death was declared. The cause of death was presumed to be due to massive intracranial bleeding within 24 hours of delivery secondary to HELLP syndrome and DIC.

Discussion

This is an illustrative clinical case to teach Regulatory Compliance. It is important to develop an awareness of patient safety issues during residency related to types of practice that residents may enter into after graduation. The case above illustrates a maternal death that resulted from failure to provide adequate care for an unknown patient, and doing so at night, with a busy practice in a level II hospital with no residents.

Regulations – Structures for Processes of Care

Regulatory oversight includes requiring state licensing to operate a healthcare facility and federal supervision

Table 23.1 Healthcare matrix of a multidisciplinary team of a case with spontaneous uterine rupture in a Jehovah's Witness patient who refused blood product transfusion.

Healthcare matrix: care of patient with abnormal fetal heart rate tracing and spontaneous uterine rupture in a Jehovah's Witness patient

Aims Competencies	Safe (Avoiding injury from care intended to help)	Timely (Reducing delays for patient and provider)	Effective (Evidence-based medicine, avoiding underuse and overuse)	Efficient (Avoiding waste of equipment, supplies, ideas, energy)	Equitable (Care does not vary based on race, ethnicity, gender, SES)	Patient-centered (Care with respect for preference, needs, values)
Assessment of Care						
PATIENT CARE (Overall assessment) Yes/No	No – We missed important factor that greatly influenced patient care	No – We did not recognize possibility of uterine rupture until delivery of fetus	No – overuse of blood draws	No – overuse of wasteful blood draws. Wasted resources	Yes	Yes – Consulted with patient and husband and minister regarding blood products during surgery
MEDICAL KNOWLEDGE and SKILLS (What must we know?)	No – NICHD guidelines for fetal heart tracing were not followed	No – Delay in delivery of fetus	No – Fetal heart tracing abnormalities suggestive of fetal hypoxia identified	Equivocal – in acute hemorrhage situation, did not have time to explore other options	Yes	Equivocal – Patient was provided full knowledge of the situation, but may not have fully understood the implications
INTERPERSONAL AND COMMUNICATION SKILLS (What must we say?)	No – Need better communication between nurses, residents, and attending staff	No – Communication should be timelier in urgent situations. Delay in care while anesthesiologist was negotiating with husband/minister	No – Residents should be more effective/assertive in communications with attending	No – Chain of command took too long	Yes – physician–patient relationship respected	Yes – Patient declined transfusions, choice upheld
PROFESSIONALISM (How must we behave?)	No – The team did not function in a manner that allowed consensus decision to prevail	Equivocal – Chain of command was utilized but not necessarily effective in final result	No – Egos over professionalism made care less effective	Chain of command was not very effective	Yes	Not sure?
SYSTEM-BASED PRACTICE (What is the process? On whom do we depend? Who depends on us?)	Important patient information not always available or noted by those who should know	Chain of command and team function needs to improve	Oxytocin overuse? System issue	Other safety mechanism in conjunction with chain of command	Care must always be equitable physicians and staff at all times	Care must always be patient-centered by all physicians and staff at all times

Improvement

PRACTICE-BASED LEARNING AND IMPROVEMENT (What have we learned? What will we improve?)						
All residents and staff on L&D must be accountable for all patients	Abnormal tracing to be identified and acted upon in timely fashion. Communicate with all members of the team to facilitate care	More effective communicators in emergent situations	Think about why we get tests/blood draws and whether it will make a difference in clinical management	Provided equitable care to the patient	Ask about personal or religious objections to receiving blood products. Pass on the information

© 2004 Bingham, Quinn Vanderbilt University

Action Plan

What needs to be done?	Who will do it?	By when?	Results
1. Early identification of fetal heart abnormalities	Everyone	Immediately	Awareness rounds with all physicians and staff, 2 times per shift Emergency protocol activation and response team
2. Chain of command – initiate sooner, speed it up	Departmental leadership	Immediately	Chain of command identification, awareness, and training
3. Resident vs. Attending; who is responsible?	Residents and staff nurses	Immediately	Chief resident and charge nurse responsible for all patients on L&D regardless of teaching status. Residents and nurses responsible for monitoring all fetal heart tracings at all times. Residents and nurses to activate Chain of command if they feel they are not being heard by attending
4. Improve physician–patient communication	Departmental leadership	By one month	In-service on improving communication with patients
5. Develop method of identifying patients with personal or religious objections to receiving blood products	Nurse manager and physician clinical leadership	By 2 weeks	Alert system created
6. Improve communication amongst all team members	Nursing, OBGYN & Anesthesia leadership	By 3 months	Organizational coaching, workshops on communications and teamwork, debriefings
7. Education on NICHD fetal heart rate guidelines, labor, uterine rupture, and Strategies in the Clinical Management of Jehovah's Witness Patients	Faculty, Program Director	By 1 week	Lectures and grand rounds given on topics

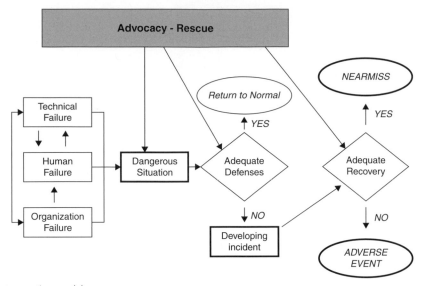

Figure 23.2 Incident causation model.

Adapted from *Patient Safety: Achieving a new standard for care.* National Academies Press, 2004, p. 228.

for Medicare reimbursement. The purposes of regulations are to: (1) protect patients by providing oversight for quality of care and safe practices; (2) survey health facilities for compliance with state and federal requirements; and (3) investigate complaints against any health facility.

Licensing, which permits (i.e., legally authorizes) a facility to provide care, is mandatory. Federal accreditation is certified by The Joint Commission and is voluntary. However, it is required to participate for reimbursement under Medicare with the Centers for Medicare and Medicaid Services (CMS) [4].

The organizational structure of a health facility includes the Governing Body, Medical Staff, and Nursing Services. The Governing Body (i.e., the Board of Directors) has the authority, responsibility, and accountability to operate a health facility. The Medical Staff is accountable to the Governing Body for the quality of care within the facility. It has oversight for all aspects of care, provides for credentialing, appointments, and privileges, performs peer review, establishes clinical departments and services, and provides oversight of non-MD providers (i.e., advanced practice nurses and allied health professionals as interdisciplinary practitioners). The Nursing Services is responsible for planning and delivering care through defined policies, implementing physician orders, and providing patient advocacy as necessary, through a defined "chain of command." Nursing Services must also assess

nurses' competency, provide for performance evaluation, and ensure appropriate staffing levels.

Regulatory violations fall under these three major domains (called "Conditions of Participation"): Governing Body, Organized Medical Staffs, and Nursing Services. Figure 23.2 illustrates the "Incident Causation Model" and the points at which clinical advocacy and patient rescue should occur to prevent an adverse outcome [5].

Complaint Investigation and Assessment for Patient Safety and Quality of Care under Regulatory Compliance

Regulatory organizations such as CMS and state licensing have the legal authority to inspect health facilities. This can be performed as a routine survey for licensing, investigation of complaints, or mandated self-reporting of "unusual occurrences," which threaten welfare, safety, and health of patients (Figure 23.3). The investigation utilizes the "tracer method," a process that tracks a patient through all the events that occur while the patient is hospitalized. The goal is to determine a facility's compliance for quality and safety in the context of the regulatory requirement.

The regulations hold the facility accountable for: (a) systems of care, and for individuals' actions within the facility; (b) the facility's own bylaws, rules, policies, and procedures; (c) standards of care as

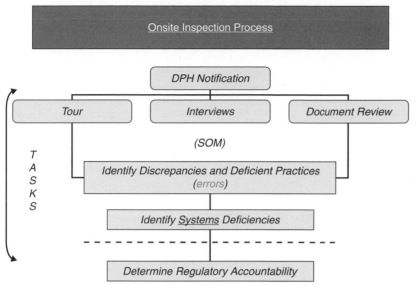

Figure 23.3 Regulatory oversight and compliance.

DPH, Department of Public Health, which in California, is the agency that conducts the investigation.

SOM, State Operations Manual, which defines the investigation process and the regulations.

Tasks, the investigative process.

Errors, clinical and other failures as defined by the regulations.

Discrepancies, variations from bylaws, policies, etc., that are unaccounted for.

Deficient practices, regulatory violations as determined by the identified discrepancies.

defined by the facility; and (d) quality/performance improvement programs [4]. The investigation process determines what the facility did, or failed to do, that led to an adverse event [6].

For trainees it is important to be aware of the institution's policies and protocols, and to follow them. If it becomes necessary to deviate from the protocol for any reason, this must be documented in the record along with the rationale for doing so [7]. Table 23.2 reviews the regulations and policies, with the associated violations from the clinical case scenario.

Using the Clinical Morbidity and Mortality Conference to Teach Patient Safety

Clinical case Scenario: The Missing Pap Smear

A 41-year-old woman, Gravida 4, Para 3 was assigned to a PGY2 resident in the resident continuity clinic. She presented with symptomatic uterine myomata. She had persistent abdominal pain and heavy periods

resulting in an iron-deficiency anemia. This occurred following conservative medical management for 6 months. She had no significant past medical history.

Physical examination and pelvic ultrasound were significant for an enlarged fibroid uterus measuring 25 cm.

The patient was counseled about surgery. The resident presented the patient to attending staff who approved the patient for surgery.

The patient underwent exploratory laparotomy and total abdominal hysterectomy. She tolerated the procedure well, and there were no complications. She had an uneventful postoperative course in the hospital and at home.

One week later at her postoperative visit she was doing well. The pathology report was obtained and was significant for a microscopic invasive cervical carcinoma with stromal invasion 2.1 mm in depth and a horizontal spread of 4.0 mm. There was no lymphovascular space involvement.

This was consistent with a FIGO Stage 1A1 cervical cancer.

On chart review, the patient's last pap smear was 5 years ago. Review of records show that a pap smear

Table 23.2 Regulatory domain violations.

Regulation/policy	Non-compliance
1: Governing body	
The governing body shall (1) Adopt written bylaws in accordance with legal requirements and its community responsibility which shall include but not be limited to provision for: Preparation and maintenance of a complete and accurate medical record for each patient	• Obstetrician: no documentation of the ante, intra, and postpartum findings and changing conditions • L&D Nursing: failure to acknowledge initial postpartum hypertension as an abnormality, or need for MD notification • Failure to document the clinical events for the seizure, Code Blue response, the administration of IV magnesium sulfate, and transfer to the ICU • ICU staff failure to fully document changing neurological and cardiopulmonary status, or MD notification
2: Medical staff	
The medical staff shall provide in its by-laws, rules and regulations for appropriate practices and procedures to be observed in the various departments of the hospital	• On-call obstetrician violated facility policies for emergency response to be "immediately available, and in a manner that is consistent with the patient's condition," when repeatedly paged for the patient's progressive clinical circumstances
The medical staff shall provide for the quality of care	• Obstetrician failed to assess an unknown patient with abnormal clinical findings and deteriorating condition over prolonged period of time • Obstetrician failed to function within scope of practice for management for preeclampsia in the ante, intra, and postpartum periods • OB MD failed to obtain facility-mandated MFM consultation for specified conditions, despite 24-hour availability, especially following seizure
3: Nursing staff	
Planning and Implementing Patient Care. The planning and delivery of patient care shall reflect all elements of the nursing process: assessment, nursing diagnosis, planning, intervention, evaluation and, as circumstances require, patient advocacy, and shall be initiated by a registered nurse at the time of admission	• Failed to review and report prenatal concerns, elevated blood pressure, and visual symptoms on admission to on-call OB MD • Failed to assess early postpartum hypertension and abdominal pain, and failed to notify MD • Failed to implement Chain of Command policy when the attending physician failed to respond to emergent nursing pages for the patient's changing clinical condition prior to the seizure • Failed to notify MD of critical value for thrombocytopenia

was done but there was no record that it was received in laboratory.

Discussion

The morbidity and mortality conference ("M&M") has historically been utilized as a tool for core resident education and department quality assurance and improvement in obstetrics and gynecology and surgery training programs [8]. An example of a standard M&M format is shown in Table 23.3. Another format is utilizing a Clinical Case Reviews Conference. In this format, the most senior resident on service selects a recent sentinel case to present. Involved professionals from all disciplines and specialties are invited to the conference. The resident presents the selected patient's presenting history, physical examination, and hospital course. This is followed by group discussion, RCA, joint identification of human and system errors, and development of an action plan to improve patient safety. This format can create a friendly, blame-free environment with successful identification of system and human errors at all levels leading to improved resident education and patient safety and quality of care [9].

Table 23.3 Educational Morbidity and Mortality Conference template.

- The conference will involve all faculty and residents
- The conference will start on time
- The conference will occur weekly
- The residents will present in teams (teams may include OBSTETRICS, GYNECOLOGY, GYNECOLOGY-ONCOLOGY, CLINIC, REI, HIGH-RISK OBSTETRICS)
- The residents' case list compilation will include:
  - High-risk obstetrics (antepartum and postpartum cases) managed by residents under faculty supervision
  - Obstetrical procedures with residents' involvement
  - Vaginal deliveries with residents' involvement
  - Surgical cases with residents' involvement
  - House staff emergency room admissions
  - GYN-ONCOLOGY: All cases managed by residents under faculty supervision
  - Ambulatory cases supervised by the chief resident and faculty
- The residents should summarize their cases on small cards that they can carry with them
- The case lists will be sent to all faculty members at least 3 days in advance
- The residents will sit in front of the room opposite the faculty during M&M conference
- Any of the faculty may ask questions about any of the cases on any of the lists
- There will be two lead faculty members who are also required to each prepare a short written learning issue on any case in the resident's case logs that the faculty feels is of important educational value
- The written learning issue will be posted on the residents' educational website after the conference
- There will be time limits to each question. It is suggested that each question and answer be kept to about 3 minutes so that up to 15 questions can be asked in 45 minutes. A bell will be used to announce the time
- The question may be directed to the team or to a specific resident; and the chief of team will select the resident who will respond
- It is expected that the objective of the faculty's questions is to assess and improve residents' fund of knowledge, clinical reasoning, and clinical management

The selected case above was discussed using the "Clinical Case Reviews Conference" format described. The patient had inadequate preoperative preparation and was incidentally found to have a cervical cancer during surgery performed for a presumed benign diagnosis. System issues were identified at multiple levels:

1. The resident did not follow up on the patient's pap smear
2. The case was presented to an attending over the telephone prior to the surgery date
3. The deposition of the Pap smear specimen could not be accounted for

An action plan was developed which included resident education for adequate preoperative preparation and cancer screening, improved resident supervision in clinic, and development of a pathology specimen book for follow-up of all specimens sent to pathology.

Illustrative clinical scenarios can be used to teach the principles and processes of patient safety and the reduction of medical errors. The healthcare matrix can be utilized to review patient management in a multidisciplinary setting based on the IOM Aims and the six ACGME competencies with the development of an appropriate action plan. Maternal and mortality conferences can allow faculty to engage residents in a blame-free environment in analyzing patient care, identifying deficiencies and developing corrective processes. Clinical cases can also be used to teach regulatory compliance, risk management and medicolegal concerns. It is important for each residency program to implement a consistent and systematic format of patient safety training for all residents.

References

1   Bingham JW, Quinn DC, Richardson MG, et al. Using a healthcare matrix to assess patient care in terms

of aims for improvement and core competencies. *Jt Comm J Qual Patient Saf.* 2005;31(2):98–105.

2   Quinn DC, Bingham JW, Garriss W, et al. Residents learn to improve care using the ACGME Core Competencies and Institute of Medicine Aims for Improvement: the Health Care Matrix. *JGME.* 2009;1(1):119–126.

3   Rad S, Ogunyemi D. Using the healthcare matrix to teach and improve patient safety culture in an OB/GYN residency training program. *J Patient Saf.* 2012;8(4):177–181.

4   State Operations Manual, Appendix A – Survey Protocol, Regulations and Interpretive Guidelines for Hospitals, Revision 78, December 28, 2011. Centers for Medicare and Medicaid Services. Available at www.cms.gov/Regulations-and-Guidance/Guidance/ Manuals/downloads/som107ap_a_hospitals.pdf (accessed June 7, 2012).

5   Aspden P, et al., eds. *Patient Safety: Achieving a New Standard for Care.* Committee on Data Standards for Patient Safety, Board of Health Care Services, Institute of Medicine. Washington, DC: National Academy Press; 2004: 228.

6   Karsh B, Alper SJ. Work system analysis: the key to understanding health care systems. In *Advances in Patient Safety: From Research to Implementation*, Vol 2. Rockville, MD: Agency for Healthcare Research and Quality; 2005.

7   Lichtmacher A. Quality assessment tools: ACOG Voluntary Review of Quality of Care Program, Peer Review Reporting System. *Obstet Gynecol Clin N Am.* 2008;35:147–162.

8   Kauffmann RM, Landman MP, Shelton J, et al. The use of a multidisciplinary morbidity and mortality conference to incorporate ACGME general competencies. *J Surg Educ.* 2011;68(4):303–308.

9   Johna S, Tang T, Saidy M. Patient safety in surgical residency: root cause analysis and the surgical morbidity and mortality conference-case series from clinical practice. *Perm J.* 2012;16(1):67–69.

Quality and Safety in Medical Education
Implementing a Curriculum of Patient Safety and Quality Improvement in Medical Education

Dotun Ogunyemi

Why Teach Patient Safety and Quality Improvement (QI)?

The Institute of Medicine has recommended team training and the implementation of team behaviors to reduce medical errors and increase patient safety, which can help improve the quality of healthcare in the United States [1,2]. The Joint Commission issued a Sentinel Event Alert in 2008, which outlined recommendations on skills-based training and coaching, relationship-building, collaborative practice, feedback on unprofessional behavior, and conflict resolution for physicians [3]. Patient safety and quality improvement training is recommended by the Association of American Medical Colleges (AAMC) and the Association of Faculties of Medicine in Canada [4]. The Accreditation Council for Graduate Medical Education (ACGME) endorses the training of these competencies and has recently started tracking teamwork and patient safety in the annual surveys distributed to all residents [5]. Patient safety and quality-improvement training is a part of the ACGME competencies of professionalism, interpersonal and communication skills, practice-based learning and improvement, and systems-based practice. Consequently, the teaching and assessment of patient safety should be a major goal in medical education. This is especially critical given the current interdisciplinary approach to healthcare delivery, the focus on evidence-based medicine, and the outcome-based model of care that must adapt to the ever-changing culture. Despite pervasive support for patient safety and QI training, only 10%–25% of medical schools in the United States and Canada currently report having a patient safety or QI curriculum [6].

Administrative processes and strategies are essential to success. It is crucial to develop and support an organizational culture that promotes patient safety with focuses on accountability, excellence, honesty,

integrity, and mutual respect, all while operating in a non-punitive way. This will not only enable effective role modeling by the faculty and leadership, but will also allow residents and medical students to learn by professional socialization [7]. To establish a curriculum in patient safety and quality improvement, institutional support, involvement, and leadership are necessary. The commitment of GME directors, departmental chairs, residency program directors, and clerkship directors is essential to building a foundation. Hospital administrators, the nursing department, human resources, and risk management personnel should also be included to ensure multidisciplinary involvement and training. Next, faculty and staff interested in QI must be identified and trained. It is vital to support and build an adequate capacity of teachers. Incentives for QI teachers should be considered, such as providing "protected time" or even creating a pathway that allows faculty members who engage in QI to be promoted on that basis [6]. To increase uniform awareness, faculty staff may be required to show a minimum degree of participation in local QI activities on an annual basis, as is expected for other professional obligations. At the residency program or clerkship level, a policy should be created outlining the curriculum. Time must be allocated in the schedules of resident and medical students for instruction and participation in QI. It is also important to create a continuum of learning at all levels of training from medical students and residents to fellows and faculty.

How Do We Teach a Curriculum in Patient Safety and Quality Improvement?

The curriculum for patient safety and QI should be delivered in clinical settings such as ambulatory care sites and inpatient hospital wards in addition to classrooms and other non-clinical settings. Didactic

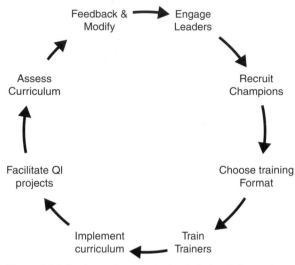

Figure 24.1 Implementing a curriculum in Patient Safety and Quality Improvement.

sessions teach the knowledge, concepts, theory, and scientific principles that can facilitate involvement of trainees in patient safety and quality of care. Small group discussions and interactive case discussions engage learners and are more effective teaching tools.

Interdisciplinary patient safety conferences are practical and integrated settings where residents and the rest of the healthcare team can engage in these topics. Situational awareness rounds can be held on the labor floor at scheduled times during the shift in which all nurses, residents, anesthesiologists, and attending faculty including non-clinical personnel such as housekeeping can meet briefly to present updates on all of the patients and any possible issues. The Morbidity and Mortality (M&M) conference is the most common educational activity incorporated into most residency programs. This conference, if done in an interdisciplinary setting and blame-free environment, can be very effective in teaching a broad range of patient safety topics through discussions of adverse events, errors, and near-misses (see Chapter 23) [8]. The healthcare matrix is a multidisciplinary meeting where participants review the potential deficiencies in the care of a patient within the framework of the ACGME competencies and the IOM aims of safety, timeliness, effectiveness, efficiency, equitable, and patient-centered care. The developed matrix encourages discussion among the participants and allows for the generation of a consensus action plan for implementation [9].

Experiential learning can impart specific skills; as such, simulation education can bridge classroom learning and real-life clinical experiences as well as strengthen individual and team performance toward improved patient safety. Simulations can be modified and adapted into multiple learning opportunities. They allow trainees to make mistakes, learn from them, and then receive detailed feedback and evaluations of their performance [2]. A major experiential learning format for trainees is to participate in quality-improvement projects. These projects allow residents to learn about the importance of quality-improvement processes, appropriate documentation, the Plan–Do–Study–Act process and its application to various clinical settings. Trainees also get hands-on experience in designing and implementing quality-improvement projects [10]. An important benefit of such projects is that they can often fulfill resident research requirements, in addition to providing opportunities to see their work implemented in a meaningful way. Several practical skills are acquired through this process, including research, leadership, and improvement methods. Training programs must carefully consider the time commitment required, because QI projects typically involve longitudinal cycles of implementation and assessment of change. Creative solutions that can improve feasibility and the quality of residents' QI projects include: scheduling QI projects during lighter rotations, establishing/building team-based systems in which resident teams work together on a project, or allow residents to sequentially pass projects from previous groups to incoming groups and/or complete one part of a larger QI project [6].

One must also keep in mind the importance of continuous teaching by role modeling and utilizing teachable moments at the patient's bedside. Faculty acting as role models will help to dispel any "hidden curriculum," in which there is a discrepancy between the concepts trainees learn in formal educational settings and what trainees observe in routine clinical practice.

Specific educational processes include developing a longitudinal curriculum in patient safety that spans residency training or medical school [11]. Utilizing electronic media such as web-based programs and videos allows for less dependence on qualified teachers in patient safety and also gives trainees the flexibility to learn at their own convenience. Trainees can also use self-reflective processes such as portfolios or case logs (Table 24.1).

Table 24.1 Curricular teaching methods for a Patient Safety and Quality Improvement Curriculum.

Teaching method	Examples
Didactics	
Formal lectures	a. Protected education time for patient safety topics b. Structured education – emphasis on error prevention, near-misses, error recognition, and error management
Small-group discussion	a. Practice of communication skills in scenarios: obtaining informed consent, sharing bad news, disclosing errors b. Role-playing as patients and providing feedback c. Analyses of sentinel events d. Incident reports as real-time experiences for review by residents
Interactive case discussions	a. Cases with optimum and adverse outcomes b. Case vignettes involving errors and near-misses c. Case studies that focus on systems problems that impact patient safety, errors, and near-misses d. Videotapes cases with trigger issues
Conferences	a. Safety rounds b. Situational awareness rounds c. Morbidity and Mortality conferences d. Quality Improvement (QI) conferences e. Near-miss conferences f. Root-cause analyses conferences g. Healthcare matrix conferences
Journal clubs Review of the current literature on patient safety topics	a. Textbooks b. Journal articles c. Selected readings
Grand Rounds	Speakers on patient safety regularly as part of departmental or GME grand rounds
Experiential learning	
Portfolios	a. Self-assessment and reflective practice b. Use of reflection in learning c. Interactive programs, with opportunities for reflection
Case log system	Systematic and ongoing assessment of clinical outcomes and impact of participation in patient safety and QI activities
Role modeling and mentoring	a. Residents participate in departmental and institutional safety committees b. Operating room and bedside teaching of patient safety concepts c. Effective teaching and role modeling of good communication and exemplary professionalism by faculty in clinical environments d. Focus on communication skills and professionalism during teaching rounds
Performance improvement projects	a. Resident participation in QI and patient safety projects using PDSA b. Resident involvement in QI teams c. Annual presentation by residents on PBLI resident projects d. Participation in failure mode and effects analyses, root-cause analyses
Simulation-based training	Cognitive and skills-based simulations coupled with specific and timely feedback
Teachable moments	a. Direct observation, with specific and timely feedback b. Review of resident clinical notes
Specific processes	
Electronic learning methods	a. Web-based educational courses b. Chat rooms and discussion groups c. CD-ROMs d. Self-paced learning tools

(continued)

Table 24.1 (*cont.*)

Teaching method	Examples
Longitudinal curriculum	Longitudinal, graded experiences of increasing complexity across the years of residency education
Special courses	a. Team training
	b. Leadership skills courses
	c. Patient safety and quality improvement
	d. Administrative and managerial responsibilities
	e. Simulation training

Wong BM, Levinson W, Shojania KG. Quality improvement in medical education: current state and future directions. *Med Educ.* 2012 Jan;46(1):107–119 [6].

Table 24.2 features a comprehensive list of topics that should be included in a didactic curriculum for trainees categorized by the six ACGME competencies. Specific elements of the proposed curriculum content will need to be prioritized and expanded by training programs.

What Specific Skills Must Trainees Learn to Improve Patient Safety and Quality of Care?

Table 24.3 lists some of the specific skills that residents require in order to provide safe patient care. Handoff training, as a component of teamwork training, is very important because many studies have shown that the transition of patient care increases the likelihood of communication errors and incomplete clinical content. The Joint Commission has included standardizing handoff communications among its National Patient Safety Goals, and the ACGME reiterates specific provisions on transitions of care in the Common Program Requirements. Handover training should include formal didactic and interactive exercises with an emphasis on two principles: face-to-face, uninterrupted communication among physicians combining verbal and written or electronic handoff information, and that data must be unambiguous and factually correct [12]. The ultimate goal of teamwork training is to optimize patient safety through development of effective communication skills, enhancing situational awareness, enabling team members to feel comfortable expressing concerns, and use of debriefing and feedback, particularly after critical events [6]. An example of this is Crew Resource Management (CRM), which focuses on interpersonal communication, leadership, and decision-making. Furthermore, specific behavioral attributes amongst trainees may be associated with providing safe

care, and emotional intelligence training using tools such as the DISC, Thomas Kilnman conflict styles or crucial conversations/confrontation workshops can improve communication efficacy and teamwork [13,14]. A readily available and extensively tested training program is Team Strategies and Tools to Enhance Performance and Patient Safety (TeamSTEPPS), available from the Agency for Healthcare Research and Quality (AHRQ). TeamSTEPPS is a teamwork system, based upon key elements of CRM adopted from the Department of Defense, designed to produce highly effective medical teams that optimize the use of information, people, and resources to achieve the best clinical outcomes for patients, and it is particularly effective in acute care settings. TeamSTEPPS includes modules on task assistance, situation monitoring, feedback, conflict resolution, two-challenge rule, and more [6]. Importantly, training must be ongoing and role models must practice these techniques in daily practice. The program has been validated in a number of settings, particularly in acute care. The Institute for Healthcare Improvement (IHI) offers several other resources for training and support of programs in quality and safety, including the Model for Improvement. There are a number of innovative learning options offered through their "Open School," as well as tuition-based courses. Other essential skill training required by residents includes surgical/technical skills training and simulation, safe medication prescribing, and discharge summary programs.

How Do We Measure Efficacy of the Curriculum?

Table 24.4 lists several assessment tools that can be used to determine residents' competencies in a QI

Table 24.2 Content of a QI and Patient Safety Curriculum based on the six ACGME competencies.

Medical knowledge	Patient care	Interpersonal and communication skills
Theory and science of patient safety: • Definitions • Impact of human factors and systems on patient safety • Epidemiology of adverse events • Risk management • Use of evidence-based medicine to promote patient safety • Specialty-specific safety principles	Risk assessment: • Assessment of error risk in clinical environments • Identification of critical situations	Principles of effective communication: • Verbal and non-verbal communication in patient care • Written communication and order writing • Technology-enhanced communications
Errors and near-misses: • Mechanisms of error occurrence • Avoidance of errors • Interplay of individuals and systems in errors and near-misses • Cognitive psychology relating to errors • Error management • Impact of errors on patients and healthcare professionals	Patient-centered care: • Needs of the patient • Needs of patient's family • Patients' perspectives • Patients' roles in safety • Continuity of care • Patient education	Transfer of care and handoffs: • Effective strategies for transfer of patient information • Ownership of patient care versus transfer of care
A safety culture: • High-reliability organizations • Attributes and benefits of a no-blame culture • Relationship between individual responsibility and organizational culture • Patient safety tools • Failure mode and effects analysis • Root-cause analysis • Error recovery and crisis management	Fatigue and duty hours: • Effects of fatigue • Compliance with resident work hour limits	Lines of supervision and chain of command: • Chain of command; who gets notified, by whom • Communication mandates for certain items or problems • Policies and protocols for delivering verbal orders • Standard nomenclature; use of Situation–Background–Assessment–Recommendation (SBAR) • Informed consent
High-risk procedures in OBGYN: • "Fetal distress" • Failure to perform a cesarean • Ruptured uterus • Stillbirth • Shoulder dystocia • Brain-damaged baby	Practice guidelines and standardized procedures	Disclosure of medical errors: • Disclosure to patients and families • Disclosure to faculty, peers, other health professionals
Error-reporting systems: • Institutional, local, and national requirements • Regulatory bodies in patient safety: The Joint Commission		Leadership and team building
Legal implications of errors		

(continued)

Table 24.2 *(cont.)*

Medical knowledge	Patient care	Interpersonal and communication skills
Professionalism	**Practice-based learning and improvement**	**Systems-based practice**
Professional self-regulation: • Mental and physical well-being • Behavior modification • Concern for peers • Acceptance of constructive feedback • Dealing with lack of professionalism of others • Strategies for handling impaired, aging, or incompetent healthcare professionals • Participation in professional organizations • Appropriate interactions with industry	Continuous quality improvement: • PDSA, FEMA, RCA • Assessing outcomes • Risk stratification, observed versus expected mortality and morbidity ratios • Practice analysis and improvement • Comprehension of volume/outcome relationships • Managing and interpreting outcomes data, and benchmarking with external standards	Systems theory: • Micro- and macrosystems in healthcare • Impact of systems on patient care and safety • Coordination and continuity of care (multiple locations, physicians, teams) • Handoffs between individuals and teams within the context of micro- and macrosystems
Elements of professionalism: • Code of Professional Conduct • Respect for all team members, avoidance of intimidation and humiliation • Recognition of capabilities and limitations of self, team, and institution • Balanced assessment of benefits of surgical versus medical treatment	Evidence-based practice	Analyses and change of systems: • Systems factors, problems, hazards • Latent conditions, and barriers • Policies and strategies to change systems to improve patient care
Handling, reporting, and dealing with consequences of medical errors: • Coping with the implications of personal errors and errors of others • Core values of transparency, disclosure of errors, ability to admit mistakes • Discussing and taking responsibility for personal errors • Ethical, legal, and institutional requirements and protocols for reporting errors	PBLI assessments: • Auditing outcomes, benchmarking with national/local standards to identify gaps in performance • Pursuit of educational opportunities and verification of knowledge and skills • Application of new knowledge and skills to practice; inclusion of preceptoring • Reassessment of outcomes to check for improvement	Patient factors and patient education: • Role of patients and families in care • Enhancement of patient safety through effective patient education • Patient advocacy
		Healthcare financing: • Billing and coding • Cost-effective practice; societal and legal issues • Social justice and appropriate resource utilization

Sachdeva AK, Philibert I, Leach DC, Blair PG, Stewart LK, Rubinfeld IS, Britt LD.Patient safety curriculum for surgical residency programs: results of a national consensus conference. Surgery. 2007;141(4):427–441 [7].

and patient safety curriculum. Standardized tests can be designed for any part of the curriculum, and pre- and post-tests can be given to assess knowledge acquisition. Faculty should provide immediate feedback on patient safety issues in the clinical setting to residents. The formal assessment of residents by faculty and 360-degree evaluations especially by nursing staff should include categories that assess the delivery of safe care. Objective Structured Clinical Examinations (OSCE) and standardized patients can be used to teach and assess students' skills at providing disclosure and obtaining informed consent [15]. Videotaping these sessions in addition to giving participants an immediate debriefing is especially useful in simulation training and emergency drills. Residents' patient safety conference presentations and quality-improvement projects

Table 24.3 Experiential training to improve patient safety and quality of care in medical education with suggested outcome measures.

Skill	Definition	Educational interventions	Outcome measures
Patient handover	Transferring responsibility for care from provider to provider	a. Development of a formal handover curriculum b. Review of the hazards associated with improper handover c. Checklist to enhance adherence to effective handover d. Role-playing handover with peers and faculty with feedback	a. Standardization of handover process b. Improved accuracy of handover information c. Fewer errors related to handover process
Disclosure of medical error	Providing open communications of medical errors to patients and family	a. Review of curriculum on principles and benefits of disclosure b. Observing and participating in disclosure process by senior faculty b. Role-playing disclosing errors to patient and family with feedback	a. Performance on OSCE station on disclosure b. Performance with Standardized patient c. Residents actually participate in disclosure
Teamwork training	Two or more individuals who have different but specific roles but are interdependent and share a common goal	a. Emotional intelligence training b. Crucial conversation and confrontation workshops d. Multidisciplinary simulation training e. Multidisciplinary team presentations and exercises f. Crew Resource Management g. TeamSTEPPS system training	a. Team members show improvements in leadership, situation awareness, communication, and mutual support b. Increased frequency of debriefing c. Decreased complaints from nurses about trainees d. Decreased complaints from trainees about faculty and nurses e. Improved evaluation of trainees by faculty on all ACGME competencies f. Improved evaluation by trainees of the program and faculty g. Improved constructive feedback
Surgical and technical skills training	Skills are learned and practiced on models and simulators as opposed to live patients Allows "low-stakes" learning for improvement and "high-stakes" testing to determine competency	a. Simulation drills of uncommon but critical events such as amniotic fluid embolism, shoulder dystocia, or eclampsia b. Simulation training to teach surgical skills such as laparoscopy, hysteroscopy, and robotic-assisted surgery	a. Improved faculty evaluation of surgical skills of trainees b. Decreased surgical complications by trainees
Safe medication prescribing	Providers write a legible, complete, and unambiguous medication order, and avoid common medication ordering errors (such as prescribing look-alike medications safely)	Didactic session and case studies with an interactive audience response system to teach safe prescribing skills	Fewer prescribing errors
Discharge summary improvement program	Discharge summaries are well-organized, accurate, comprehensive, still concise, and readable	a. Didactic lecture to outline key elements of discharge b. Summaries with feedback sessions of summaries dictated by trainees are reviewed	Improvements in elements of trainees' discharge summaries

Adapted from Wong BM, Levinson W, Shojania KG. Quality improvement in medical education: current state and future directions. Med Educ. 2012 Jan;46(1):107–119 [6].

Table 24.4 Assessment methods for patient safety curriculum for residents.

Standardized tests
Direct observations and performance evaluation by the faculty
Objective Structured Clinical Examinations (OSCEs); standardized patients (SPs)
360-degree evaluations
Standardized assessment of performance at M&M and QI conferences
Review of outcomes data
Assessment of patient safety analyses conducted by residents
Videotaping with structured debriefing
Portfolios as assessment tools
Chart audits/case/patient logs to determine outcomes and identify gaps
Evaluation of resident performance in quality improvement projects
Review of complications and their management, including the corrective actions taken by residents
Assessments in simulated environments
Assessment of performance on projects that involve analyses of errors and near-misses

should have a structured grading format report that is shared with the residents. Training programs can use chart audits, portfolios, case logs, complications, or individual patient care outcome data to provide patient safety outcome profiles for residents to increase their awareness and help with their improvement.

References

1 Kohn LT, Corrigan JM, Donaldson M. *To Err is Human: Building a Safer Health System*. Washington, DC: National Academy Press; 2000.

2 Merién AE, van de Ven J, Mol BW, Houterman S, Oei SG. Multidisciplinary team training in a simulation setting for acute obstetric emergencies: a systematic review. *Obstet Gynecol*. 2010;115(5):1021–1031.

3 The Joint Commission Sentinel Alert: Issue 40, July 9, 2008. www.jointcommission.org/SentinelEvents/SentinelEventAlert/sea_40.htm (accessed May 31, 2012).

4 Wong BM, Etchells EE, Kuper A, Levinson W, Shojania KG. Teaching quality improvement and patient safety to trainees: a systematic review. *Acad Med*. 2010;85(9):1425–1439.

5 Accreditation Council for Graduate Medical Education: (ACGME). Resident/Fellow Survey 2012. www.acgme.org/acWebsite/resident_survey/ResidentSurvekyKeyTermsContentAreas.pdf (accessed May 31, 2012).

6 Wong BM, Levinson W, Shojania KG. Quality improvement in medical education: current state and future directions. *Med Educ*. 2012;46(1):107–119.

7 Sachdeva AK, Philibert I, Leach DC, et al. Patient safety curriculum for surgical residency programs: results of a national consensus conference. *Surgery*. 2007;141(4):427–441.

8 Kauffmann RM, Landman MP, Shelton J, et al. The use of a multidisciplinary morbidity and mortality conference to incorporate ACGME general competencies. *J Surg Educ*. 2011;68(4):303–308.

9 Quinn DC, Reynolds PQ, Easdown J, Lorinc A. Using the healthcare matrix with interns and medical students as a tool to effect change. *South Med J*. 2009;102(8):816–822.

10 Nabors C, Peterson SJ, Weems R, et al. A multidisciplinary approach for teaching systems-based practice to internal medicine residents. *J Grad Med Educ*. 2011;3(1):75–80.

11 Voss JD, May NB, Schorling JB, et al. Changing conversations: teaching safety and quality in residency training. *Acad Med*. 2008;83(11):1080–1087.

12 DeRienzo CM, Frush K, Barfield ME, et al. Handoffs in the era of duty hours reform: a focused review and strategy to address changes in the Accreditation Council for Graduate Medical Education Common Program Requirements. *Acad Med*. 2012;87(4):403–410.

13 Ogunyemi DA, Mahller YY, Wohlmuth C, Eppey R, Tangchitnob E, Alexander CJ. Associations between DISC assessment and performance in obstetrics and gynecology residents. *J Reprod Med*. 2011;56(9–10):398–404.

14 Ogunyemi D, Fong S, Elmore G, Korwin D, Azziz R. The associations between residents' behavior and the Thomas-Kilmann Conflict MODE Instrument. *J Grad Med Educ*. 2010;2(1):118–125.

15 American College of Obstetrics & Gynecology. Disclosure and discussion of adverse events. Committee Opinion No. 520. *Obstet Gynecol*. 2012;119:686–689.

Index

operating room checklists *see*
    checklists
opinion leaders and innovators 87,
    125
outpatient care 25
    accreditation/certification 1, 25,
        110–111
    anesthesia 2, 26–27, 110–111
    CLIA-waived tests 109–110
    emergency response protocols 2–4
    legal environment 109–111
    medication safety 29–31
    mistaken identity 29
    procedural control 1–4, 25–29
    quality assessment 35–36
    systems failure analysis 4–6
    tracking and follow-up 4–5, 31–35,
        119
over-the-counter medications 162
oxytocin 104, 157, 162–163, 166–167

pain relief 162
Pap smears, missing 207–209
Pareto diagrams 84–85
Patient and Family Advisory
    Councils 116
patient records *see* electronic medical
    records; healthcare records
patients 120–121
    communication with the physician
        115, 116, 117, 120
        about medications 119
        disclosure of adverse events
            53–59, 119–120
        poor command of English 117,
            154–155
    consent 5, 65–66, 117
    cultural diversity 116–117, 154–155
    first impressions 115
    handoffs, *see* handoffs
    health literacy 117–119
    mistaken identity 29, 153–154
    patient-centered care 116
    response to adverse events 52–53,
        59, 120
    rights and responsibilities 119, 120
    tracking and follow-up 4–5, 31–35,
        119
PDCA/PDSA (Plan, Do, Check/Study,
    Act) cycles 35, 79, 87–88
perfection, unobtainable 65, 77–78
pharmacists 160
physicians' offices, *see* outpatient care
pilot programs 87
postpartum hemorrhage (PPH)
    case scenarios 90, 100–101
    management 104–105, 164t. 18.4b
    and rapid response teams 102–103
    and simulation training 90, 97

preeclampsia
    best-practice measures 137t. 15.2
    checklists 179
    magnesium sulfate 157, 166
prescriptions 112, 159, 166, 167,
    217t. 24.3
privileging 27
process improvement programs, *see*
    quality improvement (QI)
    programs
professional examinations 96
prostaglandins 157, 163–164, 167
ProvenCare® Perinatal model of
    integrated healthcare delivery
    139–140
    best-practice measures 133t. 15.1,
        136–137
    model overview 132–133
    outcomes 136–139
    setting up the system 136
pulse oximetry, fetal 20–21

quality improvement (QI) programs
    78–79, 81, 125
    cause and effect (fishbone)
        diagrams 83–84, 188f. 21.1
    force field diagrams 86–87
    introduction into the curriculum
        211, 212
    metrics 82, 125, 136–137
    monitoring and surveillance 88–89
    nominal group technique 85–86
    in outpatient settings 35–36
    Pareto diagrams 84–85
    PDCA/PDSA cycles 35, 79, 87–88
    run charts/control charts 82, 88
    SMART goals 82–83
    "Voice of the Customer"
        surveys 81–82
"Questions are the Answer"
    campaign 115

rapid response teams, *see* obstetric
    rapid response teams
recruitment and retention issues 47
Red Flags Rule 35
regulatory oversight and compliance
    203–208
    accreditation for outpatient
        procedures 1, 25, 110–111
reinforcement of new behaviors 88
responsibility, for an adverse event 52,
    56
resuscitation of a pregnant patient
    106–107
root-cause analysis 5–6, 185–186
    case scenario 183–184, 187
    definition 184
run charts 82, 88

S-T segment analysis 21
SCOPE (Safety Certification
    for Outpatient Practice
    Excellence) program 1, 25
second victims 53, 55, 146, 184
sedation *see* anesthesia
seizures (in eclampsia)
    103–104, 163
shared decision-making 119
shoulder dystocia 177–178
    case scenario 177
    management 105–106, 179
    simulation training 92–93, 96,
        179–181
sign-outs 192
    see also handoffs
siloization 169
simulation training
    benefits of 90–91, 179, 212
    case scenario 90, 97
    in credentialing and licensing 96
    implementation and costs 94–96
    laparoscopy 92, 94, 95, 97
    mock drills 3–4, 29, 46
    professional bodies' commitment
        to 90, 91, 96–97
    shoulder dystocia 92–93, 96,
        179–181
    and team training 94–95, 103,
        173–174
    types of simulators 92, 95
    umbilical cord prolapse 93–94
sleep deprivation
    contribution to medical errors 64,
        145
    countermeasures 145, 147–148
    effect on cognitive ability
        144, 145
    night shifts 144–146
    working after a sleepless night
        146–147
"slips" 185
SMART goals 82–83
smart infusion pumps 161
smear tests, missing 207–209
social media use 113–114
special cause variation 82
surgical checklists *see* checklists
surveys on safety 81–82, 174
Swiss cheese model (organizational
    accidents) 149, 151

"teach-back" technique 117
teams
    checklist development 66
    necessity of 78
    rapid response, *see* obstetric rapid
        response teams
    training 175